Handbook of Patient C
in Vascular Diseases

Fifth Edition

D1566942

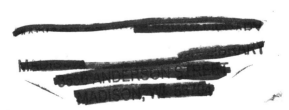

Handbook of Patient Care in Vascular Diseases

Fifth Edition

Editors

Todd E. Rasmussen, MD FACS
Chief, Vascular Surgery Services
San Antonio Military Medical Center
San Antonio, Texas
Associate Professor of Surgery
Uniformed Services University of the Health Sciences
Bethesda, Maryland

W. Darrin Clouse, MD FACS
Associate Chief, Vascular Surgery Services
San Antonio Military Medical Center
San Antonio, Texas
Assistant Professor of Surgery
Uniformed Services University of the Health Sciences
Bethesda, Maryland

Britt H. Tonnessen, MD
Attending Vascular Surgeon
Associate Program Director for General Surgery Residency
Ochsner Clinic Foundation
New Orleans, Louisiana

Wolters Kluwer | Lippincott Williams & Wilkins
Health
Philadelphia · Baltimore · New York · London
Buenos Aires · Hong Kong · Sydney · Tokyo

Acquisitions Editor: Brian Brown
Managing Editor: Julia Seto
Project Manager: Alicia Jackson
Senior Manufacturing Manager: Benjamin Rivera
Marketing Manager: Lisa Parry
Designer: Risa Clow
Cover Designer: Andrew Gatto
Production Service: Spearhead Global, Inc.

© 2008 by LIPPINCOTT WILLIAMS & WILKINS, a WOLTERS KLUWER business
530 Walnut Street
Philadelphia, PA 19106 USA
LWW.com

4/E, © 2001 by Lippincott Williams & Wilkins, 3/E © 1995 by Little Brown, 2/E © 1987 by Little Brown, 1/E © 1982 by Little Brown

Printed in the USA

Library of Congress Cataloging-in-Publication Data

Rasmussen, Todd E.
  Handbook of patient care in vascular diseases / Todd E. Rasmussen, W. Darrin Clouse, Britt H. Tonnessen. — 5th ed.
    p. ; cm.
  Rev. ed. of: Handbook of patient care in vascular diseases / John W. Hallett, Jr., David C. Brewster, Todd E. Rasmussen. 4th ed. c2001.
  Includes bibliographical references and index.
  ISBN-13: 978-0-7817-8135-0
  ISBN-10: 0-7817-8135-3
  1. Blood-vessels—Surgery—Handbooks, manuals, etc. 2. Blood-vessels—Diseases—Handbooks, manuals, etc. I. Clouse, W. Darrin. II. Tonnessen, Britt H. III. Hallett, John W. Handbook of patient care in vascular diseases. IV. Title.
  [DNLM: 1. Vascular Diseases—diagnosis—Handbooks. 2. Patient Care—Handbooks. 3. Vascular Diseases—physiopathology—Handbooks. 4. Vascular Diseases—therapy—Handbooks. WG 39 R225h 2008]
  RD598.5H35 2008
  617.4'13—dc22   2008012802

To purchase additional copies of this book, call our customer service department at (800) 638-3030 or fax orders to (301) 223-2320. International customers should call (301) 223-2300.

Visit Lippincott Williams & Wilkins on the Internet: at LWW.com. Lippincott Williams & Wilkins customer service representatives are available from 8:30 am to 6 pm, EST.

10 9 8 7 6 5 4

DRC0411

While we dedicate this Edition to our mentors, it has been our spouses (Debra, Krista, and Brian) and families who have sacrificed for its completion; and for their unwavering support we are deeply grateful.

Todd E. Rasmussen
W. Darrin Clouse
Britt H. Tonnessen

Contents

Foreword

The fifth edition of the *Handbook of Patient Care in Vascular Diseases* inaugurates the transition from one generation of authors (Hallett, Brewster, and Darling) to the next (Rasmussen, Clouse, and Tonnessen). The change in authors recognizes the need to pass the torch to the younger men and women who will lead the care of vascular patients into the future.

The first edition of the *Handbook* dates to 1982, when open surgery was well established but endovascular therapy was relatively new. Basic principles of care remain the same. However, new endovascular options, proliferating cardiovascular medicines, and developing cell therapies required a reorganization of the previous *Handbook*.

The central purpose of the original *Handbook* remains unchanged: To serve as a primer of principles that optimize patient outcomes. The authors have revised every chapter and added the latest in diagnostic and treatment approaches. They provide concise and clear suggestions to every member of the care team. Both novices and more experienced practitioners, including cardiologists, radiologists, and surgeons, will find something in these pages to help them in their daily work.

Every previous update of this *Handbook* has invited your feedback to improve future editions. Again, we encourage you to stay in touch with this enthusiastic new group of vascular specialists. They bring an exceptionally valuable handbook to you and your patients.

John (Jeb) Hallett, MD
David C. Brewster, MD

Preface

For more than two decades the *Handbook of Patient Care in Vascular Diseases* has provided health care providers at all levels a practical reference that emphasizes fundamentals and clinical concepts that "culminate in excellent outcome for vascular patients" (Darling C., First Edition). While the *Handbook* has a tradition of excellence, it finds itself in a new age of vascular care. Early editions were published in an era when information was exchanged at national meetings and in print and turned at a sluggish pace. At the time of the early editions training was dogmatic, methods of treatment changed gradually, and there were few natural history studies or randomized trials to direct vascular care.

Today there is near-instant access to a volume of clinical data often in the palm of one's hand before results are in print. Prospective trials and natural history studies guide the management of *some* vascular disease states, yet endovascular therapies are promoted on the Internet, in magazines and industry releases often without good peer review. Less invasive technologies developed by industry and favored by patients are introduced at a rapid pace. Practices and training paradigms have now evolved with an emphasis on such technology as well as proficiency through disease-specific clinical pathways.

This environment represents a challenge to those caring for patients with vascular disease. Today's provider must condense information from all directions sorting the relevant from the extraneous to develop a logical plan of care for each patient. In this setting we believe there is a role for an agile, evidence-based resource to serve as a discriminating guide and information management tool. Our hope is that this new edition of the *Handbook* represents such a resource. The Fifth Edition is structured to provide a basic understanding of vascular disease and cardiovascular risk rooted in the fundamentals of the history and physical exam. This edition incorporates noninvasive vascular testing and new clinical guidelines into the patient evaluation and provides a basic but thorough review of endovascular technologies and devices. Finally the Fifth Edition culminates in logical care outlines for eight areas of vascular disease encountered by trainees, nurses, and physicians.

With mentorship from two of the original authors we are privileged to continue this time-honored endeavor and hopeful that you will find the *Handbook* a useful resource to assist in the management of vascular disease.

T. E. R.
W. D. C.
B. H. T.

Acknowledgments

The authors would like to acknowledge John P. Reilly, MD, Associate Director, Cardiac Catheterization Laboratory, Ochsner Clinic, New Orleans, Louisiana, as sub-editor for Section IV, Catheter-Based and Endovascular Concepts. His experience in and expertise with endovascular technologies and procedures is greatly appreciated.

We would also like to thank Barbara Siede of Medical Illustrations, Ochsner Clinic Foundation, New Orleans, Louisiana, for her numerous innovative and artistic contributions to this edition. Her talent knows no bounds.

Finally, we would also like to acknowledge Kevin S. Franklin, RVS, Technical Director, San Antonio Military Vascular Laboratories for his dedication as an overall vascular specialist, especially in the field of noninvasive vascular testing.

Handbook of Patient Care in Vascular Diseases

Fifth Edition

SECTION I

Vascular Pathophysiology and Hypercoagulable Disorders

BASIC CONCEPTS

Like other disease processes, a number of basic principles guide the management of most vascular problems. These include *obtaining a history, performing a physical examination,* and *gathering information from other diagnostic testing.* Following these principles, one can provide logical and appropriate patient care; neglect one of these steps and a clinical scenario may become confusing and the patient's care misguided. In the first two chapters of this handbook, we outline and emphasize these basic concepts. Because the handbook covers both arterial and venous diseases, we have organized the basic concepts around these two disease groups. Each chapter is subdivided under the headings "Magnitude of the Problem," "Anatomy," "Etiology," "Pathophysiology," and "Natural History."

CHAPTER 1

Arterial Disease

I. Magnitude of the problem. Peripheral arterial disease (PAD) is a leading cause of death worldwide. As an age-related process, PAD will become much more prevalent in decades to come. Specifically, the first of the 82 million Americans in the "baby boom" demographic turned 60 years old in 2006, and the number of people over the age of 65 is anticipated to increase 100% by 2032. Perhaps as important as mortality is the disability resulting from PAD. For example, approximately 750,000 Americans have strokes annually, and many are left with a permanent neurologic deficit, which is devastating to both the patient and the family. Patients with arterial disease may also be limited by chest pain (angina pectoris), exertional leg pain (claudication), extremity ulceration (tissue loss), and even amputation (Chapter 14).

Advances in the diagnosis and successful treatment of PAD have occurred rapidly, and now include broader use of noninvasive duplex ultrasonography (US) and minimally invasive endovascular techniques (Chapters 10, 11, and 12). Significant progress has also been made in the identification of clinical risk factors and development of new classes of medications that allow prevention or reduction of arterial disease in many patients (Chapter 7). Despite these advances, many patients are unwilling to modify their lifestyles or comply with medication use. Thus, arterial disease will remain a leading health problem during the career of most physicians practicing today.

II. Anatomy. The peripheral arterial system refers to noncardiac arteries, including the thoracic and abdominal aorta and branches thereof, as well as arteries of the extremities. The arterial network is a complex organ system that must withstand the stress of pulsatile flow for the life of an individual. The wall of the artery consists of three layers, or tunics, referred to as the *tunica intima, tunica media*, and *tunica adventitia* (Fig. 1.1). Each of these layers plays a unique part in arterial function to allow delivery of oxygenated blood throughout the body. Although the makeup of each layer varies slightly, depending on the location of the artery in the body, all must function and remain intact in the setting of health.

   A. The intima. The inner lining of the artery is a single layer of endothelial cells called the **intima**. Endothelial cells of the intima perform unique functions via receptors on their cell surfaces by secretion of proteins, such as endothelin, and other substances, such as nitric oxide, which regulate vessel tone and affect platelet aggregation and formation of thrombus. Like other cells in the body, the cells of the intima require oxygen for survival and function, and receive this from the flowing blood (i.e., luminal blood supply). Underlying the intima is a thin matrix of elastic fibers called the **internal elastic lamina**.

   B. The media. The middle layer of the artery is formed by a circumferential layer of smooth muscle cells and variable amounts of elastin and collagen. The amount of elastic tissue within the media decreases proportionally to the smooth muscle content as arteries become more peripheral (e.g. further from the heart). Central arteries such as the thoracic aorta with greater elastic content are termed *elastic arteries* while *muscular arteries,* such as the femoral or carotid arteries, have greater smooth muscle content in the media. The media primarily responds to signals from endothelial cells of the nearby intima. Under normal conditions, the media provides structure to the vessel and is responsible for variations in vessel tone. In the setting of injury or disease, the media is the main location for cellular response including proliferation of smooth muscle cells and migration of other cell types into the media (e.g., macrophages and fibroblasts). The media has a dual source of nourishment receiving oxygen via diffusion from the circulating blood (luminal oxygen supply) and by small vessels that penetrate the outer wall, which are termed **vasa vasorum** (abluminal oxygen supply). A second **external elastic membrane** encloses the outer border of the media and separates it from the adventitia.

   C. The adventitia. The outermost layer of an artery is called the adventitia and is composed mainly of the long fibrous structural protein called collagen as well as autonomic nerves that supply the smooth muscle cells of the media. Additionally,

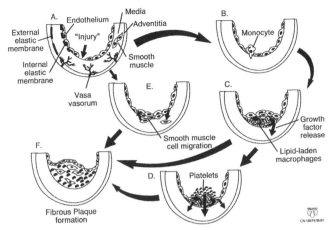

Figure 1.1.   Pathogenesis of atherosclerosis. Endothelial "injury" or dysfunction can be initiated by a variety of forces: hyperlipidemia; free radicals caused by cigarette smoking, hypertension, and diabetes mellitus; genetic alterations; elevated plasma homocysteine. Monocytes (**A**) attach to injured endothelium (**B**), secrete growth factors (**C**), and finally migrate into the subendothelial layer. Lipid-laden macrophages become part of the fatty streak. Endothelial disruption attracts platelets (**D**) that secrete platelet-derived growth factor (**PDGF**). Smooth muscle cells in the proliferative atheromatous lesion may also secrete growth factors such as PDGF. Increased endothelial turnover results in enhanced growth factor production. Smooth muscle cells are stimulated to migrate into the intimal layer (**E**). Smooth muscle and "injured" endothelial cells turn up their growth factor production. Fibrous plaques (**F**) evolve from fatty streaks. Atheromas develop from fatty streaks to fibrous plaques that can degenerate eventually into complicated plaques with surface ulceration, hemorrhage, and embolization. This fibrous plaque rupture and ulceration appear to be related to macrophages releasing proteolytic enzymes. (Adapted from Ross R. Atherosclerosis—an inflammatory disease. *N Engl J Med*. 1999;340:115-126.)

the vasa vasorum courses along and through the adventitia. Although the adventitia may appear thin and without substance, it is a key element in the total strength of the arterial wall. In muscular arteries the adventitia may be as thick as the media itself. In such arteries, surgical closure of the arterial wall or anastomosis of a synthetic graft to the vessel should incorporate the adventitial layer; failure to do so may result in anastomotic breakdown.

III. Etiology. The etiology of nearly all acquired arterial disease is **atherosclerosis**. The term atherosclerosis comes from the Greek terms *athero,* meaning gruel or paste, and *sclerosis,* meaning hardening. Arteriosclerosis refers to any hardening of the artery or loss of its elasticity, and is often used interchangeably with atherosclerosis, although technically atherosclerosis is a form of arteriosclerosis.

The etiology of atherosclerosis is a complicated immune-mediated process that begins at the interface of endothelial cells and the circulating blood. The etiology has not been linked to a single causative factor, but rather to a combination of *mechanical* (e.g., shear stress and hypertension), *circulating* (e.g., lipids, glucose, or insulin), and *environmental* (e.g., tobacco use) factors. Together these factors reach a threshold in certain genetically predisposed persons and initiate the disease process of atherosclerosis. The etiology of atherosclerosis may be thought of generally in two stages.

A. Response to injury. Under normal circumstances the endothelial lining of the blood vessel provides a nonsticky surface through which circulating blood may flow. However, this fragile layer of cells may be damaged by mechanical forces such as hypertension or circulating factors such as metabolites from cigarette smoke or oxidized lipids. Damage to the endothelial cells causes the lining of the vessel to become sticky, and white blood cells (monocytes and T cells) and platelets (thrombocytes) begin to adhere in an attempt to patch the injury (Fig. 1.1 A and B).

Experimental and clinical observations also indicate that early endothelial injury is more prone in areas of blood-flow separation and low **shear stress** (Fig. 1.2). The layer of blood

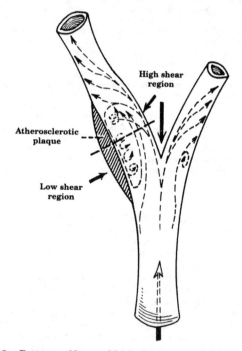

Figure 1.2. Patterns of low and high shear stress. Atherosclerotic plaques, which usually localize to the outer wall at arterial bifurcations, tend to develop at areas of boundary layer separation and low shear stress. (Adapted from Malek AD, Alper SL, Izumo S. Hemodynamic shear stress and its role in atherosclerosis. *JAMA.* 1999;282:2035-2042.)

adjacent to the intima is referred to as the **boundary layer** and, although flow in the center of the artery is **laminar**, this outer area of boundary layer separation has slower, more disturbed currents. These areas of low shear force (<4 dyne/ cm^2) have also been shown to induce endothelial dysfunction and generally occur at the outer walls of arterial branch points. Depending upon the magnitude and length of time over which any one of these insults occurs, the process may be self-limiting and result in healing of the vessel lining.

Alternatively, and in more severe or chronic cases, the injury process continues and alters the permeability and activity of the endothelial cell layer. From this point, adherent cells as well as the endothelial cells secrete substances that initiate an *immune-directed* process within the media of the vessel wall— immune-directed in the sense that inflammatory cells of various types (monocytes, T cells, and macrophages) and the factors that they secrete (cytokines) play a central role in directing the process. In response to cytokines, cells not typically in the media, such as macrophages, T cells, and fibroblasts, migrate into the media in the area of injury (Fig. 1.1 C-E). Smooth muscle cells in the media proliferate and alter their function with regard to production of the extracellular matrix and calcium metabolism, while macrophages engulf oxidized lipids and become lipid-laden macrophages, or **foam cells**. While the intent of this reaction is to "heal" the vessel damage, the result is formation of the earliest atherosclerotic lesion referred to as an atherosclerotic plaque or "fatty streak." These early atherosclerotic lesions or fatty streaks can occur early in life and are composed primarily of inflammatory cells, cholesterol, low-density lipoproteins, and calcium. Whether or not these early lesions progress to more advanced pathologic lesions depends upon several of the clinical, environmental, and genetic factors already noted. Research has shown that cigarette smoking accelerates formation and progression of these early lesions and that exercise, risk-factor modification, and medications such as statins cause such lesions to remain stable or regress.

B. Advanced atherosclerosis. In instances where the vascular injury response advances, it is thought that, for various reasons, the immune response remains "turned on." This may be due to local factors, such as foam cell death and increased oxidative stress; circulating factors, such as elevated lipids, glucose levels, or metabolites of cigarette smoke; or genetic factors related to the immune-response genes. Additionally, the observation that advanced atherosclerotic plaques occur mostly at *arterial branch points* suggests that differences in local shear stress related to turbulent flow may also act as an accelerating factor. Whatever the cause, the end result is propagation of the immune response within the wall of the artery, leading to deposition of calcium between the vessel layers and formation of an intermediate lesion termed the **fibrous cap** (Fig. 1.1F). Capped fatty deposits, also termed **atheromas**, can extend into the lumen of the artery, causing the artery to narrow or become unstable and open or rupture, releasing debris into the bloodstream (embolization). Atheromas are also active as they secrete cytokines, which lead to a condition termed **vascular remodeling**. Remodeling is a process in which smooth muscle cell proliferation continues and activates a set of enzymes (**matrix matalloproteinases**) able to destroy the structural proteins of the vessel wall. One or two specific metalloproteinases cause breakdown of the structural proteins in the media and adventitia resulting in weakening of the artery and dilation of the arterial segment. While such dilation initially compensates for the luminal narrowing (stenosis) caused by atheroma or plaque, the process leads to arterial aneurysm formation if unchecked. In such chronic and advanced atherosclerotic lesions, the elasticity of the arterial wall is lost and the process eventually narrows the vessel lumen or continues to break down the structural components of the arterial wall to form an aneurysm.

Although intimal thickening and calcification (hardening) of the arteries are to some degree a "normal aging process," the variability or spectrum of disease among individuals is a topic with many unanswered questions. Why is it that in the same patient one may find early and complicated lesions as well as arterial segments completely unaffected? Why is it that atherosclerosis appears to lead to occlusive lesions in some individuals but arterial aneurysms in others? Why are some arterial segments prone to aneurysm formation while others appear protected against aneurysm formation?

IV. Pathophysiology. To keep the pathophysiology of atherosclerosis simple, one may think of three main categories of clinical outcome:

1. Formation of a flow limiting blockage within the artery (*significant stenosis*)
2. Dilation of the artery (*aneurysm formation*)
3. Release of atheroma down the arterial stream (*embolization*)

A. Occlusive disease. Atherosclerosis becomes symptomatic by gradual occlusion of blood flow to the involved extremity or end organ. Symptoms occur when a **critical arterial stenosis** is reached. Blood flow and pressure are not significantly diminished until at least 75% of the cross-sectional area of the vessel is obliterated (Fig. 1.3). This figure for cross-sectional area can be equated with a 50% reduction in lumen diameter. The formula for the area of a circle (area = $3.14 \times \text{radius}^2$) explains the relationship between vessel diameter and cross-sectional area.

Factors other than radius also influence the significance of an arterial stenosis, but to a lesser extent (**Poiseuille's Law**). These include the length of stenosis (i.e., longer segments become critical earlier), blood viscosity, and peripheral resistance. In situations where resistance is decreased beyond a fixed stenosis (vasodilation), velocity and turbulence across that stenosis increase, resulting in a decrease in pressure across the lesion (**Bernoulli's principle**) (Table 1.1). Evidence also suggests that a series of subcritical stenoses can have an additive effect, similar to a single critical stenosis although not linear. Thus, three subcritical stenoses (30%, 40%, and 10%) may not have the same effect as a single 80% narrowing of a vessel.

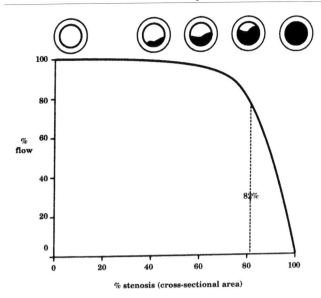

Figure 1.3. Critical arterial stenosis. Blood flow remains relatively normal across an arterial stenosis until at least 75% of the cross-sectional area is obliterated (50% diameter reduction).

The hemodynamic concepts pertaining to the velocity of blood across fixed stenoses are critical to our understanding of patient symptomatology and physical examination findings. For example, these concepts help in the diagnosis of patients who complain of extremity pain with exertion, yet have normal examinations, including ankle-brachial indices (ABIs), while at rest in the office. In such patients a basic understanding of hemodynamics allows us to recognize the value of a provocative test, such as walking or treadmill ABIs, in confirming or excluding the diagnosis of vascular claudication.

Under normal conditions (i.e., no arterial stenoses) a person's ABIs will increase with and immediately following walking. However, if the patient in the above scenario has significant arterial occlusive disease (stenoses), the ABIs will *decrease* in the symptomatic extremity with exercise. In this situation, Bernoulli's principle shows that with exertion comes vasodilation in the extremity, which increases velocity and turbulence across any fixed stenoses and results in a pressure decrease across the same area. This decrease in arterial pressure during exertion manifests as decreased exercise ABIs and symptoms of claudication. Hence, a stenosis may be noncritical at rest but critical with exercise used as a provocative maneuver.

B. Aneurysmal disease. Arterial aneurysms arise as a consequence of the loss of structural integrity of the vessel wall, namely degradation of the network of structural proteins such as elastin and collagen in the mid and outer layers of the

Table 1.1. Basic principles of fluid dynamics

Principle	Definition	Equation	Terms of Equation
Bernoulli's	Relationship between pressure, gravitational (potential) energy, and kinetic energy in an idealized fluid system. In moving blood through arteries, the portion of total fluid energy lost is dissipated in the form of heat.	$P_1 + \rho gh_1 + \frac{1}{2}\rho\vartheta_1^2 = P_2 + \rho gh_2 + \frac{1}{2}\rho\vartheta_2^2 + \text{heat}$	P = pressure ρgh = gravitational potential energy $\frac{1}{2}\rho\vartheta_2^2$ = kinetic energy
Law of LaPlace	Arterial wall stress and therefore risk of aneurysm rupture is directly proportional to vessel diameter and arterial pressure.	$\text{Wall stress} = P \times d/t$	P = systolic blood pressure, d = vessel diameter; t = vessel wall thickness
Poiseuille's	Relationship between flow and the pressure difference across the length of a tube, its radius, and the fluid viscosity. The most important determinant of flow is radius.	$Q = \pi r^4 (P_1-P_2)/8L\eta$	Q = flow r = radius of vessel P_1-P_2 = potential energy between 2 points L = distance between 2 points η = viscosity coefficient
Reynolds number	A dimensionless quantity that defines the point at which flow changes from laminar (streamlined) to turbulent (disorganized). If Re >2,000, disturbances in laminar flow will result in fully developed turbulence. In normal arterial circulation, Re is usually <2,000.	$Re = \rho\vartheta d/\eta$	Re = Reynolds number d = tube diameter ϑ = velocity ρ = specific gravity η = viscosity
Resistance (rearranged Poiseuille's law)	Analogous to Ohm's equation of electrical circuits (resistance = pressure/flow)	$R = P_1-P_2/Q = 8\eta L/\pi r^4$	R = resistance P_1-P_2 = pressure drop Q = flow η = viscosity L = length of tube r = radius of tube

arterial wall. Over time, this weakening results in dilation and aneurysm formation (*aneurysm = 1.5 times the normal diameter of the vessel*). Once an aneurysm forms, laminar flow is disturbed in this irregularly shaped vessel, turbulent blood flow increases, and there is accumulation of **mural thrombus** (i.e., clot) within the aneurysm. Although the amount of mural thrombus can at times be considerable, it does not offer strength to the aneurysm or prevent expansion or rupture, and is in fact a risk for embolization or even aneurysm thrombosis (occlusion).

The etiology of arterial aneurysms is not fully understood but shares pathways with the etiology of atherosclerosis already discussed in this chapter (Fig. 1.4). Unique to aneurysm formation, however, is the important role of the proteolytic enzymes referred to as **matrix metalloproteinases** (MMPs) and **temporary inhibitors of matrix metalloproteinases** (TIMPs). The balance between the activity and inhibition of these enzymes appears to be negatively altered in predisposed individuals. This phenomenon, in association with the inflammatory response associated with atherosclerosis, results in loss of arterial wall structural integrity and leads to aneurysm formation.

The tendency for arterial aneurysms to form in certain locations, such as the abdominal aorta, can be partially explained by differences in arterial content and hemodynamic factors. It is accepted that the elastin content of arteries is greatest during childhood and that the more distal abdominal aorta has proportionally less elastin content than the paravisceral or thoracic aorta. Consequently, in individuals affected by atherosclerosis, the abdominal aorta is proportionally more susceptible to elastin degradation and, therefore, aneurysm formation when compared to other arteries higher in either elastin or smooth muscle content.

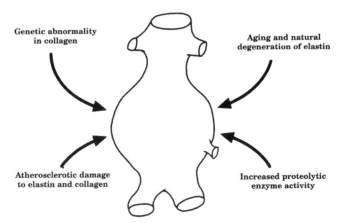

Figure 1.4.   Factors contributing to the multifactorial pathogenesis of arterial aneurysms.

Additionally, it is known that a pulse wave arrives at any vessel bifurcation and that a portion of this pressure is reflected back against the arterial wall proximal to the bifurcation. Minimal reflections occur when the sum of the cross-sectional areas of the daughter arteries (e.g., iliacs) to the parent artery (i.e., aorta) is 1.15 or greater. With advancing age, this sum decreases even in aortas without atheromatous change, and so more pressure is reflected back to the wall of the infrarenal abdominal aorta. The result is a partial standing wave in the abdominal aorta, the chronicity of which may contribute to the relative commonality of aneurysms in this and other locations.

Lastly, it is proposed that there is a relative paucity of vasa vasorum in the abdominal aorta, which also may contribute to its relative susceptibility to aneurysm formation. It is hypothesized that the blood supply to the media and adventitia of the aorta is adversely affected by the atherosclerosis, specifically through obliteration of these vasa vasorum. Areas in which the concentration of these nutrient vessels is less, such as the abdominal aorta, are considered more susceptible to structural weakening of the artery and aneurysm formation. Congenital defects in the integrity of the vessel collagen and elastic content are found in certain connective tissue disorders, such as Marfan syndrome and Ehlers-Danlos syndrome type IV; these unique conditions will be described in later chapters.

The risk of aneurysm rupture is described by the **Law of LaPlace**, which places arterial wall stress in relation to vessel diameter and arterial pressure: Wall stress $= P \times d/t$. Aneurysm rupture occurs when the intralumenal pressure exceeds the tensile strength of the wall of the artery. The risk of rupture, therefore, is proportional to aneurysm diameter (d) and intralumenal or systolic blood pressure (P) and inversely related to wall thickness (t).

V. Natural history. Peripheral arterial disease is considered a diffuse, slowly progressive "polyvascular" disease; polyvascular in the context that, if present, atherosclerosis affects all arteries of the body to some degree. During early adult life, arterial disease usually remains asymptomatic and undiagnosed. However, if the diagnosis is made, the disease process should be considered to be present in multiple circulations, most notably the coronary. It is now accepted that coronary death is the most common cause of mortality in patients with symptomatic and asymptomatic atherosclerotic disease, and should therefore be considered in all patients with arterial disease, even if it is only apparent in the legs.

Additionally, if atherosclerosis is diagnosed in one area of the vasculature, a careful history and physical examination will often reveal evidence of significant disease at other peripheral sites. For example, a patient may present with calf claudication but have an unknown abdominal aortic aneurysm palpable on routine physical examination. The diffuse nature of atherosclerosis requires that the initial patient evaluation include a baseline examination of the entire vascular system.

The natural history of atherosclerosis is variable. Some patients are minimally bothered by its presence, while others are incapacitated. Although atherosclerosis may follow a progressive course, the natural history can be altered favorably in most cases by appropriate risk-factor modification, use of select medication, and invasive treatment in certain cases. Although not curative, properly selected arterial interventions can offer excellent palliation of the atherosclerotic process. Subsequent chapters will emphasize specific aspects of the natural history of atherosclerosis, so that clinicians can select patients who are most likely to benefit from medical, endovascular, and open surgical intervention.

SELECTED READING

Ailawadi G, Eliason JL, Upchurch GR, Jr. Current concepts in the pathogenesis of abdominal aortic aneurysms. *J Vasc Surg.* 2003;38:584-588.

Bhatt D, Steg P, Ohman E, Hirsch A, Ikeda Y, Mas J, et al. International prevalence, recognition and treatment of cardiovascular risk factors in outpatients with atherthrombosis. *JAMA.* 2006; 295:180-189.

Frangos SG, Chen AH, Sumpio B. Vascular drugs in the new millennium. *J Am Coll Surg.* 2000;191:76-92.

Goessens BMB, van der Graaf Y, Olijhoek JK, Visseren LJ, SMART Study Group. The course of vascular risk factors and the occurrence of vascular events in patients with symptomatic peripheral arterial disease. *J Vasc Surg.* 2007;45:47-54.

Hackman DG. Cardiovascular risk prevention in peripheral arterial disease. *J Vasc Surg.* 2005;41:1070-1073.

Hobeika MJ, Thompson RW, Muhs BE, Brookes PC, Gagne PJ. Matrix metalloproteinases in peripheral vascular disease. *J Vasc Surg.* 2007;45:849-857.

Norgren L, Hiatt WR, Dormany JA, Nehler MR, Harris KA, Fowkes FGR. Intersocietal concensus for the management of peripheral arterial disease (TASCII). *J Vasc Surg.* 2007;45(suppl S):S5A-S67.

Ross R. Atherosclerosis—an inflammatory disease. *N Engl J Med.* 1999;340:115-126.

CHAPTER 2

Venous Disease

The spectrum of venous disorders ranges from unsightly (spider veins) to uncomfortable (varicose veins) to disabling (chronic venous insufficiency). Although many venous problems are chronic, thromboembolic events are acute and life-threatening. A solid understanding of the basic principles of venous disease can help the clinician effectively diagnose and treat these challenging patients.

I. Magnitude of the problem. The magnitude of venous disease is widespread, with at least 15% of the U.S. population affected by simple varicose veins, and an even greater prevalence among women and the elderly. Another 5–10% are afflicted by **chronic venous insufficiency**, defined by skin changes in the leg related to prolonged venous hypertension in the deep and/or superficial venous system. Acute **deep venous thrombosis** (DVT) affects several hundred thousand people annually. A spectrum of **postphlebitic syndrome**, defined by symptoms of leg pain, edema, and/or ulceration, exists in all patients to some extent in the years following DVT. **Pulmonary thromboembolism** is a potential life-threatening consequence of untreated DVT, and is the most common preventable cause of death in hospitalized patients.

Chronic venous disease is classified by the **CEAP grading system** (Table 2.1), a standardized reporting method used worldwide. Four key features of venous disease are included: clinical signs, etiology (congenital, primary, or secondary), anatomic location (superficial, deep, or perforator), and pathophysiology (reflux, obstruction, or both). This system was established in 1995 by an international Ad Hoc Committee of the American Venous Forum to encourage uniform reporting of venous disease and promote clinical study including natural history and treatment strategies.

**Table 2.1. Basic CEAP classification
of chronic venous disease**

Clinical	Anatomy
C_0 no signs of venous disease	As superficial veins
C_1 telangiectasias or reticular veins	Ap perforator veins
C_2 varicose veins	Ad deep veins
C_4 pigmentation or eczema	
C_5 healed venous ulcer	Pathophysiology
C_6 active venous ulcer	Pr reflux
	Po obstruction
Etiology	Pr,o reflux and obstruction
Ec congenital	
Ep primary	
Es secondary (post-thrombotic)	

II. Anatomy. Descriptions of venous anatomy have been historically limited by a lack of standardized nomenclature. The current consensus nomenclature should be utilized uniformly.

A. The superficial venous system (Fig. 2.1) of the lower extremity includes the **great saphenous vein (GSV)**, **small saphenous vein,** and their tributaries. The GSV is occasionally duplicated in the thigh or calf. In the thigh, an anterior accessory GSV is the most constant branch. At the knee, the **saphenous nerve** becomes superficial and joins the great saphenous vein as it courses down the leg, an anatomic proximity that is relevant in instances where intervention on the

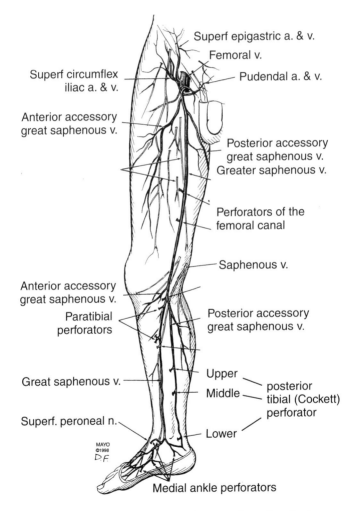

Figure 2.1.   **Anatomy of the great saphenous vein and perforators.**

great saphenous vein is considered. Below the knee, the posterior accessory saphenous vein drains into the great saphenous vein. Numerous medial perforating veins connect the deep calf veins with the great saphenous system and are called **perforating veins**. The small saphenous vein (formerly the lesser saphenous vein) ascends along a posterior course in the calf to join the popliteal vein in the popliteal fossa in the majority of limbs (Fig 2.2). As a normal variant, the small saphenous vein may continue cephalad to join the great saphenous or femoral vein.

B. The deep veins of the lower extremity are the paired posterior tibial, peroneal, and anterior tibial veins in the calf, which ascend with their correspondingly named arteries. The popliteal vein becomes the **femoral vein** in the adductor canal. The **profunda femoris vein** drains the lateral thigh

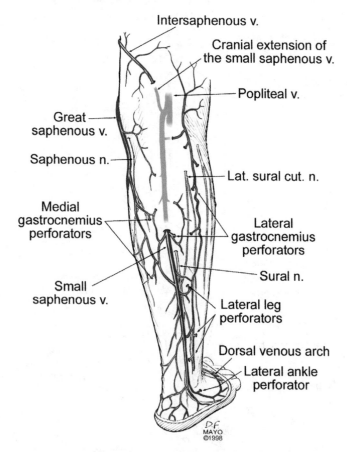

Figure 2.2.   Anatomy of the small saphenous vein. Note the proximity of the small saphenous vein to the sural nerve. (Reprinted with permission from the Mayo Foundation.)

muscles, joining with the femoral vein to become the common femoral vein in the groin. The external iliac vein begins above the inguinal ligament, before its confluence with the internal iliac vein at the sacroiliac joint which then becomes the common iliac vein.

C. Perforating veins connect the superficial with either the deep veins (direct perforators) or with venous sinuses in the calf (indirect perforators). Abundant perforating veins normally direct flow from the superficial toward the deep network via a system of **venous valves**. The more anatomically constant direct perforators are located in four general locations: *medial calf* (**paratibial** and **posterior tibial perforators**), *lateral calf*, *thigh*, and *foot*. Perforators have often been assigned eponyms, but in modern nomenclature are described according to their anatomic location.

D. Venous sinuses comprise a thin-walled, valveless, large capacitance system located in the calf musculature. When the calf muscles contract, pressures in excess of 200 mm Hg are created, propelling venous blood toward the heart. A normally functioning calf-muscle pump displaces >60% of venous blood within that leg into the popliteal vein with a single contraction.

E. Venous valves. A unique histologic feature of many veins is the presence of valves. These bicuspid, endothelialized structures direct "one-way" flow of venous blood from the extremity toward the heart, and by their closure prevent reflux. Present throughout the column of venous blood from the foot to the inguinal ligament, these valves work to equalize pressure throughout the venous system. Valves are present in the both superficial and deep veins. In the lower extremity the greatest number are located below the knee, decreasing in frequency until the inguinal ligament. A single valve in the common femoral vein or external iliac that may protect against "spillover" reflux into the great saphenous vein is absent in one-third of the population. The common iliac, vena cava, and portal venous system are devoid of valves.

F. The vein wall is comprised of the same concentric layers discussed in the previous chapter (intima, media, and adventitia), although their composition and function differ slightly in the venous circulation. These differences include (a) a thin wall that is one tenth to one third as thick as an artery, (b) less elastic tissue, (c) an attenuated media comprised of smooth muscle and adventitia, and (d) a thickened adventitia comprised of fibroelastic connective tissue. Although veins possess vasa vasorum, they receive most of their nourishment by diffusion from the bloodstream.

G. Upper extremity. As with the lower extremity, anatomic variations are far more common in the venous than in the arterial system. The **cephalic**, **median antebrachial**, **brachial**, and **basilic** veins constitute the venous system of the arm (Fig. 2.3). The cephalic and median antebrachial veins are generally considered superficial veins of the arm while the basilic and brachial veins are subfascial or deep. The superficial or deep location of upper extremity veins is particularly important as one considers formation of arteriovenous circuits (*arteriovenous fistula*) for hemodialysis access in the arm (Chapter 20). At the elbow fossa, the **median cubital vein**

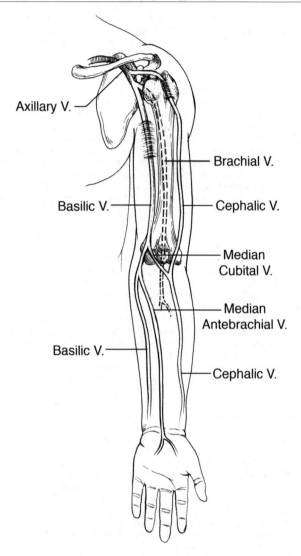

Figure 2.3.   Anatomy of the veins of the upper extremity. Anatomic variations in the upper-extremity veins, as with those of the lower extremity, are common.

joins the cephalic with the basilic vein, and also receives a deep communicating branch from the forearm. The paired **venae comitantes** course with the arteries in the forearm, becoming the paired brachial veins in the upper arm. The medial brachial vein and basilic vein typically join at the axillary vein, which then becomes the subclavian vein at the border of the first rib. In contrast, the cephalic vein joins the sub-clavian vein at the **delto-pectoral groove** of the anterior shoulder.

III. Etiology.

A. Venous insufficiency or reflux results from a failure of one or more of the valves within the venous system, resulting in loss of the balance of venous pressure. In the setting of reflux, the venous system below the abnormal segment is exposed to high venous pressures from pooling of blood due to gravity. Under these circumstances, venous pressure in the lower extremity in a person who is standing can be chronically elevated and sustained as high as 150–200 mm Hg (as long as the individual is on his or her feet). This condition preferen-tially affects the most dependent parts of the extremity and over time leads to venous distention, seeping of blood compo-nents into the interstitial space, and the sequelae of **chronic venous insufficiency**. Venous reflux can affect any combina-tion of the superficial, perforator, and deep veins, and can be the result of a degenerative process, as is commonly seen in varicose veins. From the histological standpoint, varicose veins possess less elastin and less contractile force and, as a result, are more prone to dilate and become varicose in a setting of chronic venous hypertension.

Valvular dysfunction may also be acquired after a throm-botic event damages the valves, resulting in a fibrous contrac-ture of the cusps (**postphlebitic syndrome**). **Deep venous insufficiency** usually follows thrombosis (DVT) and is some-times a result of primary degeneration or congenital defect in the valves. Thrombosis not only adversely affects the valves of the venous system but also damages the endothelium of the deep veins, rendering it ineffective at preventing future clot formation. Postphlebitic syndrome develops years after a DVT and is a result of valvular and endothelial dysfunction of the deep veins. Postphlebitic syndrome is a clinical spectrum pres-ent in all patients who have had DVT and can, in its most severe form, lead to venous hypertension, edema, subdermal scarring (**lipodermatosclerosis**), and venous ulceration. Venous ulcers occur most commonly at the medial and lateral malleoli of the leg (e.g., the most dependent), where venous pressures over time are the greatest.

B. Venous obstruction may be due to either intrinsic or extrinsic venous disorders. Failure of the deep vein to reopen (recannulize) after thrombosis can lead to reflux as well as out-flow obstruction. The most severe clinical symptoms of post-thrombotic syndrome occur in limbs with a combination of reflux and obstruction. **Klippel-Trénaunay syndrome** is a congenital triad of *capillary hemagiomas* (port-wine stains), *limb hypertrophy*, and *varicose veins*. Patients with this condi-tion may have venous obstruction as a consequence of complete (aplasia) or partial (hypoplasia) development of the deep venous system. The etiology of extrinsic venous compression can be pelvic malignancy, retroperitoneal fibrosis, and iatro-genic or congenital factors. A condition known as **May-Thurner syndrome** results from compression of the left common iliac vein underneath the right common iliac artery. This anatomic relationship is asymptomatic in most adults, but a small fraction may manifest edema, subtle leg asymmetry, or venous thrombosis. It is speculated that the anatomic proximity of the left iliac vein underneath the right iliac artery is responsible for the higher prevalence of left lower extremity venous thrombotic events compared to the right.

C. Acute venous thrombosis may result from a combination of three factors that comprise **Virchow's triad**: stasis, intimal injury, and hypercoagulability.

   1. Venous stasis may result from immobilization, such as in patients in a postoperative situation. Slow movement of blood, particularly through valve cusps, may predispose to leukocyte adhesion and local hypoxia, triggering endothelial injury and hypercoagulable factors.

   2. Minor endothelial injury and the ensuing cascade of platelet migration and fibrin adherence is usually balanced out and overcome by the intrinsic fibrinolytic system. However, significant injury, as may be associated with an indwelling catheter, or in combination with other permissive factors, may result in thrombosis.

   3. Hypercoagulable states that predispose to venous thrombosis may be genetic (hereditary) or acquired (Chapter 2). Common acquired states include the postoperative condition (transient decrease in fibrinolysis and increase in procoagulant factors), trauma, malignancy, pregnancy, and oral contraceptives. Genetic hypercoagulable states may contribute to 50–60% of unexplained DVTs, and should be investigated in those patients with iatrogenic, familial, or recurrent thrombosis (Chapter 2).

D. Pulmonary thromboembolism results from dislodged venous thrombi, which travel to the right heart and through the tricuspid and pulmonic valves of the heart to lodge in the pulmonary arteries. The majority come from untreated lower extremity thrombosis, but may also come from pelvic and upper extremity veins.

IV. Pathophysiology.

A. Normal physiology. Venous pressure at the ankle measures the weight of the column of blood to the level of the right atrium. Normal pressures in the standing position are 90–100 mm Hg, depending on height. With exercise, the calf muscle propels blood from the leg, *reducing* the venous pressure by over 70% after about 10 steps. The recovery time to refill the calf with venous blood upon cessation of exercise normally exceeds 20 seconds (mean 70 seconds) (Fig. 2.4).

B. Superficial venous insufficiency. Patients with varicose veins may only be able to reduce their ambulatory venous pressure by 30–40%. As much as one fifth to one fourth of the total femoral outflow is refluxed into the incompetent saphenous system, back down the leg in a "circus" motion.

C. Deep venous insufficiency. With deep venous insufficiency, ankle pressures may decrease less than 20% with exercise and calf refill time is abnormally fast. Limbs with combined deep and perforator reflux in particular may develop significant venous volume pooling in the calf at rest and an inefficient calf-muscle pump with activity.

D. Deep venous obstruction. Ambulatory venous pressures may not decrease with exercise and may even increase. Signif-

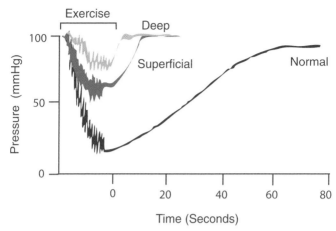

Figure 2.4. Ambulatory venous pressures. Normally, leg exercises cause lower-extremity venous pressures to drop approximately 70% because the musculovenous pump propels blood toward the heart and competent venous valves prevent reflux. Normal return to baseline venous pressure after exercise with refilling of the calf muscle is greater than 20 seconds. Varicose veins (superficial veins) are associated with a 30–40% venous pressure reduction with exercise because a portion of deep venous return is refluxed down the incompetent saphenous vein. Deep venous valve incompetence results in less initial drop in venous pressure, but a more rapid restoration of venous pressure in the leg with cessation of exercise. (Adapted from Schanzer H, Peirce EC II. Pathophysiologic evaluation of chronic venous stasis with ambulatory venous pressure studies. *Angiology.* 1982;33:183-191.)

icant venous outflow obstruction may lead to **ambulatory venous hypertension** and **venous claudication**, a characteristic "bursting" sensation in the leg with ambulation. The presence of venous collaterals may diminish the symptoms of venous obstruction.

E. Pulmonary embolism. The main physiologic consequence of acute pulmonary embolism is hypoxemia, which is primarily the result of mechanical blockage of the pulmonary arteries. Significant pulmonary emboli to either pulmonary artery (or certainly a **saddle embolus** that straddles the main pulmonary arteries) cause outflow obstruction from the right heart and right heart strain or failure. Large pulmonary emboli may lead to sudden cardiovascular collapse from hypoxia as well as right heart failure. Smaller or recurrent emboli can also be fatal, particularly in people with underlying cardiopulmonary disease who are unable to compensate.

V. Natural history. Although venous thrombosis can acutely threaten life, many venous disorders are chronic problems. It is important that both the patient and physician understand this chronicity. In most cases, the natural history can be altered so that the patient remains productive and comfortable.

A. Varicose veins and telangiectasias (spider veins) are nearly universal. Natural history may range from the asymptomatic unsightly appearance, to achiness and heaviness after prolonged standing, to swelling and itching in the limb. Superficial thrombophlebitis may occur, but is rarely complicated by deep venous thrombosis or pulmonary embolism. Large varicosities can cause overlying ulceration of the skin and (rarely) bleeding, especially in elderly or debilitated people.

B. Postphlebitic syndrome is present in all individuals who have had DVT. For the first year or two following a DVT event, it consists of mild chronic leg discomfort and mild edema. Five years after the DVT, however, 50% of patients have developed significant leg edema, induration, and stasis dermatitis at the ankle. Another 5–20% of individuals develop venous ulceration. By 10 years, more than 90% have lower extremity symptoms. The natural history of post-thrombotic syndrome can be altered by compression therapy with heavy support hose (40 mm Hg). Thrombolytic therapy (**catheter-directed thrombolysis**) for acute, symptomatic DVTs in the proximal circulation of the extremity may favorably alter the natural history of postphlebitic syndrome by more quickly reducing clot burden, preventing venous obstruction, and reducing valvular damage.

C. Acute deep venous thrombosis. The most serious consequence of deep venous thrombosis is thromboembolism to the lung. Pulmonary embolism seldom occurs when the thrombus is located below the knees, and is more common with iliofemoral thrombosis. The natural course for many patients with simple deep venous thrombosis, even without anticoagulation, is resolution of the acute tenderness and swelling. Over a period of 3–6 months, the deep veins usually recanalize. Without appropriate anticoagulation, about 30% of untreated patients have recurrent thrombosis or pulmonary embolism with a high mortality. Most limbs with acute venous thrombosis are normal in color or have a cyanotic appearance. In contrast and in more severe cases, **phlegmasia alba dolens** (turgid, white, painful leg) occurs with extreme acute venous outflow obstruction. A more severe manifestation of venous thrombosis is **phlegmasia cerulea dolens** (turgid, blue, painful leg), in which massive swelling can lead to arterial compromise and venous gangrene.

D. Pulmonary embolism. Because many episodes of deep venous thrombosis probably go undetected, the incidence of thromboembolism to the lungs is difficult to ascertain. Estimates indicate a pulmonary embolism rate of 5% even in adequately treated patients. Approximately one patient in 10 with a symptomatic pulmonary embolus dies within an hour. The remaining patients who are adequately treated with anticoagulants usually follow a course of complete resolution and return to good cardiopulmonary function within several weeks. The most important factor predicting a poor prognosis is pre-existing heart disease. A minority of patients develop recurrent emboli and pulmonary hypertension with **cor pulmonale** (right heart failure).

SELECTED READING

Eklof B, Rutherford RB, Bergan JJ, et al. Revision of the CEAP classification for chronic venous disorders: Consensus statement. *J Vasc Surg*. 2004;40:1248-1252.

Gloviczki P, Yao JST, eds. *Handbook of Venous Disorders: Guidelines of the American Venous Forum.* 2nd ed. London: Arnold Publishers; 2001.

Lindner DJ, Edwards JM, Phinney ES, et al. Long-term hemodynamic and clinical sequelae of lower extremity deep vein thrombosis. *J Vasc Surg.* 1986;4:436-442.

Mozes G, Glovicski P. New discoveries in anatomy and new terminology of leg veins: Clinical applications. *Vasc Endovasc Surg.* 2004;38:367-374.

Schanzer H, Peirce EC II. Pathophysiologic evaluation of chronic venous stasis with ambulatory venous pressure studies. *Angiology.* 1982;33:183-191.

Silverstein MD, Heit JA, Mohr DN, Petterson TM, O'Fallon WM, Melton JL. Trends in the incidence of deep vein thrombosis and pulmonary embolism: A 25-year population-based study. *Arch Int Med.* 1998;158:585-593.

CHAPTER 3

Hypercoagulable Disorders

The opening chapters of this handbook address the basic concepts of the arterial and venous systems in health and disease. Because hypercoagulable conditions play such a significant role in the management of patients with arterial and venous disease, this chapter is included as a basic tenet of vascular pathophysiology. The medical term **thrombosis** refers to the formation of clot, and **thrombophilia** describes a physiologic state in which blood has an increased tendency to form clot. This chapter provides a summary of inherited (i.e., genetic) and acquired hypercoagulable conditions, their prevalence in the populace, and basic concepts related to their management.

Hypercoagulable conditions in the formation of clot (thrombogenesis) were acknowledged around the year 1860 by Rudolph Virchow, who recognized them as a part of the triad (**Virchow's triad**) of factors contributing to thrombosis (*hypercoagulable condition*, *endothelial injury*, and *stasis of blood*). It is estimated that nearly 2 million persons in the United States die annually from arterial or venous thrombosis. Inherited disorders and/or acquired factors causing hypercoagulability are responsible for more than half of these events. Genetic factors are recognized as *primary hypercoagulable states*, while acquired disorders are considered *secondary forms of hypercoagulability* (Tables 3.1 and 3.2).

I. Mechanisms. The **coagulation cascade** consists of the intrinsic and extrinsic pathways. The *extrinsic pathway* includes tissue factor, and factors VII, X, V, and II, and fibrin. The *intrinsic pathway* consists of factors, all of which are contained in the blood, specifically, high molecular weight kininogen, prekallikrein, and factors XII, XI, IX, VIII, X, and V, as well as prothrombin (factor II) and fibrinogen. The extrinsic pathway is viewed as the primary pathway of coagulation and is triggered by vascular damage and exposure of tissue factor to blood. Thrombin, created by the extrinsic pathway, activates factor XI of the intrinsic pathway in a positive feedback manner, assuring that clot will be formed independently of tissue factor.

Table 3.1.   Inherited thrombophilia disorders

Antithrombin III deficiency

Protein C deficiency

Protein S deficiency

Activated protein C resistance

Factor V R506Q (Leiden) mutation

Homocystinemia

Prothrombin gene variant (20210A)

Hypoplasminogenemia

Dysfibrinogenemia

Controls within this system exist to prevent excess thrombin formation and undesired thrombosis. Specifically, plasma proteins and endothelial receptors act to counterbalance the coagulation cascade. **Antithrombin III** acts as an inhibitor of thrombin and other coagulation factors to a lesser degree. The activity of antithrombin III is enhanced by **heparin** and heparin-like molecules (polysaccharides) exposed on the endothelium of blood vessels. Also exposed on the endothelial cell is the receptor **thrombomodulin**. Thrombin binds to thrombomodulin and loses its procoagulant potential. It then participates, with thrombomodulin, in the activation of the **protein C system**. Protein C is a proenzyme of a serine protease, which inactivates the clotting factors Va and VIIIa. **Protein S** is a cofactor to protein C and greatly accelerates its activity, thereby further preventing clot formation. As factor V is a central coagulation factor common to both the intrinsic and extrinsic pathways, its inactivation by protein C is especially important in controlling hypercoagulability and excess clot formation.

II. Inherited hypercoagulability. Of all patients with a hypercoagulable condition, a genetic or familial cause can be identified nearly 40% of the time. Discovery of antithrombin III deficiency and characterization of the protein C and protein S systems identified an important but very small percentage of individuals and families affected by familial thrombosis. Protein C and S and antithrombin III deficiencies are autosomal dominant forms of inherited hypercoagulability and were among the first of this category to be described; however, they are responsible for only 5% to 10% of cases of familial thrombosis (Table 3.1).

In 1994, a point mutation in factor V of the coagulation pathway was identified by Bertina et al. in Leiden (the Netherlands). This genetic mutation was found to cause *activated protein C resistance* and an associated hypercoagulable condition. This mutation at position 506 of the factor V polypeptide is called *factor V Leiden* and leads to an activated protein C resistance (APC resistance). Factor V Leiden is absent in certain ethnic groups but is present in up to 15% of some Caucasian populations. In contrast to the relative rarity of the protein deficiencies, APC resistance has been described in up to 60% of patients with familial thrombosis. Importantly, some individuals may be affected by more than one genetic disorder and usually present early in life with one or more thrombotic events.

A. Antithrombin III deficiency. Antithrombin III deficiency is an autosomal dominant disease, and its prevalence in the population is one in 2,000 to 5,000 people. Antithrombin III is synthesized by liver cells (hepatocytes) and inactivates thrombin as well as other coagulation factors. Its activity is greatly enhanced by heparin. Two types of antithrombin III deficiency exist, the most common resulting from decreased synthesis of a biologically normal molecule. These patients have functional levels of circulating antithrombin III that are only 50% of normal. The second type of antithrombin III deficiency is less frequent and results from a functional deficiency associated with specific molecular abnormalities in the molecule involving the heparin or thrombin-binding domains.

Antithrombin III deficiency is suspected when patients have recurrent, familial, and/or juvenile deep vein or mesenteric venous thrombosis. Such an event frequently occurs in conjunction with another recognized predisposing event such as trauma, immobilization, pregnancy, or oral contraceptives. Deficiency may also be suspected by the inability to anticoagulate a patient with intravenous heparin. Such patients may require unusually large doses of heparin to achieve anticoagulation or may actually require treatment with fresh frozen plasma (FFP) that contains antithrombin III along with intravenous heparin in order for the heparin to be active.

Acquired antithrombin III deficiency may also be seen with liver and kidney disease, sepsis, oral contraceptives, and some chemotherapeutic agents.

B. Deficiencies in protein C and S system. The protein C and S system is a major regulator of blood fluidity. Its actions are particularly important at the capillary level where there exists a relatively high concentration of thrombomodulin receptors on endothelial cells. These deficiencies are also inherited as autosomal dominant traits and are most frequently heterozygous. The prevalence of protein C deficiency is one in 200 to 300. Homozygous forms of protein C or S deficiency are associated with extreme, highly lethal forms of thrombosis in infancy, termed **purpura fulminans.** Both forms of protein C or S deficiency have also been associated with a condition referred to as **warfarin-induced skin necrosis.** In this disorder, skin necrosis begins within days of initiation of warfarin therapy (Coumadin). Its pathogenesis is related to a transient, severe hypercoagulable state related to an exaggerated protein C deficiency caused by warfarin. It is treated with intravenous heparin, administration of vitamin K, and/or plasma protein C concentrates.

Acquired protein C and S deficiencies occur with activation of inflammatory response syndromes, such as severe sepsis. In such conditions the complement system is upregulated and C4b binding protein (present in the activated complement system) binds and inactivates protein S, creating a relative protein S–deficient state. Acquired deficiencies may also be present in liver disease, pregnancy, postoperative states, and nephrotic syndrome.

C. Activated protein C resistance. One of the most prevalent hereditary hypercoagulable states is APC resistance. Also called factor V Leiden, the prevalence of this hypercoagulable condition varies widely from one population to another but has been demonstrated in 40% to 60% of patients with familial thrombosis. Factor V Leiden is considered the most common form of hypercoagulable condition in people of European and Asian descent. A limitation in identifying individuals who have activated protein C resistance is the inability to accurately perform testing in patients who are anticoagulated (i.e., taking Coumadin). However, testing for the factor V genetic mutation (position 506 of the factor V polypeptide) is not affected by Coumadin or heparin and allows for more accurate identification of patients with this condition.

Similar to protein C or protein S deficiencies, patients who are homozygous for factor V Leiden have a much higher risk of thrombosis than patients who are heterozygous for the mutation. The most common manifestation of APC resistance is *deep venous thrombosis* (DVT), and, in contrast to persons who are homozygous for protein C or protein S deficiency, some persons homozygous for factor V Leiden never experience thrombosis.

As with other inherited hypercoagulable conditions, the development of thrombosis in APC resistance is affected by the coexistence of other genetic or circumstantial risk factors (Virchow's triad). The most common risk factors affecting APC-resistant individuals are oral contraceptive use, pregnancy, trauma, and surgery. Women who are heterozygous for factor V Leiden and use oral contraceptives have a near 30-fold increase in risk for venous thrombosis; women who are homozygous have a several hundred–fold increase in risk for similar events. Although our understanding of this condition is relatively new, the factor V Leiden mutation appears to be more commonly associated with venous thrombotic events than with arterial thrombosis.

D. Hyperhomocysteinemia. Abnormalities in the metabolism of homocysteine result in increased circulating levels of this sulphur-containing amino acid (>14 μmol/L). Additionally, acquired hyperhomocysteinemia may occur as a result of deficiencies of vitamin B_6, vitamin B_{12}, or folate. Hyperhomocysteinemia is present in 5% of the population and is associated with early atherosclerosis and, less commonly, venous thrombosis. Elevated homocysteine levels act primarily by causing endothelial dysfunction and platelet activation. Circulating homocysteine levels have been shown to alter favorably with B-vitamin and folate supplementation; screening individuals who have premature atherosclerosis is recommended. Recently, however, the role of B-vitamin and folate supplementation in preventing early atherosclerosis in this setting has been called into question and its clinical effectiveness remains unsettled.

E. Prothrombin gene variant (20210A). A genetic mutation on position 20210 of the prothrombin gene was discovered in 1996 and is referred to as the *prothrombin variant*. This mutation results in overproduction of the clotting factor **prothrombin** (**factor II**) causing an increased tendency to form clot. Heterozygous prothrombin mutations are found in about 2% of the Caucasian population and 0.5% of the African American population and are present in 20% of patients with familial venous thrombophilia. Having the prothrombin mutation primarily increases one's risk of venous thrombosis and thromboembolism (by two to three times) but may also predispose to arterial thrombosis, although to a lesser degree.

F. Other primary hypercoagulable states. Other less common inheritable hypercoagulable syndromes exist and consist mostly of disorders related to **plasminogen** synthesis or release. Plasminogen is a pro-enzyme that is released into the bloodstream and converted to the active form **plasmin** by an enzyme called **tissue plasminogen activator** (**tPA**). Plasmin plays an important role in maintaining blood fluidity by breaking down fibrin clots in an action referred to as **fibrinolysis**. Individuals with disorders of the plasminogen and fibrinolysis pathways have high rates of venous and arterial thrombosis often at an early age.

Table 3.2.   Causes of acquired hypercoagulable disorders

Cigarette smoking
Pregnancy
Oral contraceptives
Hormone replacement therapy
Heparin-induced thrombocytopenia
Antiphospholipid syndrome
Malignancy
Antineoplastic medications
Myeloproliferative syndromes
Hyperhomocysteinemia
Inflammatory bowel disease

III. Acquired hypercoagulability (Table 3.2).

A. Smoking. The nicotine and carbon monoxide in cigarette smoke cause endothelial dysfunction with increased platelet deposition and lipid accumulation. Smoking decreases the production of prostacyclin, a potent vasodilator and inhibitor of platelet aggregation, and increases blood viscosity. These and other effects make smoking the *most common acquired hypercoagulable condition* and contributor to arterial and venous thrombosis.

B. Heparin-induced thrombocytopenia occurs in 2% to 3% of patients who undergo therapy with unfractionated heparin. This acquired condition results from the formation of antiplatelet antibodies after exposure to heparin. Patients who have heparin-associated antiplatelet antibodies have extreme platelet aggregation and thrombosis when exposed to heparin (**heparin-induced thrombocytopenia and thrombosis**, or **HITT**). The development of antibodies to heparin is independent of patient age, gender, or amount or route of heparin exposure. All forms of heparin, including low-molecular weight heparin, can result in antibody formation. Clinical presentation of heparin-induced thrombocytopenia and thrombosis includes decreasing platelet count, resistance to anticoagulation with heparin, and often severe thrombotic events. Management includes avoidance of all forms of heparin, initiation of platelet inhibition with intravenous administration of Dextran 40 or Abciximab (ReoPro), and/or use of one of the **direct thrombin inhibitors (DTIs)** Argatroban, lepirudin (Refludin), or bivalirudin (Angiomax), depending upon the clinical scenario and thrombus burden.

C. Oral contraceptives/pregnancy. Exogenous estrogens are associated with an increased risk for venous thrombosis as well as coronary and cerebral arterial thrombotic events. Estrogens are associated with decreased antithrombin III and protein S activities and increases in activated factors VII and X. Estrogens have also been associated with decreased levels of thrombomodulin and a subsequent reduction in protein C activity. The combination of the factor V Leiden mutation plus the use of certain oral contraceptives places the patient at a nearly 30-fold increase for venous thrombosis.

Pregnancy is associated with an increase in nearly all of the clotting factors, an increased platelet count, and a decrease in protein S activity. In addition, pregnancy is associated with decreased antithrombin. These factors combined with venous stasis from the uterus compressing venous drainage of the legs lead to at least a fivefold increase in venous thrombosis during pregnancy.

D. Antiphospholipid syndrome (APS) is also referred to as **Hughes syndrome** after the rheumatologist Graham R.V. Hughes, who described the syndrome while working at St. Thomas's Hospital in London. APS is present in 1% of the population, is more common in women than in men, and increases in prevalence with age. Antiphospholipid syndrome is caused by circulating antibodies to negatively charged proteins that bind to phospholipids in the bloodstream and can be diagnosed using the assay for either **anticardiolipin antibody** or **circulating lupus anticoagulant.** The main target for the anticardiolipin antibody appears to be a negatively charged protein called B_2 Glycoprotein-1, while the target for the lupus anticoagulant is prothrombin (factor II). The assay for anticardiolipin antibody is most sensitive and specific for the diagnosis of APS. Circulating lupus anticoagulant may be independent of an underlying collagen vascular disorder (primary APS) or part of the connective tissue disease such as *systemic lupus erythematous (SLE),* in which case it is referred to as secondary APS. As many as 50% of individuals with SLE or lupus-like disorders have either the circulating lupus anticoagulant or antiphospholipid antibodies.

The most common arterial event in patients with APS is ischemic stroke, while the most common venous event is DVT. Antiphospholipid antibody syndrome is also known to cause pregnancy-related complications, including late-term miscarriage likely due to a thrombotic event. The pathogenesis of thrombosis in individuals with APS is not well understood but has been suggested to involve autoantibodies that inhibit endothelial cell prostacyclin or that interfere with thrombomodulin-mediated protein C activation.

E. Malignancy. The association of malignancy and venous thrombosis is well recognized. One of the first recognized patterns of this association was that of superficial thrombosis in patients with adenocarcinoma of the bowel or pancreas or cancers of the lung (**Trousseau's syndrome**). Patients who develop deep venous thrombosis and have no other identifiable risk factors have a 10% chance of having an undiagnosed malignancy. The hypercoagulable state associated with malignancy is due to interaction of tumor cells and their products with host cells. This interaction leads to elimination of normal protective mechanisms that the host employs to prevent thrombosis.

Tumor cells may induce procoagulant properties such as secretion of tissue thromboplastin, which is a constituent composed of protein and phospholipid that is widely distributed in many tissues. Tissue thromboplastin serves as a cofactor with factor VIIa to activate factor X in the extrinsic pathway of blood coagulation, and its secretion in the setting of malignancy may contribute to a relative hypercoagulable condition.

Additionally, tumor cells may cause the release of proteases, which activate clotting factors. Patients with malignant disease may also have increased levels of factors V, VIII, IX, and X. Cancer patients frequently have other risk factors that place them at risk for thrombosis, such as chemotherapeutic treatment, in-dwelling central venous catheters, and limited mobility.

F. Antineoplastic drugs. Chemotherapeutic agents have been associated with vascular abnormalities such as thrombotic thrombocytopenic purpura, **Budd-Chiari syndrome**, myocardial infarction, and venous thrombosis. Thrombotic events are related to hypercoagulable states caused by the effect of these drugs or their metabolites on vascular endothelium.

G. Myeloproliferative syndromes. At least three myeloproliferative disorders have been associated with thrombosis and hypercoagulable conditions likely secondary to increases in whole blood viscosity. The disorders, **polycythemia vera**, **essential thrombocythemia**, and **agnogenic myeloid metaplasia**, may also affect platelet function either directly or indirectly. In addition to association with extremity venous thrombosis, the myeloproliferative disorders predispose individuals to mesenteric, hepatic, or portal venous thrombosis. This type of hypercoagulable state rarely manifests as arterial thrombosis unless combined with other thrombotic risk factors previously described.

IV. Management. The management of patients with identified hypercoagulable states is highly individualized and often hinges on the decision whether or not to anticoagulate an individual in a prophylactic manner. Unfortunately these clinical decisions are not yet guided by prospective clinical studies. **Hypercoagulability is now viewed as a multigenic or multi–risk factor disease.** Except for a few rare inherited homozygous conditions, thrombophilia exists in patients with one or more additive risk factors that in combination may or may not reach a thrombotic threshold. The decision to anticoagulate rests on the number of identified risk factors in a given patient and whether or not that patient has experienced one (or more) thrombotic events. This decision should involve a multidisciplinary approach and include internists, hematologists, vascular medicine specialists, and vascular surgeons. Generally, asymptomatic patients are not anticoagulated unless additional risk factors such as surgery are anticipated.

Long-term prophylaxis with warfarin is considered when a patient with an identified hypercoagulable condition has experienced two or more thrombotic events or a single life- or limb-threatening event. This general guideline may be modified in patients with prosthetic grafts, heart valves, or, specifically, certain identified hypercoagulable conditions. Immediate therapy for acute thrombosis consists of unfractionated or low molecular weight heparin with initiation of oral warfarin (see Chapter 21). In select instances, there may be a role for catheter-directed thrombolysis of symptomatic extremity thrombosis or use of direct thrombin inhibitors in cases of HITT. **Given the risk of warfarin-induced necrosis in patients with protein C or S deficiency, it is recommended that warfarin therapy be** initiated with the patient fully anticoagulated with intra-venous unfractionated heparin or therapeutic doses of low molecular weight heparin.

SELECTED READING

Auerbach AD, Sanders GD, Hambleton J. Cost-effectiveness of testing for hypercoagulability and effects on treatment strategies in patients with deep venous thrombosis. *Am J Med*. 2004;116:816-828.

Falanga A, Rickles FR. Pathophysiology of the thrombotic state in the cancer patient. *Semin Thromb Hemost*. 1999;25:173-182.

Gerotziafas GT. Risk factors for venous thromboembolism in children. *Int Angiol*. 2004;23:195-205.

Johnson CM, Mureebe L, Silver D. Hypercoagulable states: a review. *Vasc Endovasc Surg*. 2005;39:123-133.

Kroegel C, Reissig A. Principle mechanisms underlying venous thromboembolism: epidemiology, risk factors, pathophysiology and pathogenesis. *Respiration*. 2003;70:7-30.

Merrill JT. Diagnosis of the antiphospholipid syndrome: how far to go? *Curr Rheumatol Rep*. 2004;6:469-472.

Page C, Rubin LE, Gusberg RJ, Dardik A. Arterial thrombosis associated with heterozygous factor V Leiden disorder, hyperhomocysteinemia and peripheral arterial disease: importance of synergistic factors. *J Vasc Surg*. 2005;42:1014-1018.

Wakefield TW. Treatment options for venous thrombosis. *J Vasc Surg*. 2000;31:613-620.

Examination of the Vascular System

INITIAL PATIENT EVALUATION

The interview and physical examination provide information that directs the need for additional diagnostic testing and treatment of patients with vascular disease. Today's noninvasive vascular testing and imaging technologies tend to divert attention from the importance of talking to and examining the patient. These diagnostic tests add valuable hemodynamic and anatomic data but **do not replace the need for a careful history and physical examination as the first step in optimal patient care.** Even in this era of specialized imaging, the adage that "the patient will tell you what's wrong, if you're willing to listen" remains true.

The initial history and physical examination serve several purposes. The process enables the clinician to establish a **clinical impression** or preliminary diagnosis. Vascular diseases manifest physical changes that are apparent by inspection, palpation, and auscultation. Interviewing and examining the patient often provide enough information for a good clinical impression. Diagnostic tests can then be ordered in a more appropriate and efficient manner to further hone the clinical impression.

The history and physical also allow the clinician to determine the **urgency for treatment.** Although some vascular problems require urgent intervention, most entail elective evaluation and treatment. This important distinction must be made on the basis of the history and physical exam and not the appearance of vascular disease on an imaging study. Additionally, the history and physical provide an opportunity to assess the physiologic age of the patient. Comorbidities such as pulmonary, cardiac, or renal dysfunction heavily influence management strategies and outcomes in patients with vascular disease. One should not underestimate the value of the "eyeball test" and review of systems and functional status as one considers the best treatment plan. An astute clinician would also be mindful that the vascular patient may harbor an occult nonvascular disease such as gastrointestinal or pulmonary malignancy.

Finally, the initial interview establishes a **rapport or relationship** between the patient and provider, which is particularly valuable in caring for patients with vascular disease. Through this process the provider gains the trust to reassure the patient and family and to obtain insight into the patient's overall living situation. For example, the patient's vocation, level of independent living, and whether he or she drives an automobile all weigh heavily in the management decisions related to vascular disease.

The following chapters outline the techniques of the **arterial and venous examination** of the following anatomic regions: neck, upper extremity, abdomen, and lower extremity. A stethoscope, manual blood pressure cuff, and continuous wave Doppler are needed to perform the physical exam, and a marker can be handy to note location of arterial signals or even varicose veins.

CHAPTER 4

History and Physical Examination of the Arterial System

I. General Examination. Age-related arterial disease is a diffuse process. Therefore, the exam, regardless of complaint, should include the entire arterial system in order to identify unrecognized atherosclerotic disease and should include the following:

1. Checking of heart rate and rhythm.
2. Measurement of blood pressures in both arms.
3. Neck auscultation to listen for carotid bruits.
4. Cardiac auscultation to listen for arrhythmias, gallops, and murmurs.
5. Abdominal palpation to assess for a pulsatile mass (e.g., aortic aneurysm).
6. Abdominal auscultation to listen for bruits.
7. Palpation of peripheral pulses.
8. Auscultation of the femoral region to listen for bruits.
9. Full length inspection of upper and lower extremities to assess for ulcers, gangrene, or evidence of distal embolization in the toes and/ or fingers (**blue toe syndrome**).
10. Measurement of leg pressures using a continuous wave Doppler and manual blood pressure cuff to calculate the **ankle-brachial index (ABI)**.

II. Head and neck. Vascular disease in the head and neck relates mostly to atherosclerosis of the carotid arteries, which is a common cause of stroke (Chapter 13). Patients should be questioned about previous stroke or **transient ischemic attack** (TIA), carotid artery intervention (endarterectomy or stent), and prior duplex ultrasound of the carotid arteries. If a carotid intervention or duplex ultrasound has been performed in the past, the indications and results are important to understand. Symptoms of TIA or stroke typically relate to episodes of *unilateral* extremity weakness or paralysis. Stroke or TIA may also manifest as an inability to initiate speech (**aphasia**), inability to form words (**dysarthria**), or facial weakness or slurring of speech. The clinician should also inquire about episodes of **transient monocular blindness (amarousis fugax)**, which would suggest occlusive disease of the carotid artery on the same side (ipsilateral) as the ocular symptoms. Amaurosis (also described as a "descending curtain or shade") results from temporary occlusion of a retinal arteriole from emboli originating from the carotid bulb passing through the **ophthalmic artery**. The differential diagnosis of amaurosis is broad, and includes migraine headache, papilledema, and giant cell arteritis.

The *differential diagnosis* of stroke or TIA originating from the carotid arteries in the neck includes **seizure disorder**, which more commonly causes global or bilateral symptoms followed by somnolence (postictal period). Severe hypertension can lead to **small vessel cerebral infarct** or **hemorrhagic stroke**, which can be differentiated from embolic stroke from the patient's history and presentation. **Brain tumors** or **brain aneurysms** may also cause neurologic deficits but are often accompanied by other symptoms such as headache. Diffusion-weighted magnetic resonance imaging (DW-MRI) is useful in differentiating primary intracranial disease (small vessel cerebral infarct or brain tumor) from embolic TIA or stroke originating from carotid disease in the neck. Syncope, lightheadedness, and dizziness are common in the elderly and are referred to as **posterior circulation** or **vertebral artery symptoms**. These symptoms are rarely related to carotid disease and are more commonly due to fluctuations in blood pressure, cardiac arrhythmias, disease within the middle ear (vestibular system), or **subclavian steal syndrome**.

A. Inspection. Normally, the carotid pulsation is not visible. However, it may be prominent at the base of the right neck in thin patients with longstanding hypertension. Such patients are often referred for concerns of aneurysm, when in fact they have a tortuous or prominent common carotid artery. **Carotid artery aneurysm** and **carotid body tumor** occur near the bifurcation and can be visualized in the middle or upper aspect of the anterior neck.

Another observation related to carotid occlusive disease is a bright reflective defect or spot on the retina referred to as a **Hollenhorst plaque**. These plaques seen on funduscopic exam of the eye were described by a Mayo Clinic ophthalmologist in the 1960s, and represent cholesterol emboli originating from atherosclerotic disease of the carotid arteries.

B. Palpation. The common carotid pulse is palpable low in the neck between the midline trachea and the anterior border of the sternocleidomastoid muscle. Even in the setting of internal carotid artery occlusion, there is generally a palpable common carotid pulse as the external carotid often remains patent. A diminished or absent common carotid pulsation suggests significant proximal occlusive disease at the origin of the carotid artery in the chest. The presence of a temporal artery pulse anterior to the ear indicates a patent common and external carotid artery. Palpation itself cannot differentiate between carotid aneurysm and carotid body tumor, both of which may present as a pulsatile mass in the neck. Enlarged lymph nodes often have similar findings, and differentiation in the setting of a pulsatile neck mass requires duplex ultrasonography, computed tomography (CT), or magnetic resonance imaging (MRI).

The vertebral artery is not accessible to palpation as it lies deep at the posterior base of the neck and is surrounded by cervical bone for most of its course. Pulsatile masses at the base of the neck or in the supraclavicular fossa generally originate from the **subclavian artery**.

C. Auscultation. The stethoscope is placed lightly over the middle and base of the neck while the patient suspends respirations. **Cervical bruits** are an abnormal finding and may originate from carotid stenosis or lesions of the aortic valve or arch vessels. A bruit from a carotid stenosis is usually loudest at the midneck over the carotid bifurcation. Transmitted bruits or cardiac murmurs tend to be loudest over the upper chest and base of the neck.

The presence of a cervical bruit does not necessarily mean that a carotid stenosis is present. In fact, only half of patients with carotid bruit will have stenoses of 30% or more and only a quarter will have stenoses of more than 75%. Additionally, **the severity of underlying carotid stenosis does not correlate with the loudness of the bruit**. Duplex ultrasound is standard in determining the significance of a cervical bruit and is noninvasive, inexpensive, and readily available. Carotid arteriography is not used as a screening tool in the setting of an asymptomatic bruit as it is invasive and carries a risk of stroke (Chapter 13).

III. Upper extremity. Although atherosclerosis is less common in the upper than the lower extremity, arterial lesions of the subclavian and axillary arteries can develop (Chapter 18). Upper-extremity occlusive or aneurysm disease may cause claudication or signs of embolization in the arm or hand. For reasons that are not fully understood, arterial occlusive lesions of the subclavian artery are more common on the left than the right side. In instances where a subclavian stenosis is *proximal* to the origin of the vertebral artery, the patient can develop a condition known as **subclavian steal syndrome**. In these cases exertion of the arm results in a pressure decrease across the stenosis that leads to reversal of flow in the vertebral artery ("steal") causing posterior circulation symptoms (Fig. 4.1). Acute arm ischemia is most often the result of an embolus from a proximal arterial or even cardiac source. Acute thrombosis of a chronic subclavian or axillary artery aneurysm or stenosis may also result in acute arm ischemia.

A variety of nonatherosclerotic vascular diseases can affect the upper extremity (Chapter 18). **Takayasu's arteritis (pulseless disease)** is an inflammatory condition of the arteries that occurs predominantly in young Asian women. The early stage of Takayasu's disease is characterized by an acute inflammatory response that often includes fever, malaise, and muscle aches. The later stages occur after the acute arteritis has been treated and can result in fibrotic arterial stenoses or even arterial occlusion. **Giant cell arteritis (GCA)** occurs most commonly in mature Caucasian women and can affect aortic arch vessels and axillary and brachial arteries. Other symptoms associated with GCA include headaches, monocular blindness, and jaw claudication. Episodic coolness, pain, and numbness of the hand suggest **small vessel vasospasm or Raynaud's syndrome,** which is often triggered by an identifiable event such as exposure to the cold. The etiology may be idiopathic (Raynaud's disease) or associated with other systemic collagen vascular diseases or prior frostbite (Raynaud's phenomenon).

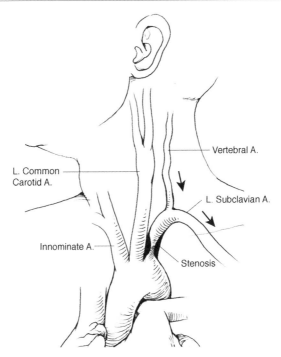

Figure 4.1. A proximal left subclavian stenosis or innominate artery stenosis can result in the syndrome of subclavian steal. Flow is "stolen" retrograde from the ipsilateral vertebral artery to supply the upper extremity. Symptoms related to posterior circulation insufficiency such as ataxia, dizziness, syncope, and visual disturbances may develop and are exacerbated by arm activity.

Thoracic outlet syndrome (TOS) may affect the upper extremities, causing vascular compromise from repetitive use of the arm. Pure vascular TOS is uncommon (10% of cases) and results from compromise of the subclavian artery or vein at the thoracic outlet (Fig. 5.1). At this location, the first rib, the scalene and subclavius muscles, and the clavicle form an often tight space through which the subclavian vessels pass (Chapter 18). This condition is especially common in young muscular individuals such as weight lifters, pitchers, and swimmers. Over 90% of TOS is related to or has a neurologic component involving brachial plexus.

A. Inspection. Inspection of the upper extremity provides information about arterial perfusion. Pink fingertips with a capillary refill time of less than 3 seconds are a sign of good perfusion. In contrast, the acutely ischemic upper extremity is pallid, and may have neurologic compromise in the form of motor or sensory deficits. The main change in appearance of the extremity with chronic arterial ischemia is muscle atrophy, especially in the forearm and proximal hand. Embolization or small-vessel disease may be recognized by painful mottled areas or ulcerations of the fingertips. Raynaud's phenomenon presents as a triphasic color change (white, blue, red) in the hands and fingers following an inciting event such as cold exposure or emotional stress. The fingers first appear pallid or white, then cyanotic or blue, and lastly hyperemic or red as circulation is restored.

B. Palpation. Normally, upper-extremity pulses can be palpated at three locations: the upper medial arm in the groove between the biceps and triceps muscles (axillary and proximal brachial artery); the antecubital fossa just medial to the biceps tendon (brachial artery); and the wrist over the distal radius (radial) or distal ulna (ulnar). In young women with absent upper-extremity pulses, **Takayasu's disease** (pulseless disease) should be suspected.

Skin temperature also can be assessed by palpation, especially using the more sensitive back of the examining hand or fingers. The level of skin temperature demarcation in the acutely ischemic arm is immediately distal to the level of the arterial occlusion.

Arterial aneurysms of the upper extremities are detectable if they occur in regions where the pulse is accessible to palpation. While larger subclavian and axillary artery aneurysms may be palpable above or below the clavicle or in the axilla, smaller aneurysms in these locations may go undetected. Aneurysms of the brachial artery are most commonly due to the artery having been accessed during an arteriogram. Aneurysms of the ulnar artery can occur in laborers as a result of repetitive trauma to the artery, which is in close proximity to the hamate bone in the wrist (**hypothenar hammer syndrome**).

Several bedside tests are available to provide information related to the diagnosis of TOS. **Adson's test** is performed by having the patient rotate the head toward the tested arm and letting the head tilt backward (to extend the neck) while the examiner extends the patient's arm. A positive test is indicated by reduction in or disappearance of the radial pulse. This test may be positive in as much as 10% to 20% of the normal population. During the elevated arm stress test (**EAST test**), the arms and hands are raised to the level of the head and the hands are repeatedly opened and closed for 3 minutes. Symptoms of numbness, pain, or weakness on the affected side suggest neurogenic or arterial TOS. Neither of these tests in and of itself is diagnostic. Rather, findings from these provocative maneuvers should be used in conjunction with other findings from the history, physical exam, and other testing when considering the diagnosis of TOS.

C. Auscultation. Auscultation of upper-extremity arteries should include comparison of blood pressure in both arms and examination of the supraclavicular fossa for bruit. A difference in arm pressures of more than 10 mmHg indicates a hemodynamically significant innominate, subclavian, or axillary artery stenosis on the side with the diminished pressure. Because collateral flow to the arm is extensive, a proximal subclavian stenosis may be present in an asymptomatic individual with palpable pulses at the wrist. If the patient has symptoms suggesting arm claudication, the arm should be exercised for 2 to 5 minutes and the brachial pressures rechecked. With this provocative maneuver, the brachial pressure will decrease if a significant arterial stenosis exists. When pulses are not palpable, continuous wave Doppler can be used to assess arterial signals and measure arm and forearm pressures. Doppler signals can normally be heard over the thenar and hypothenar eminences, as well as over the palmar arch of the hand.

IV. Abdomen. Most vascular pathology in the abdomen is asymptomatic and the history may not provide insight into the diagnosis. The majority of patients with **abdominal aortic aneurysms** (AAAs) are asymptomatic (Chapter 15). The acute onset of severe back or abdominal pain in a patient with a known AAA is considered a ruptured aneurysm until proven otherwise. Patients with **chronic mesenteric ischemia** relate a subtle history of postprandial pain, weight loss, and sitophobia (fear of food) (Chapter 17). **Acute mesenteric ischemia** causes diffuse abdominal "pain out of proportion" to examination. Poorly controlled hypertension in association with worsening renal function may be evidence of **renal artery stenosis**. Occlusive aortoiliac disease can manifest as bilateral hip and buttock claudication, absent femoral pulses, and impotence (**Leriche's syndrome**). In patients with prior aortic surgery, it is important to determine the original pathology for which the operation was performed (e.g., occlusive or aneurysmal disease). Ulcerated aortoiliac atherosclerosis is associated with mottled, painful blue toe syndrome, and abdominal bruit. Sudden, bilateral leg pain, coldness, paresthesias, and paralysis are caused by **acute aortic occlusion** from thrombosis of an existing aneurysm or occlusive process, saddle embolus from a cardiac source, or aortic dissection.

   A. Inspection. Inspection of the abdomen is the most limited part of the examination of the abdominal aorta and its branches. The normal aortic pulsation usually is not visible. However, a large abdominal aortic aneurysm may be seen pulsating against the anterior abdominal wall, especially in thin patients.

   B. Palpation. Palpation remains the simplest and most common technique to detect an abdominal aortic aneurysm. Although its sensitivity is limited in larger patients, palpation of the abdomen should be a part of the routine physical exam. Similarly, **palpation and comparison of femoral pulses** is the quickest way to confirm a clinical history suggestive of aortoiliac occlusive disease (**in-flow disease**). Although numeric grading systems for quantification of femoral pulse strength are useful, description of the pulses may also be simply described as *normal, diminished,* or *absent* and *symmetric versus asymmetric* in relation to the pulse on the other side.

   Certain anatomic features related to the aorta and iliac arteries should be considered when one palpates the abdomen. The aorta bifurcates into the common iliac arteries at about the level of the umbilicus and, in order to assess the infrarenal aortic segment, one must palpate deeply above this surface landmark. Having the patient bend the knees, relax the abdominal musculature, and exhale slowly and fully can facilitate the exam. It should also be remembered that, unless the patient is obese, an aortic pulse should normally be palpable above the umbilicus, especially if the abdominal wall is relaxed. The normal aorta is approximately the width of the patient's thumb or 2 cm in diameter.

An aortic aneurysm should be suspected when the aortic pulse feels expansile and larger than 4 cm. Elderly patients may have a tortuous, anteriorly displaced aorta that can be mistaken for an aneurysm. Because the sensitivity of abdominal palpation is limited, an aortic ultrasound should be ordered as an easy, noninvasive test in patients in whom there are any questions about aortic diameter. In addition to size, other characteristics of an aneurysm may be identified by palpation. If the enlarged aorta extends high to the xiphoid or costal margins, a suprarenal or thoracoabdominal aortic aneurysm should be suspected. Aneurysm tenderness with palpation is a sign indicating pending rupture, aneurysm leak, or the presence of an **inflammatory aneurysm**. Because of the anatomic location of the iliac arteries deep within the pelvis, aneurysms in this location are often not palpable. Occasionally a large **internal iliac artery aneurysm** may be palpable on digital rectal examination.

C. Auscultation. Auscultation commonly reveals bruits when significant occlusive disease of the aorta or its branches is present. Aortoiliac occlusive disease causes bruits in the middle and lower abdomen and the femoral region. Bruits secondary to isolated renal artery stenosis are faint and localized in the upper abdominal quadrants lateral to the midline. Mesenteric artery occlusive disease may be associated with epigastric bruits.

Asymptomatic abdominal bruits are an occasional incidental finding on abdominal examination of young adults, especially thin women. If the patient is not hypertensive and does not have intestinal angina or leg claudication, these bruits may be considered benign. The bruits may originate from impingement of the diaphragmatic crura on the celiac axis.

V. Lower extremities. Evaluation of leg circulation may appear overwhelming at first with a seemingly unlimited number of possible diagnoses. To simplify and organize the process, an initial priority is to **categorize the temporal presentation into either acute or chronic lower-extremity ischemia**. This determination allows the examiner to focus on a limited number of diagnoses and to understand the urgency of the problem. Clinical decision making in the setting of acute ischemia is based on the status of the limb, while chronic lower-extremity ischemia is further broken down into two subcategories: **claudication** and **critical ischemia**. The question, "does this process fall into the acute or chronic category?" should be asked in every instance in which the clinician is called to evaluate lower-extremity circulation. If the process is chronic, the next question should be, "does this condition represent claudication or critical ischemia?" Nearly all patients with lower-extremity arterial disease fall into one of these categories and, once the determination is made, the diagnostic and management process becomes more focused and clear (Chapter 14).

1. **Acute lower-extremity ischemia.** Acute lower-extremity ischemia most often presents as sudden onset of symptoms in a patient without a prior history of extremity vascular dis-

ease. Because the arterial occlusion occurs suddenly without time to develop collateral circulation, there is limited ability to compensate and the limb may be quite ischemic. Acute ischemia in any extremity, upper or lower, classically manifests the **5 Ps: pulselessness, pain, pallor, parathesia, and poikilothermia.**

2. **Chronic lower-extremity ischemia: Asymptomatic.** Some patients with diminished or even absent lower-extremity pressures or pulses may not have symptoms. Persons with a sedentary lifestyle may not be active enough to experience the symptoms of occlusive disease. The significance of asymptomatic peripheral arterial disease (PAD) relates more to the cardiac risk of the patient over time than it does to the well-being of the leg(s) (Chapters 8 and 14).

3. **Chronic lower-extremity ischemia: Claudication.** Claudication is leg pain that occurs with ambulation as a result of poor blood flow to a muscle group distal or beyond an arterial stenosis. This symptom often occurs at a fixed and reproducible walking distance or level of exertion, and resolves when the patient stops the activity (e.g., stops walking). It is essential to determine whether or not the symptoms of claudication are **lifestyle-limiting.** Occupational or recreational restrictions may occur as a result of exertional leg pain in some, while others may be aware of the symptoms but not limited in daily activities. The relatively benign natural history of claudication is important to communicate to patients and their families. With risk factor modification and exercise programs, claudication is stable or improved in 50% of patients. Only 25% of individuals with claudication ever require surgery and less than 5% require amputation over time.

4. **Chronic lower-extremity ischemia: Critical ischemia.** Critical lower-extremity ischemia, also referred to as "limb threat," represents the minority of patients with leg ischemia and may present in two forms: **ischemic rest pain or ischemic tissue loss** (ischemic ulcers or gangrene). These patients have severe arterial disease affecting multiple levels in the lower extremity and are at risk of amputation without revascularization. Ischemic rest pain typically is described as a burning pain on the dorsum of the foot or in the toes. This pain becomes most noticeable at night or with the leg elevated, and may be relieved by dangling the limb to enlist the help of gravity to improve perfusion.

The *differential diagnosis* of lower-extremity ischemia is extensive, and includes neurogenic and musculoskeletal conditions. Discomfort in the leg(s) that is positional or occurs without exertion is suggestive of **lumbar disk disease** or **spinal stenosis**, and commonly occurs in those with concomitant back pain. These conditions often occur with prolonged standing and cause leg weakness and numbness relieved by change of position (e.g., leaning forward). **Osteoarthritis of the hip and knee joints** commonly occurs in the elderly and can be distinguished from vascular disease by the location and nature of the pain.

Symptoms of **diabetic neuropathy** such as parasthesia, burning pain, and numbness that affects the foot and toes may mimic ischemic rest pain. Symptoms of neuropathy are bilateral and may also involve the fingertips, while ischemic rest pain is commonly unilateral and limited to the forefoot and toes. **Nighttime leg cramps** and **restless leg syndrome** are often misinterpreted as "rest pain" because they technically occur at rest. However symptoms from these conditions occur in the thigh and calf muscles and not in the distribution of ischemic rest pain and are not related to vascular disease. **Neuropathic ulcers** of the foot or toes occur in patients without protective sensation in these areas. These ulcers commonly arise in diabetic patients prone to infection as a result of poorly fitting shoes that cause foot trauma. Importantly, not all neuropathic ulcers are ischemic, as ulceration of the foot or toe may be present in patients with normal lower-extremity perfusion.

    A. Inspection. Inspection of the leg and foot may reveal important signs of acute and chronic arterial insufficiency. Acute insufficiency will produce definite changes of pallor followed by cyanosis or skin mottling. In addition, muscle weakness or paralysis, especially of the foot dorsiflexors (anterior compartment), may become obvious. After 24 hours of acute ischemia, the leg often becomes swollen and the skin may blister.

    Chronic claudication may have no findings on inspection other than mild muscle atrophy and/or hair loss on the leg or foot. Critical lower-extremity ischemia, however, is associated with **elevation pallor** and **dependent rubor** of the forefoot. Additionally, skin breakdown in the toes or forefoot tissue may occur and nonhealing ulcers or gangrene will appear. Neuropathic ulcers are difficult to distinguish from those that are primarily ischemic by inspection alone, as they both occur in the same distribution. Dry gangrene with black tissue or wet gangrene with draining purulence and foul odor may be present in the setting of neuropathic and ischemic ulcers, and often there is a mixed component.

    B. Palpation. Pulses are normally palpable in four locations on each lower extremity. The femoral pulse is palpated just below the inguinal ligament, two fingerbreadths lateral to the public tubercle. In obese patients, external rotation of the hip may facilitate palpation of the artery. The popliteal pulse is more difficult to feel as it lies in the popliteal space. With the patient supine and the knee slightly flexed, the examiner should hook the fingertips of the hands around the medial and lateral knee tendons and press the fingertips into the popliteal space. The pulse usually lies slightly lateral of midline. The dorsalis pedis is a terminal branch of the anterior tibial artery and is found in the mid-dorsum of the foot between the first and second metatarsals. The posterior tibial is found behind the medial malleolus, while the peroneal artery terminates at the ankle and is not palpable on physical exam.

    Grading of pulses is subjective, and a simple method is to describe the pulses as normal, diminished, or absent and symmetric versus asymmetric in relation to the other side. Numbered grading systems can also be used, although these may vary among institutions. An example of a pulse grading system is: 0, absent; 1+, diminished; 2+, normal; 3+, prominent, suggesting local aneurysm. **If a pulse is not palpable, further assessment with a continuous wave Doppler should be pursued.** Doppler signals should be qualified as triphasic, biphasic, or monophasic with the triphasic signal considered normal. In the absence of a palpable pulse, biphasic and monophasic signals correlate with moderate and severe arterial occlusive disease, respectively. In severe cases of acute lower-extremity ischemia or chronic critical ischemia, the only Doppler signal in the foot may be a soft continuous venous signal.

Palpation is also helpful in the assessment of acute-extremity ischemia. Skin coldness and the level of temperature demarcation can be detected by palpation with the back of the examiner's hand and fingers. Acute ischemia also may be associated with tenderness and tenseness of the calf muscles, especially the anterior compartment. In addition, acute ischemia may cause sensory nerve damage, detectable by pinprick sensory examination or testing of proprioception in the toes.

The **ABI** is a simple and necessary extension of the vascular exam and can be performed at the bedside. To measure the ABI, the strongest Doppler signal is identified at the ankle and a blood pressure cuff is placed around the calf and inflated until the signal disappears. The cuff is slowly released and the pressure at which the signal returns is recorded as the numerator of the ABI equation. The same maneuver is performed to assess the occlusion pressure of the brachial artery of both arms, the higher of which is recorded as the denominator of the ABI equation. The index may be falsely elevated in the setting of diabetes mellitus or renal failure, either of which can lead to medial calcinosis and poor compressibility of the tibial vessels. A normal ABI is greater than 0.9 while an index between 0.4 and 0.9 is characteristic of patients with chronic **claudication**. An ABI of less than 0.4 is generally suggestive of **critical ischemia** of the extremity. Not only does the ABI provide an idea of the severity of occlusive disease in the extremity, it is also useful for following extremity perfusion over intervals of time (Chapter 14).

C. Auscultation. Auscultation of lower-extremity arteries is most useful in the femoral area, where bruits indicate local femoral artery disease or more proximal aortoiliac disease with bruits transmitted to the groin. If there is a question about the presence of a femoral bruit, walking the patient for 25 to 50 steps at the bedside often will increase lower-extremity flow enough to increase the severity of the bruit. Auscultation is also important when an arteriovenous fistula is suspected, which generally has a characteristic continuous to-and-fro bruit.

CHAPTER 5

History and Physical Examination of the Venous System

Venous disease is usually localized to one anatomic area, unlike arterial disease, which is more diffuse. The lower extremities are most commonly involved, although venous problems can impair function of the upper extremities as well.

I. Upper extremities. The most common venous conditions to affect the upper extremities are superficial and deep venous thrombosis. **Superficial thrombophlebitis** can result from intravenous access, which causes endothelial damage, local vein thrombosis, and subsequent inflammation of a peripheral vein. This condition rarely progresses to deep venous thrombosis and is most often self-limited, requiring local treatment in the form of warm compresses applied directly to the affected vein. Acute or chronic thrombosis of the axillary, subclavian, or innominate veins represents the upper-extremity equivalent of **deep venous thrombosis (DVT)** and represents a serious condition. The clinician should assess for a history of prior central venous catheter or peripherally inserted central catheter (PICC lines), as these are a risk factor for the development of central venous thrombosis. The chief complaint in most cases is arm swelling. A diffuse aching pain frequently accompanies the swelling and is worse with use or dependency of the arm.

Paget-Schroetter syndrome is synonymous with **effort thrombosis,** and refers to the development of axillary or subclavian vein thrombosis in the setting of repetitive upper extremity exercise. Usually this form of axillo-subclavian vein thrombosis occurs acutely as a result of thoracic outlet syndrome, in which compression of the subclavian vein between the subclavius muscle underlying the clavicle and the first rib is present (Fig. 5.1). Chronic compression of the axillary or subclavian vein in these circumstances results in underlying endothelial injury and is a contributing factor to the thrombosis. Chronic arm swelling may also be the result of lymphatic obstruction, which usually is associated with a previous operation (e.g., node dissection for breast cancer), infection, or irradiation that involved the axillary lymph nodes. Distinguishing between venous obstruction and lymphedema may be difficult, although the clinical setting suggests the most likely etiology in most cases.

A. Inspection. The examiner should inspect the arms for scars from previous indwelling venous lines or procedures and note limb size discrepancy, edema, discoloration, deformity (e.g., clavicular fracture), or venous collaterals. Subclavian vein thrombosis causes swelling of the entire arm and hand and will often result in superficial venous collateral formation across the shoulder region. Acutely, the arm may appear bluish or cyanotic, although rarely does subclavian-axillary venous thrombosis result in phlegmasia or venous gangrene.

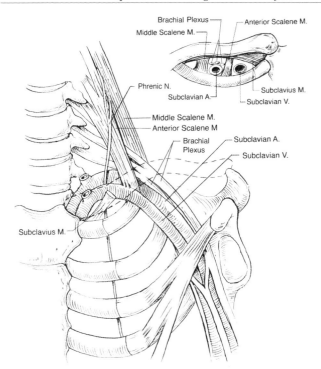

Figure 5.1. The thoracic outlet is a complex anatomic area with potential neurovascular compromise. The larger illustration depicts the left shoulder with associated neurovascular and bony structures of this area. The smaller inset depicts a view if the right thoracic outlet through a transaxillary view (i.e., the right arm raised). Note the important relationship of the subclavian vein and artery to the anterior scalene muscle, first rib, and clavicle.

Patients in whom upper-extremity venous thrombosis leads to phlegmasia often have an underlying malignancy or hypercoagulable condition such as heparin-induced thrombocytopenia and thrombosis (Chapter 3). Following upper-extremity DVT, the arm generally does not develop venous stasis dermatitis that accompanies post-thrombotic syndrome in the lower extremities.

Another cause of acute arm swelling is placement of a hemodialysis fistula or graft in the arm that has an unrecognized venous stenosis or occlusion in the proximal or central venous outflow (Chapter 20). In such cases, completing the arterial-venous circuit for dialysis increases venous flow and pressure, which exacerbates a previously asymptomatic central venous stenosis.

B. Palpation. The palpable cord associated with superficial thrombophlebitis of the arm is typically warm and tender. Fluctuance or purulent drainage from the cord upon palpation suggests the diagnosis of **suppurative** or **infected throm-**

bophlebitis, which may require operative drainage. The internal and external jugular veins are occasionally palpable if inflamed or thrombosed, while the axillary and subclavian veins are not palpable because they lie deep to the clavicle. Arm edema, which is pitting upon palpation, is more often associated with lymphatic obstructions, while chronic venous edema tends to be nonpitting in nature. A palpable thrill over any area of the upper extremity suggests the presence of an arteriovenous fistula.

C. Auscultation. Normally, venous sounds are not audible with a stethoscope. If arm swelling follows a penetrating injury or operation of the arm, listening over the scar or entrance wound may reveal a bruit caused by an arteriovenous fistula.

II. Lower extremities. The most common venous problems of the legs are *superficial varicose veins* and *DVT* with subsequent *post-thrombotic syndrome*. Although occasionally these conditions are asymptomatic, they are more frequently associated with some degree of leg pain and swelling (Chapter 2). Superficial venous reflux and postphlebitic syndrome resulting from DVT can lead to chronic leg swelling and ulceration months or years after diagnosis. Physical exam is the primary method of evaluating varicose veins and post-thrombotic syndrome, as they both cause visible changes on the surface of the leg. In contrast, history and physical examination alone are limited in making the diagnosis of DVT. In fact, only 50% of patients who are initially thought to have DVT by history and physical will have an abnormal duplex ultrasound. Some cases of lower extremity DVT, especially those in the tibial and distal popliteal veins, may be silent or nearly asymptomatic, presenting with only subtle leg swelling. Although there is a risk of pulmonary embolus and postphlebitic syndrome in these cases, the risk is low given the distal location and limited extent of thrombosis. In rare instances, the first sign of lower-extremity DVT can be pulmonary embolus. The complexity of lower-extremity venous disorders emphasizes the need for a careful and complete history and physical exam as well as the liberal use of the duplex ultrasound as a diagnostic adjunct.

A. Inspection should be done with both legs exposed from the groin to the feet. Important findings may be recognized by comparing the abnormal to the normal extremity and, when possible, the patient should stand so that superficial veins fill. We prefer that the patient stand on a short stool while the examiner sits on a chair or stool. If good overhead lighting is not available for illumination of all aspects of the leg, an adjustable lamp is useful. The entire leg should be examined as the patient turns 360 degrees.

Varicose veins are dilated, saccular, and compressible unless thrombosed. Some healthy, thin patients may have prominent superficial veins that may be incorrectly thought to be varicose. Varicose veins most commonly involve the great saphenous vein on the medial side of the leg and tributaries often course around the upper calf to appear on the posteromedial aspect of the leg. Tributaries of the small saphenous appear on the posterior calf from the knee to the ankle. The location of the varicosities may suggest the etiology. For example, a dilated great saphenous vein from the groin to the ankle is typical of **familial valvular incompetence**. In contrast, varicosities that begin at or below the knee may be secondary to incompetent perforating veins from the deep venous system. A rare congenital pattern of varicosities is present in **Klippel-Trénaunay syndrome,** which is a triad of capillary hemagiomas (port-wine stains), limb hypertrophy, and varicose veins. Importantly, these patients may have persistent lateral embryologic veins and absent or abnormal deep venous systems. **Telangiectasias** or "spider veins" are 0.1–2.0 mm dilated vessels of the dermis that appear red or blue in color and tend to arborize. Reticular veins are slightly larger and act as feeding veins to the telangiectasias.

Several bedside tests can help the examiner better identify the underlying pathophysiology of lower-extremity varicosities.

Trendelenburg test: The patient lies supine, and the leg is elevated to empty all varicosities. A soft rubber tourniquet or the examiner's hand is used to compress the thigh at the saphenofemoral junction, and the patient stands. If the lower leg varicosities fill slowly with the tourniquet in place, but then dilate rapidly after release, the great saphenous vein is incompetent. In contrast, incompetent deep and perforating veins will cause immediate filling of the varicosities when the patient stands, despite the tourniquet (Fig 5.2).

Perthes' test checks for obstruction of the deep veins. The patient stands to fill the varicosities, and a soft rubber tourniquet is applied to the midthigh. The patient then ambulates or performs repetitive calf muscle contractions (tiptoe maneuvers). Normally the veins collapse, implying competence of the deep and perforating veins. If the veins remain distended, the deep and perforating veins are incompetent. If the varicosities become more distended or painful, deep venous obstruction is present.

Acute deep venous thrombosis. Most limbs with acute venous thrombosis are normal in color or have a slightly cyanotic appearance. Extremity swelling is the most common sign and usually is limited to the lower leg, although thrombosis of the more proximal iliac and femoral venous circulations can lead to thigh and even buttock edema. **Phlegmasia alba dolens** (turgid, white, painful leg) or **phlegmasia cerulea dolens** (edematous, cyanotic, and painful leg) can be seen in cases of severe proximal vein thrombosis (Chapter 2). In these instances the degree of swelling should be documented by measurement of calf and thigh diameters at a distance above or below a bony landmark to allow close and accurate serial examination of the leg.

Inspection also helps with the differential diagnosis of acute leg pain and swelling. Superficial thrombophlebitis often is evidenced by a localized erythematous streak along the course of the vein, usually a tributary or the great saphenous vein. A break in the skin with surrounding erythema and induration suggests cellulitis. A localized ecchymosis over the thigh or calf may indicate that the leg pain is caused by a muscle contusion or hematoma. Diffuse, nonpainful leg edema with a thick "pigskin" appearance (peau d'orange) is typical of lymphedema.

Deep venous insufficiency, usually as a result of postphlebitic syndrome, is associated with specific changes in the appearance of the leg, including hyperpigmentation from

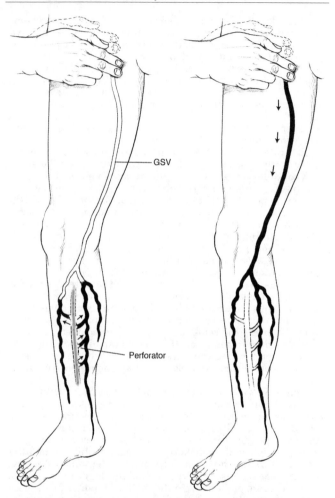

Figure 5.2. Trendelenburg test. The leg is elevated to empty the varicosities. Then, the saphenofemoral junction is compressed with the patient upright and non–weight-bearing. Superficial varicosities fill from incompetent deep and perforating veins when the proximal saphenous system is compressed (*left*). The varicosities fill immediately with release of proximal compression, implying superficial venous insufficiency (*right*).

hemosiderin deposition occurring at the medial malleolus. **Lipodermatosclerosis** is a more severe manifestation of chronic venous hypertension, with the development of thickened and contracted skin and subcutaneous fat around the ankle. Stasis dermatitis may be complicated by skin ulceration, classically on the medial lower leg at the site of the perforating vein. **Venous ulcers** are usually shallow, with apparently healthy granulation tissue that bleeds with manipulation. It is important when inspecting a venous ulcer to regularly measure the dimensions and depth, and to assess surrounding skin integrity, as well as the quality of granulation tissue. The onset of a new odor or change in color, or erythema of the surrounding skin, suggests infection of the ulcer or even transformation to an epidermoid skin cancer. It is important to note that these cutaneous changes of the leg may also occur with chronic, severe superficial venous insufficiency as well.

Chronic diffuse lower-limb swelling without stasis dermatitis may be caused by iliac vein obstruction, deep valvular incompetence, or lymphedema. Compression of the left common iliac vein by the right common iliac artery (**May-Thurner syndrome**) can result in venous intimal fibroplasia, obstruction, and progressive left leg swelling. In contrast, primary or secondary lymphedema can result in chronic leg swelling that typically has a pitting or "pigskin" appearance and does not resolve with bedrest at night. Venous edema, on the other hand, most often resolves with bed rest and worsens with dependency. Lipedema, the deposition of fat in the lower extremity, can easily be confused with other causes of edema, but characteristically spares the feet. Bilateral lower-extremity edema can also result from right heart failure, valvular heart disease, and nephrotic syndrome, and should prompt a search for other signs of systemic disease (e.g., rales, S3 gallop).

B. Palpation can distinguish soft and compressible varicosities from those that are firm and thrombosed. Tenderness, heat, and induration over a firm varicosity define superficial thrombophlebitis. The "tap test" can be used in order to identify connections between varicose segments. With the patient standing, the examiner sharply percusses over a varicosity, while using the other hand to feel for an impulse from the vein at a lower level. The impulse should be felt if the intervening segment is open and incompetent. The examiner should palpate for fascial defects on the medial aspect of the calf. These may represent sites of deep, incompetent perforating veins or saphenous tributaries emerging from the superficial fascia.

Calf tenderness may be present in acute deep venous thrombosis, but is not specific. Such tenderness may occur with muscle strain, contusion, or hematoma. Forceful dorsiflexion of the foot elicits calf pain in 35% of patients with acute deep venous thrombosis (**Homans' sign**). However, this test is also positive with muscular strains and lumbosacral disorders.

Palpation may help determine the cause of leg swelling. Occasionally, chronic venous obstruction is secondary to extrinsic compression by a pelvic, femoral, or popliteal mass, and so these regions should also be examined for aneurysms or tumors. The inability to tent the skin over the interdigital webs (**Stemmer's sign**) is characteristic of lymphedema.

C. Auscultation. Except in the cases of arteriovenous fistula in which an audible bruit may be present, a stethoscope does not provide much information about superficial or deep venous flow. In contrast, a continuous wave Doppler unit is a helpful adjunct in the bedside examination of lower-extremity veins. While holding the continuous wave Doppler over the vein of interest, normal respiratory variation of the Doppler signal should be present if the vein is patent with normal flow. Additionally, if patent, flow through the vein will be audibly increased (augmentation) if the examiner's other hand squeezes the leg distally. With release of distal compression, flow will cease as competent valves snap shut. If the vein is incompetent, prolonged flow will be heard after release. Although continuous wave Doppler is quite a useful adjunct, it does not provide images or velocity measurements of flow. Duplex ultrasound, which combines B mode imaging and pulsed wave Doppler, should be used frequently in the evaluation of symptomatic venous disease to allow more detailed examination of venous anatomy and provide useful physiologic information.

CHAPTER 6

Noninvasive Vascular Testing

This chapter summarizes the basic principles of selecting, performing, and interpreting noninvasive hemodynamic studies for both arterial and venous problems. It should be emphasized that these noninvasive tests do not replace but **supplement** a thorough patient history and physical examination (Chapters 4 and 5). In some situations, the results of noninvasive studies help the clinician determine the need for an invasive study such as an arteriogram. In addition, noninvasive tests provide a physiologic baseline before therapy and an objective assessment of outcome after treatment. The use of noninvasive testing has grown exponentially, as the safety and ease of testing is increasingly attractive to clinicians. The temptation to order noninvasive tests without a justifying history and physical exam should be resisted, as unnecessary studies can lead to unnecessary procedures. Additionally, redundant noninvasive tests add to the cost of patient care.

I. The vascular laboratory. The laboratory should be in a quiet area and located for convenient use by both inpatients and outpatients. A medical sonographer or registered vascular technologist (RVT) usually performs the tests, which are then reviewed by a physician. The setup in a vascular laboratory may be very basic or quite sophisticated, depending on the clinical demand. Consistency and quality assurance should be the goal of all vascular laboratories. Accreditation can be obtained by meeting the standards outlined by the **Intersocietal Commission for the Accreditation of Vascular Laboratories**.

II. Instrumentation. The following list of equipment is sufficient for the evaluation of most arterial and venous problems in the noninvasive laboratory. Their basic functions are briefly described.

1. Continuous-wave Doppler system. The Doppler effect states that flow velocity is proportional to the frequency shift in sound waves that are transmitted toward moving blood cells and reflected back to the Doppler-receiving crystal (Fig. 6.1). A handheld Doppler probe is placed over the course of the blood vessel being examined and is coupled to the skin with an acoustic gel. Skin lubricants other than an acoustic gel do not have the proper electrolyte content and can damage the probe crystal. Transmitted sound waves strike moving blood cells and are reflected back to the Doppler probe. An amplifier filters the sound and gives a flow signal or tracing that is proportional to the blood velocity. Just as palpable pulses can be graded with regard to strength, the audible Doppler signal can also be qualified with regard to strength and phasicity.

The normal Doppler signal is **triphasic** in a high-resistance arterial bed, such as the lower extremity. A triphasic signal has three audible components, corresponding to the forward flow of systole, early reverse flow in diastole, and the later forward flow of diastole. In a

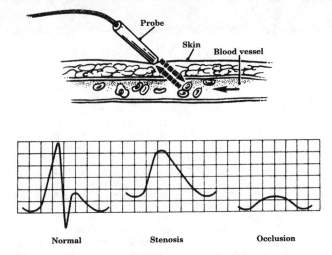

Figure 6.1.   Doppler arterial examination. The Doppler probe is coupled to the skin with acoustic gel and angled toward the direction of arterial flow. The normal Doppler arterial signal is triphasic. Stenosis and occlusion cause diminished monophasic signals.

low-resistance arterial bed, such as the internal carotid or lower extremity after exercise, flow normally remains forward or prograde. Without reversal of flow in diastole, there are only two components (**biphasic**) for these signals. With increasing degree of stenosis, wave morphology becomes weak, lower-pitched, and **monophasic**.

In practice, a continuous-wave Doppler unit (range, 5–10 MHz) is most commonly used for performing basic noninvasive tests such as segmental pressures. A handheld version is a valuable asset to the bedside arterial and venous exam. Some Doppler units are bidirectional; that is, they can detect direction as well as velocity of flow. **Pulsed Doppler,** when combined with brightness mode (B-mode) ultrasound, comprises **modern duplex**. In this setting, pulsed Doppler differs from continuous wave in two ways: (a) bursts of sound waves are emitted, and (b) a distinct portion of flow within a vessel can be selected with the B-mode image of the vessel for Doppler sampling. This technique provides more accurate measurement of frequency (velocity) of flow through the vessel. The velocity pattern correlates with the degree of stenosis, in that a higher velocity suggests a greater stenosis. Although continuous-wave Doppler can also analyze velocity patterns, they collect all velocities from within the vessel and may also receive other signals from adjacent arteries or veins, making signal interpretation more difficult.

2. **Plethysmography** was one of the earliest means of measuring blood flow in an extremity, using the principle of volume change in an organ or body region. Various techniques of plethysmography have been used, but only a few

remain popular. Both air plethysmography (APG) and photoplethysmography (PPG) are commonly utilized techniques in the noninvasive laboratory. The basic tools for APG are a blood pressure cuff, inflated to optimize contact with the leg, a transducer, and recording instrument. PPG uses a probe that emits infrared light into the superficial skin layers and a photoelectric detector that measures the reflected light. The amount of light absorbed depends on the blood volume in the skin. A waveform is transduced and recorded corresponding to the blood flow.

3. Duplex ultrasound combines two technologies for the evaluation of blood vessels. Real-time, B-mode ultrasound provides black and white (gray-scale) images of the vessel and **pulsed wave Doppler** is used to sample flow velocity in a selected area of the vessel. The angle of insonation should be kept close to 60°, which provides the best return signal for spectral analysis and velocity measurement.

Spectral analysis pertains to the spectrum of different velocities of blood cells and particles traveling in the vessel and provides insight into the degree of narrowing as well as the degree of perfect (**laminar**) versus imperfect (**turbulent**) flow. The parameters used for this are (a) spectral width during systole, (b) peak systolic velocity, and (c) end diastolic velocity. A normal spectrum (Fig. 6.2) consists of a relatively low systolic peak velocity (e.g., less than 125 cm/s in the internal carotid) and a narrow band of frequencies during systole, resulting in a clear region or window beneath the systolic peak. In this case, blood cells and particles are

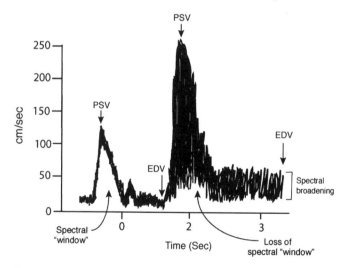

Figure 6.2.   Arterial spectrum analysis. The Doppler spectrum analysis allows classification of the degree of stenosis. The most common parameters used for this classification are spectral broadening (with loss of the normal "spectral window"), elevation in peak systolic velocity (PSV; normal <120 cm/sec), and elevation in end diastolic velocity (EDV).

traveling the same velocity within the vessel with limited turbulent flow. With even a minimal stenosis, turbulent flow is detected, resulting in **spectral broadening** during the deceleration phase of systole. Further stenosis results in increased spectral broadening until the entire window beneath the systolic peak is filled, followed by increased peak systolic and then end diastolic velocities. Spectral broadening in these cases reflects the many different velocities of flowing cells and particles within the vessel resulting from the disorderly or turbulent flow.

A third mode, color flow imaging, is helpful in identifying the presence and direction of flow. Red indicates flow toward the transducer, and blue is away. Lighter shades are associated with higher flow and darker shades with lower flow. Laminar flow is uniform in color while a stenosis results in a bright "flow-jet" of color and a mosaic distal to the stenosis reflective of turbulent flow. Color flow is particularly useful for tracing tortuous vessels and identifying areas of ulceration.

4. A **treadmill** at speeds of 1.5 to 2.5 miles per hour at a 10% to 12.5% grade is used for exercise testing.

5. Transcutaneous oximetry requires a transcutaneous electrode probe and calibrated instrument for measuring oxygen tension on the skin, which is used as a surrogate marker for blood flow.

6. Blood pressure cuffs of various sizes, including miniature cuffs for digital pressures, should be available.

III. Lower-extremity arterial occlusive disease. Noninvasive laboratory evaluation of the lower extremities is useful in the setting of chronic intermittent claudication (tiring or pain in the extremity with walking) as well as more severe critical leg ischemia (ischemic rest pain or tissue loss). Noninvasive vascular testing documents the severity of disease, provides a baseline for follow-up, and can help predict potential for healing ulcers. Testing can sometimes help the clinician clarify whether leg pain is related to peripheral vascular disease or nonvascular etiologies in patients with atypical symptoms. However, no amalgamation of vascular tests is a substitute for a thorough history and physical examination.

A. Ankle-brachial index (ABI) provides useful information about lower-extremity perfusion as a supplement to the physical exam. This test can be performed at the bedside with a handheld Doppler and a manual blood pressure cuff. The Doppler probe is placed over an arterial signal at the foot, typically the dorsalis pedis or the posterior tibial artery (Fig. 6.3). A blood pressure cuff on the calf is inflated until the arterial signal occludes or disappears. As the cuff is deflated, the pressure at which the signal is again audible is recorded. The test should be performed in the supine position and the greater of the two pressures at the foot selected as the numerator in the ABI equation. Next, the pressure of each arm is recorded in a similar manner and used as the denominator in the equation. If there is more than a 10 mm Hg difference between arm pressures, the higher pressure should be selected, keeping in mind that a diminished arm pressure could indicate a subclavian artery stenosis. Normally, the pressure in the leg is

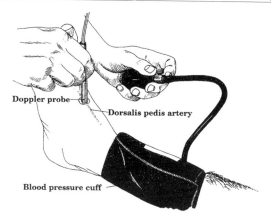

Figure 6.3.   Measurement of ankle blood pressure with a standard blood pressure cuff and a handheld continuous-wave Doppler unit. This ankle pressure can be compared to the brachial (arm) blood pressure to calculate the ankle-brachial index (ABI).

slightly higher than that in the arm, due to a higher resistance in the lower extremities and the **normal ABI ≥1.0**.

When performed in the noninvasive lab, ABIs may be combined with a plethysmograph for pulse volume recordings. In this setting ABI measurements provide more complete and standardized data that can be used as part of the clinical assessment over time of patients with lower-extremity occlusive disease. ABIs should also be performed following an open or catheter-based revascularization in order to confirm improvement and establish a new baseline. A change in an ABI value of more than 0.15 over time or following revascularization is generally termed a significant change in perfusion.

Lower-extremity circulation is often divided into three levels: aortoiliac, femoropopliteal, and tibial (Chapter 14). In limbs with one level of occlusive disease, the ABI is usually 0.5–0.85, while an index of less than 0.5 indicates multilevel disease. ABIs may be falsely elevated or even noncompressible in patients with longstanding diabetes or end-stage renal disease. Patients with these medical conditions may develop **medial calcinosis** of the tibial vessels, which render them difficult or impossible to compress with a manual blood pressure cuff. In some cases the Doppler signal in the foot will not occlude despite inflating the cuff to pressures that are well above the systolic blood pressure and are uncomfortable for the patient. In such instances, the ABI calculation should not be pursued but simply be termed **noncompressible**. In this situation, combining PVRs with ABIs can provide more complete information. Table 6.1 lists common clinical scenarios found in association with several categories of ABIs. However, it must be remembered that many patients with abnormal ABIs do not fall in these allotted categories. Over two-thirds of patients with abnormal ABIs are asymptomatic, as a result of well-developed collaterals or a sedentary lifestyle.

**Table 6.1.   Categories of clinical severity
for the ankle-brachial index (ABI)**

ABI Measurement	Clinical Correlation
1.2–2.0 or greater	Medial calcinosis or noncompressible
0.95–1.2	Normal
0.5–0.95	Claudication
0.2–0.5	Rest pain
0.0–0.2	Tissue loss or gangrene

B. Toe pressures are useful in patients with medial calcinosis of the tibial vessels, as digital vessels of the toes are often spared from the process. A 2 cm cuff is applied to the great toe and a PPG sensor is placed on the tip because the area is too small to assess with a standard Doppler. The greatest value of toe pressures may be in their ability to predict healing of ischemic foot ulcers or toe or foot amputation sites. A toe–brachial index <0.7 is abnormal in diabetics and nondiabetics and an absolute toe pressure of less than 30 mm Hg suggests insufficient perfusion to heal an open wound of any type.

C. Pulse volume recording (PVR) is a form of APG, developed by Raines and Darling at Massachusetts General Hospital, in which lower-extremity pulsatility is used as an indirect measurement of arterial flow. In order to perform the test, an air-filled blood pressure cuff of appropriate size is placed on the lower extremity, usually on the calf, and inflated to a baseline pressure of about 65 mm Hg. The cuff is attached to the plethysmograph, and small fluctuations in limb volume as a result of pressure changes are then recorded as arterial contours. The contour provides qualitative information about the arterial blood flow, closely corresponding to the direct intra-arterial pressure waveform recording at that level.

Characterized by a sharp upstroke (**anacrotic slope**), distinct pulse peak, and rapid decline (**catacrotic slope**), the normal PVR tracing becomes progressively flattened and prolonged with increasing stenosis (Fig. 6.4). PVRs can be quantified by amount of chart deflection, but laboratories often use different scales. The greatest emphasis is placed simply on qualitative wave morphology. A severely attenuated or flat PVR tracing at the ankle correlates with poor healing. PVRs are particularly useful when combined with ABIs or segmental pressures in order to provide a more complete picture of the limb blood flow. For example, patients with medial calcinosis may have falsely elevated ABIs, such that the PVRs provide a better estimate about the severity of disease (Fig 6.5). The PVR can also be helpful in evaluating the young patient whose claudication may be due to **popliteal artery entrapment** by the medial head of the gastrocnemius muscle. Such patients usually have normal ankle PVR tracings at rest. With active plantar flexion or passive dorsiflexion of the foot, the gastrocnemius contracts and compresses the popliteal artery, so that the real-time PVR tracing flattens.

D. Segmental pressures can be useful in patients with abnormal ABIs in order to better approximate the level and

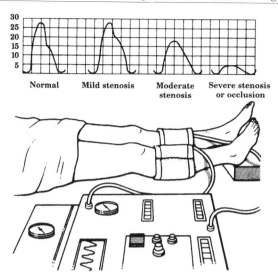

Figure 6.4.   Pulse volume recordings. The normal pulse volume recording becomes progressively flattened and prolonged with increasing arterial stenosis.

degree of arterial obstruction. Measurements are obtained by the same technique as ABIs, except that blood pressure cuffs are placed at several levels—thigh, upper calf, and ankle. The Doppler probe is always placed over the best arterial signal at the ankle level. Two standard 10–12 cm diameter cuffs can be used on the upper and lower thigh. Alternatively, a single large cuff (18–20 cm diameter) can be placed as proximal as

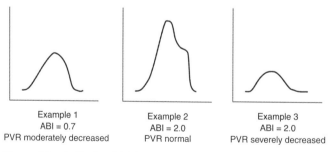

Example 1	Example 2	Example 3
ABI = 0.7	ABI = 2.0	ABI = 2.0
PVR moderately decreased	PVR normal	PVR severely decreased

Figure 6.5.   Ankle brachial index (ABI) and pulse volume recording (PVR) are complementary, as shown in these examples. In example 1, the ABI of 0.7 is decreased with a correspondingly dampened PVR waveform, suggesting more proximal peripheral arterial occlusive disease (PAOD). In example 2, the ABI of 2.0 is well above the normal range indicating incompressible tibial vessels due to medial calcinosis. However, the PVR in this example is normal suggesting no significant PAOD. In example 3, the ABI is 2.0 in conjunction with a severely dampened PVR, consistent with both medial calcinosis and severe PAOD.

possible on the thigh. In general, the larger thigh-to-cuff ratio will result in higher pressures in the thigh than the ankle, so that the normal thigh–brachial index is 1.3 to 1.5.

Some decrease in pressure from proximal thigh to ankle is normal, but a pressure decrease of 15–30 mm Hg between adjacent segments suggests an intervening stenosis. Segmental pressures should also be compared at the same level between legs, as a lack of symmetry implies arterial disease in the leg with lower pressures. Figure 6.6 provides examples of arterial occlusive disease at various anatomic levels.

PVRs are usually combined with segmental pressures at each level to improve accuracy, especially in patients with falsely elevated pressures from calcified vessels. Segmental PVR tracings normally show augmentation from the thigh to calf, caused by differences in cuff volume and a high ratio of well-vascularized calf muscle. Therefore, the calf PVR should have greater amplitude than that of the thigh. If it does not, a superficial femoral artery lesion should be suspected. Disease in the common or proximal superficial femoral artery can mimic aortoiliac disease by causing a decrease in the thigh pressure, particularly if a single large cuff is used on the thigh. Of course, simple palpation of the femoral pulse can also distinguish between aortoiliac and superficial femoral artery occlusion. Segmental pressures can also be misleading when collateral blood flow is so well developed that a significant gradient is not present across an occlusive segment. These limitations of segmental leg pressures emphasize that results must be combined with findings on physical exam for accurate detection of the occlusive lesions.

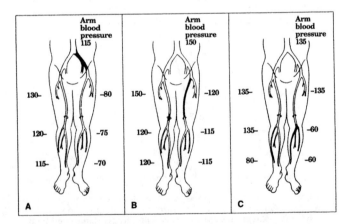

Figure 6.6.   Segmental leg pressures. (A) Segmental leg pressures in a normal lower extremity (*right*) and one with isolated left iliac artery occlusion (*left*). (B) Segmental leg pressures with a distal occlusion of the superficial femoral artery (SFA) at Hunter's canal (*right*), compared to proximal occlusion of the SFA (*left*). (C) Segmental leg pressures with distal tibial artery occlusions (*right*) and tibial disease extending into the proximal popliteal artery (*left*).

E. Exercise or treadmill ABIs can unmask the presence of arterial occlusive disease in a select group of patients with ambulatory leg pain. Treadmill ABIs are useful in the subgroup of patients with symptoms of exertional pain that have normal pulses and only mildly decreased ABIs at rest. In these cases a mild arterial stenosis does not result in a measurable pressure decrease while the patient is sitting at rest in the office. *Remember: his or her symptoms are with ambulation.*

Under normal circumstances, the treadmill ABI will increase slightly and remain elevated for a few minutes following ambulation as blood flow into the extremity increases with exertion. However, in patients with a proximal arterial stenosis, vasodilation of the leg musculature results in an increase in velocity of blood across the stenosis as the body attempts to supply the leg with blood. This phenomenon results in a decrease in pressure distal to the stenosis with a decreased exercise ABI and a delay in return to baseline. Insight into this basic concept of hemodynamics is provided in part by **Bernoulli's principle**, which states that with increased velocity across a fixed stenosis there is loss of kinetic energy distal to the stenosis and a necessary decrease in pressure.

Resting ABIs are performed first, and then the patient is asked to walk on a treadmill at a rate of 2 mph at a 5–10° incline for 5 minutes or until the leg pain becomes significant. In addition to measurement of ABIs after exercise, recording of the time to onset of pain, recovery from the pain, and the location of pain is important, as it defines the overall effect on the patient. At the same time, the general cardiac and respiratory reserve of the patient can be observed. Exercise should be terminated if the patient complains of chest pain, dyspnea, or dizziness.

Exercise testing may be most helpful if there is confusion about whether the leg symptoms are caused by arterial occlusive disease versus a musculoskeletal or neurologic condition such as **spinal stenosis**. Normal treadmill pressures in these cases effectively exclude arterial occlusive disease and point to a musculoskeletal or neurologic condition. It is the authors' opinion that there is no additional diagnostic value in performing treadmill ABIs in patients with obvious arterial occlusive disease, typical claudication, and reduced ABIs at rest.

F. Transcutaneous oximetry ($TcPO_2$) provides local measurement of skin oxygen tension, which indirectly reflects arterial perfusion to the foot. The principle of transcutaneous oxygen determination involves heat application (45°C) to the skin, which produces hyperemia and oxygen excess. Since oxygen diffuses along a concentration gradient from the capillaries to the tissues, it can diffuse across the skin where it is measured by a modified **Clark platinum oxygen electrode**. Local vasodilation allows for $TcPO_2$ to accurately approximate arterial PO_2.

The transcutaneous electrode is applied to the skin at various levels on the lower extremity. Normal $TcPO_2$ exceeds 55 mm Hg, but levels of less than 30 mm Hg suggest a degree of arterial ischemia. Critical ischemia manifested by ischemic tissue loss or ischemic rest pain is associated with forefoot

$TcPO_2$ levels of 0 to 10 mm Hg. $TcPO_2$ measurements can also help predict healing of ischemic foot ulcers, with levels greater than 20 mm Hg necessary for healing. $TcPO_2$ is generally only accurate if local infection has been controlled and edema in the foot has been minimized.

$TcPO_2$ can be particularly useful in evaluating patients with longstanding diabetes and/or peripheral neuropathy, in whom the origins of resting foot or toe pain or ulcerations may be unclear. In such cases, ABIs will often be noncompressible as a result of medial arterial calcinosis, and the $TcPO_2$ provides a measure of perfusion that may help distinguish whether the pain or ulceration is the result of arterial insufficiency or neuropathy (Tables 6.2, 6.3).

G. Duplex ultrasound is an accurate noninvasive method for evaluating lower-extremity circulation and can be used to create a "road map" of arterial disease. Duplex ultrasound provides visual information about plaque morphology as well as physiologic information about the speed and flow of blood within the vessel. Together this information can help characterize and quantify degrees of stenosis. Arterial occlusion is identified by absence of color-flow imaging and collaterals may be visualized proximal and distal to an occlusion or stenosis. A jet on color-flow imaging suggests a stenosis and velocities are then measured using pulsed Doppler proximal to, at the stenosis, and distal to the stenosis. The **systolic velocity ratio (SVR)** is calculated by dividing the peak systolic velocity (PSV) at or within the stenosis by the PSV proximal to the stenosis. An SVR of >2.5 or an absolute PSV >200 cm/sec has been shown to correlate with a >50% stenosis. However, there are limitations to duplex ultrasound of the lower extremities. A complete exam is time-consuming and accuracy is operator-dependent compared with the "gold standard" of arteriography. Obesity and overlying bowel gas limit visualization of the iliac arteries, and tibial vessels can be difficult to image if there is severe calcification, overlying skin disorders, or edema.

Surveillance duplex following lower-extremity revascularization can identify failing bypasses otherwise not detected by history and physical and help preserve the **primary patency** of such bypasses. In fact, recurrent leg symptoms or significant decreases ABI (0.15 or more) detect a failing bypass in only 50% of cases. **Technical defects**, **myointimal hyperplasia**, and **recurrent atherosclerosis** can result in stenoses, following a leg bypass, that threaten the durability and primary patency of the revascularization. Identification of the "at-risk" bypass prior to its failure (e.g., thrombosis) allows for intervention on and salvage of the bypass (**assisted primary patency**) with improved limb salvage in certain groups of patients.

Duplex criteria have been developed to identify the "at-risk" lower-extremity bypass graft and include grafts with a focal *PSV >300 cm/sec, a systolic velocity ratio of >3.5* at a stenosis, or *low velocities throughout the graft (<40–45 cm/sec)*. A typical surveillance program is every 3 months in the first year after surgery, and every 6–12 months thereafter. It is possible to follow endovascular interventions such as femoropopliteal, balloon angioplasty, stenting, and/or atherectomy with duplex

Table 6.2. Criteria for ischemic rest pain

Noninvasive study	Unlikely	Probable	Likely
Ankle pressure (mm Hg)			
Nondiabetic	>55	35–55	<35
Diabetic	>80	55–80	<55
Ankle PVR category	Normal	Moderately decreased	Severely decreased or flat
$TcPO_2$ (torr)	>40	10–20	0–10

Table 6.3. Criteria for healing ischemic foot lesions

Noninvasive study	Unlikely	Probable	Likely
Ankle Pressure (mm Hg)			
Nondiabetic	<55	55–65	>65
Diabetic	<80	80–90	>90
Ankle PVR category	Severely decreased or flat	Moderately decreased	Normal
$TcPO_2$ (torr)	<20	40–50	>50
Toe pressure (mm Hg)	<30	30–50	>50

Note: The higher ankle pressure criterion in diabetics is due to false pressure elevation secondary to decreased compressibility due to medial calcinosis. PVR, pulse volume recording; $TcPO_2$, transcutaneous oxygen tension.

although data on the effectiveness of such surveillance programs is currently scarce.

IV. The renal arteries. These can also be evaluated for stenosis in the noninvasive vascular laboratory by duplex ultrasound. Testing should be considered for those patients with resistant hypertension and/or renal insufficiency. A lower frequency probe (2–3 MHz) is used for deeper penetration of the abdomen than for the peripheral vessels. Evaluation can be limited by obesity and overlying bowel gas, and is dependant upon the skill and experience of the vascular technologist. Inadequate visualization of the renal arteries may occur in 5–15% of studies and the presence of multiple or accessory renal arteries decreases the sensitivity of the examination.

PSV is measured in the renal artery and compared against PSV in the aorta (**renal-aortic ratio, or RAR**). Typical criteria for a greater than 60% stenosis of the renal artery are **PSV >200 cm/sec and RAR of >3.5**. Atherosclerotic renal artery disease usually occurs at the renal orifices, whereas **fibromuscular dysplasia** often affects the mid segments of the renal arteries. Although renal artery duplex has a high level of accuracy, a negative test does not definitively rule out the presence of a significant stenosis. Ultimately, the clinician's pretest probability of disease is the most important factor in determining who should undergo further testing with magnetic resonance arteriography (MRA) or arteriography.

V. Mesenteric occlusive disease. The presence of this disease, involving the **superior mesenteric artery (SMA)** and **celiac** arteries may also be effectively assessed with duplex. Chronic mesenteric ischemia is characterized by *post-prandial pain, weight loss, and sitophobia (food fear)*. Patients with suspected acute mesenteric ischemia should not undergo duplex ultrasound, and are typically better served with CT angiography, arteriography, or laparotomy in the operating room (Chapter 17).

Duplex ultrasonography of the mesenteric vessels should be conducted in the fasting state. The examination is rarely limited by abdominal girth, as patients with true CMI are generally quite thin. The SMA, celiac artery, and their branches are interrogated. **A PSV >275 cm/sec for the SMA and >200 cm/sec for the celiac artery is predictive for >70% stenosis**. As with renal artery stenosis, CMI from atherosclerosis usually affects the orifices of these vessels. Retrograde flow in the gastroduodenal or common hepatic artery is suggestive of severe celiac artery disease. The inferior mesenteric artery (IMA) should be interrogated for patency or occlusion. Isolated disease of the IMA in the absence of SMA or celiac disease does not result in CMI, but can be associated with ischemic colitis when inadequate collateral flow is present. When there is a high index of suspicion for CMI, an inadequate or negative duplex study should be followed by further imaging such as CTA, MRA, or angiography.

VI. Noninvasive vascular testing of the upper extremities. This is quite useful for a variety of atherosclerotic and nonatherosclerotic diseases that affect the circulation of the arms and hands. PPG can be used to assess digital blood flow with the probe placed on the fingertips and arterial waveforms recorded. A qualitative examination of waveform morphology is helpful on its own, and can be combined with digital pressure measurements if desired. **Raynaud's syndrome** causes an intense transient vasospasm of the digital vessels and is most often diagnosed clinically (Chapter 18). Patients with vasospastic Raynaud's will have normal digital pressures, and PPGs may be normal or have a "peaked pulse" pattern as a result of increased distal resistance. A number of nonatherosclerotic conditions (e.g., Buerger's disease, autoimmune disease, repetitive vibratory trauma) can cause actual occlusions of the forearm and digital arteries. End-stage renal disease and longstanding diabetes can lead to calcification and obstruction of the distal arteries. As a result, decreased digital pressures and dampened PPG waveforms are seen in the affected fingers.

A fraction of patients with upper-extremity hemodialysis access, develop **upper-extremity vascular steal** (Chapter 20). In such cases the arteriovenous fistula or graft "steals" more flow from the hand than is physiologically tolerable, resulting in ischemic pain, coolness, cyanosis, and, in severe cases, tissue loss. Finger PPGs in the affected hand will be dampened in comparison with the other hand and with manual compression of the fistula, the steal is reversed and the PPGs return to normal. Persistently abnormal PPGs with fistula compression imply intrinsic arterial disease of the forearm and hand.

Thoracic outlet syndrome (TOS) that results in arterial compromise is less common than neurogenic or venous TOS. Arterial compression at the thoracic outlet can result in stenosis, aneurysm, or even thrombosis of the subclavian artery. Provocative maneuvers such as hyperabduction and external rotation of the arm can result in diminished digital blood pressures and PPGs (Chapters 4 and 18). Duplex ultrasound can also reveal a thrombosed subclavian artery or aneurysm. The noninvasive lab findings should be correlated with clinical symptoms and additional workup such as angiography to make the diagnosis of arterial TOS.

Proximal arterial disease in the upper extremity can be differentiated from distal disease by palpation of pulses. A difference of more than 10 mm Hg in arm pressures (left vs. right) suggests a proximal arterial stenosis that is *more frequent in the left subclavian artery than the right*. Duplex can be used to diagnose suspected arterial disease in the upper extremity in a manner similar to the lower extremity. This test is used less commonly in the upper extremities, due to a lower prevalence of atherosclerotic disease in the arms compared to the legs. Additionally, disease of the subclavian artery is difficult to detect because of the position of the artery within the chest and behind the clavicle. A proximal subclavian stenosis can result in a condition referred to as **subclavian steal syndrome**. In such cases, exertion of the arm results in distal vasodilation with increased velocity across the stenosis. The increased velocity across the fixed stenosis results in a pressure decrease distally. In this case, the decrease in pressure results in reversal of flow in the vertebral artery distal to the subclavian stenosis. Abnormal retrograde or bidirectional flow in the vertebral artery can be seen on duplex at baseline and is a sign of proximal subclavian occlusive disease.

VII. Carotid arterial disease.

    A. Duplex ultrasound is the test of choice for the initial evaluation of extracranial carotid disease. Developed in the mid-1980s, this method of evaluation was rapidly embraced because it allowed accurate, inexpensive, and noninvasive evaluation of the carotid arteries. Although contrast arteriography was and still is useful in select instances, it is invasive and has an associated risk of stroke. It also introduces risk related to the use of contrast agents and to the puncture or access site. Currently, the most common reasons for carotid duplex are the presence of a cervical bruit or the history of neurologic symptoms such as a transient ischemic attack or stroke (Chapter 13).

Similar to the use of duplex in other vascular distributions, B-mode imaging is combined with pulsed Doppler to provide a visual image and physiologic evaluation of the common, internal, and external carotid arteries. Using the B-mode image, the Doppler signal is positioned in the center of blood flow within the vessel at an optimal **angle of insonation** to allow (a) *spectral analysis* and (b) *measurement of velocities*. The first indication of an abnormal flow disturbance is turbulence, which may not be reflected by elevated velocities but instead by the phenomenon of **spectral broadening** discussed previously (Fig. 6.2). As the amount of disease worsens and a stenosis develops, velocities become elevated, first the PSV and eventually the end diastolic volume, until the stenosis is so great there is only a trickle of flow through the vessel or it occludes (Fig. 6.7; Table 6.4).

In addition to spectral analysis and velocity measurement, carotid plaque morphology and color-flow analysis provide useful information. Carotid plaques may be characterized as smooth, irregular, or ulcerated, and the degree of calcification is also noted. A heterogeneous or mixed plaque contains a combination of echolucent and echodense signals and can indicate pending intraplaque hemorrhage. Color-flow analysis not only identifies of areas of turbulence but is also useful for mapping tortuosity of the carotid artery.

Carotid stenoses were originally categorized according to criteria developed by Dr. Eugene Strandness and a group at the University of Washington in Seattle in the 1980s. Duplex criteria were defined or validated by comparing thousands of

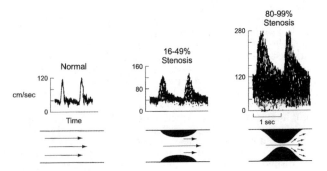

Figure 6.7. Internal carotid artery Doppler spectrum patterns. (The criteria are summarized in Table 6.4.) The percentage refers to the degree of stenosis.

Table 6.4.   Criteria for carotid artery disease based on duplex ultrasonography

ICA stenosis	PSV	EDV	Ratio ICA/CCA
1–39%	<115 cm/sec	<40 cm/sec	<1.8
40–59%	<130 cm/sec	>40 cm/sec	<1.8
60–79%	>130 cm/sec	>40 cm/sec	>1.8
80–99%	>250 cm/sec	>100 cm/sec	>3.7
Occluded	No ICA signal	No ICA signal	—

Note: the quality of the plaque is noted to be homogeneous (uniform echo pattern) or heterogeneous (complex echo pattern).
CCA, circumflex carotid artery; EDV, end diastolic volume; ICA, internal carotid artery; PSV, peak systolic velocity.

duplex ultrasounds to the "gold standard" of the day, carotid arteriography. Specifically, spectral analysis and velocity measurements were compared to the relationship between the greatest point of narrowing versus the estimated normal diameter of the carotid bulb on arteriography (degree of stenosis). Specific spectral patterns and velocity ranges were then correlated with increasing degrees of carotid stenosis and criteria established for a range of duplex findings from A (normal carotid with no disease) to D+ (high-grade, preocclusive stenosis) (Table 6.4).

Growing experience has confirmed that carotid duplex is accurate, especially in the mid to high range of stenosis (50–99%) where the sensitivity and specificity are over 95%. In some instances, duplex may have limitations in differentiating a very high-grade stenosis from internal carotid occlusion. In such cases flow beyond the stenosis may be so sluggish or limited that it is not detected or recognized by the sonographer, and the findings are interpreted as occlusion. Depending upon the clinical setting, additional diagnostic studies such as arteriography may be necessary to differentiate stenosis versus occlusion in these cases.

Duplex also provides useful information about the vertebral arteries in patients with nonlateralizing, posterior cerebral symptoms such as dizziness, vertigo, blurred vision, and ataxia. In most instances, the proximal vertebral (V_1 segment) can be studied directly and flow-limiting stenosis visualized and quantified. Indirect assessment of the vertebral is also made by determining the direction of flow (antegrade, retrograde, or bidirectional), which may indicate proximal arterial disease of the subclavian or innominate arteries. The more distal vertebral segments (V_2–V_4) are surrounded by the vertebral bodies and cannot generally be assessed by duplex.

In most cases, carotid duplex is the only imaging modality necessary for surveillance prior to endarterectomy. Additional imaging is only needed when duplex cannot provide complete information because of clinical factors related to the patient's presentation or technical factors related to performance of the duplex. In such instances other noninvasive studies such as

CT angiography (CTA) and MRA complement duplex by providing images of the proximal and distal carotid circulations and of the brain (Fig. 6.8). Contrast arteriography carries a low but finite risk of stroke and access site complications (1–2%) and is typically reserved for cases when duplex, CTA, and MRA are unable to provide complete information.

Limitations of duplex exist in its inability to examine the proximal intrathoracic vessels (aortic arch and supra-aortic trunk) and distal cervical and intracranial carotid circulation. Additionally, the quality and reliability of duplex is directly related to the training level and experience of the vascular sonographer. As such, additional imaging may be indicated depending upon experience level of the lab and specifically in cases of high carotid bifurcation precluding visualization of the distal carotid artery. Additional imaging may also be necessary if there is suspicion of tandem stenoses in the aortic arch, proximal common, or distal intracranial carotids. Lastly, in cases of unilateral carotid occlusion, duplex may overestimate the degree of the contralateral carotid disease. This phenomenon occurs as velocities through the patent carotid contralateral to the occlusion become elevated as a compensatory mechanism to maintain cerebral perfusion and not because of high degrees of stenosis.

B. Transcranial Doppler (TCD) is a noninvasive method to assess the intracranial circulation. TCD devices emit pulses of ultrasound from a 2 MHz probe through specific bony "windows" to the intracranial arteries. By placing the probe superior to the zygomatic arch, one can insonate the distal internal carotid siphon, anterior cerebral artery A1 segment, middle cerebral artery M1 segment, and posterior cerebral artery P1 and P2 segments. The ophthalmic artery and a portion of the internal carotid siphon may be assessed with the transorbital approach, and the suboccipital window is used to insonate the distal intracranial segment of the vertebrobasilar system.

A variety of clinical applications have been established for TCD that can be of use to the vascular specialist. The intracranial circulation can be assessed for collateral flow patterns in cases with severe bilateral carotid artery stenosis or occlusion. During carotid endarterectomy, TCD has been used to monitor for microembolic events, and intracranial stenosis or occlusions can also be detected. However, the total impact of TCD on the current evaluation of cerebrovascular disease remains relatively small compared to the role of extracranial carotid duplex ultrasonography.

VIII. MRA and CTA. These are noninvasive tests performed in the radiology department, outside of a traditional vascular laboratory. As has been discussed, these modalities, in combination with duplex, provide a definitive diagnosis of vascular pathology without standard arteriography in most cases. In preparation for vascular and endovascular interventions, MRA and CTA are being used increasingly as adjunctive tests or sometimes as the sole imaging modality. The choice whether or not to utilize this technology, and if so which kind, depends largely on the availability and quality of these studies at a particular institution.

Magnetic resonance imaging (MRI) relies on the principle that hydrogen nuclei (protons), when subjected to a magnetic field, align themselves in the direction of the field's poles. However, bursts of radio waves of appropriate frequency will alter this alignment (excitation). Following each radio frequency burst, the protons realign themselves with the magnetic field. This realignment (relaxation) is associated with the emission of a faint radio signal. A computer translates these signals into an image of the scanned area, which reveals varying densities of protons that correlate with different tissues (e.g., soft tissue and bone).

The physics of MRI are well suited for imaging vascular disease. In rapidly moving blood, the hydrogen nuclei do not line up in the applied magnetic field and thus produce little or no signal when stimulated by a radio frequency burst. The result is a natural contrast between the blood and the vessel wall. Several techniques of MRI have evolved in order to optimize resolution of blood vessels, but the use of contrast-enhanced MRA is most popular among vascular specialists. Gadolinium is a heavy metal analog that is injected intravenously in order to enhance the clarity of MR arterial images.

Spiral or helical CT scanners have the ability to collect a volume of data by continuously rotating 360 degrees over the entire area of interest. Three-dimensional reconstructions can be created based upon coronal, sagittal, and axial images. Visualization of the vasculature is enhanced by the use of 100–200 cc of iodinated contrast for a typical CTA. Nonionic contrast is preferable due to decreased pain with injection and lower risk of contrast nephropathy in patients with renal insufficiency. However, the greater expense of the nonionic contrast has limited it from everyday use at many hospitals.

All of the major vascular beds can be interrogated by CTA or MRA. Imaging of intracranial vessels and parenchymal disease with either modality provides high-quality images and visually appealing three-dimensional reconstructions. Computer software advances have brought brachiocephalic imaging with these techniques to a level comparable to standard contrast arteriography. MRI is superior to CT scanning in evaluating cerebral edema, and has the potential to accurately stage strokes and to determine the optimal time for any cerebrovascular operation in such patients. Mesenteric or renal artery stenoses can also be visualized by either modality with sensitivity and specificity approaching that of invasive angiography. The timing of the contrast bolus is key to providing good visualization of these vessels. These imaging studies are also very useful with the coexistence of an aortic aneurysm, dissection, or other abdominal pathology. Although small abdominal aortic aneurysms are followed with ultrasound, enlarging or larger aneurysms are usually imaged with CT (Chapter 15). The greatest experience with preoperative planning and postoperative surveillance for endovascular aneurysm repair has been with CTA and not MRA.

Lower-extremity arterial occlusive disease is frequently evaluated by CTA or MRA. Images similar to arteriography can be created with post-processing techniques. By and large, arteriography is considered the gold standard prior to lower-extremity bypass. However, some authors have found that high-quality MRA can identify obscure distal target vessels not seen on angiography. MRA may be obscured by venous artifact, if timing is not optimal. A particular strength of MR is the ability to simultaneously visualize muscular and tendinous structures. For example, popliteal artery entrapment from surrounding musculature can be diagnosed with positional stress. MR has also shown great promise in diagnosing venous thrombosis and obstruction, and is of the most value in areas inaccessible by ultrasound such as the abdominal, pelvic, and innominate veins. Protocols have been developed for the CT diagnosis of DVT, which can be combined with lung scan to detect pulmonary thromboembolus.

Certain limitations exist that are specific to each MRA and CTA, the major one being cost. In addition, patients with metallic life-support systems (e.g., pacemakers) are excluded from MRI, since the magnet creates problems with their function and some intracranial arterial aneurysm clips preclude accurate MRI. Finally, some patients become quite claustrophobic during MRI and are unable to tolerate its completion. CTA involves exposure to ionizing radiation, and iodinated contrast can cause allergic reactions and anaphylaxis, albeit uncommonly. Of even greater concern is the potential damage to the kidneys caused by the contrast agents used during CTA (contrast nephropathy), particularly in the elderly and in those with existing diabetes mellitus or renal insufficiency. An advantage of MRA has been that the use of gadolinium-based contrast does not have such a strong propensity to contrast nephropathy. However, the U.S. Food and Drug Administration has issued warnings regarding reports of renal fibrosis after gadolinium injection in patients with severe renal insufficiency. Vascular specialists can therefore no longer rely on MRA as a diagnostic tool in this subgroup of renal patients. CTA can be limited by the presence of vessel wall calcification that can obscure the lumen, whereas calcium does not cause artifact on MRA. More so than CTA, MRA is more difficult to interpret in areas with prior metallic stents, which can cause a loss of signal within the stent. Therefore, stents may give the false appearance of a stenosis or occlusion, although nitinol stents produce fewer artifacts. MRA also has a greater tendency to overestimate native artery stenosis. Some authors also caution that less expensive but effective methods of vascular imaging such as duplex ultrasound must not be abandoned during the current rapid proliferation of these diagnostic modalities.

IX. Venous disease. Symptoms of venous disease are nonspecific, and therefore can be difficult to diagnose by physical examination alone. The indications to assess for venous reflux may include leg swelling, varicose veins, and venous ulceration. The clinical signs of DVT are notoriously insensitive, and patients may in fact be entirely asymptomatic. Accurate diagnosis of venous diseases in the noninvasive vascular laboratory is therefore essential in establishing a diagnosis and can be potentially life-saving in the setting of DVT. Although the diagnosis of DVT by venography is primarily of historical interest, contemporary treatment with **catheter-directed thrombolysis** has witnessed a resurgence of this procedure.

   A. Venous insufficiency (reflux) can be measured physiologically by **APG.** With this technique, a recording pneumatic cuff is inflated minimally on the calf to hold it in place. The leg is elevated to empty it of venous blood. Alternately, the patient can perform toe raises to contract the calf muscle, which also leads to emptying of the venous system. Then, the patient stands without bearing weight on that leg (so the calf muscle will not eject blood). The venous refill volume into the calf over time is determined. Patients with venous reflux will have shorter refill times. Deep venous reflux will have a more profound effect than superficial reflux. This technique can be modified to assess for chronic venous outflow obstruction. A separate thigh cuff is then inflated to 60–80 mm Hg to occlude the venous outflow. Arterial flow continues to fill the calf over several minutes. The thigh cuff is then released. The recording calf cuff measures the venous outflow, which will be much slower in limbs with more proximal venous outflow obstruction (Fig. 6.8). Because it measures the physiologic function of the lower-extremity venous system, APG is not helpful in determining the presence of acute DVT.

B. Duplex ultrasound is an extremely valuable tool in the diagnosis of venous reflux and thrombosis. Venous reflux should be assessed with the patient in the standing position and the examiner's hand used to periodically squeeze the calf to augment venous flow towards the heart. When compression from the hand is then released, the vein of interest should be interrogated with duplex. Reflux will result in prolonged retrograde flow towards the foot and prolonged **valve closure times** (>1.0 sec). Using a pneumatic cuff on the calf that can be inflated and rapidly deflated helps to standardize the test, while freeing up the examiner's hands. The Valsalva maneu-

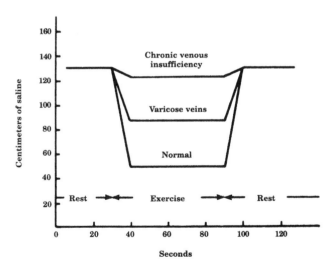

Figure 6.8.   Venous plethysmography. Blood is ejected from the calf by tiptoe maneuvers. A recording cuff on the calf measures the residual volume (RV) at the nadir. Patients with no reflux have a low RV, due to efficient calf muscle ejection. Chronic deep venous insufficiency is associated with the highest RV due to pooling of blood in the calf. Superficial reflux from varicose veins results in an intermediate RV.

Table 6.5. Duplex criteria for acute
deep venous thrombosis

Incompressible vein in transverse plane
Visualization of thrombus
No flow by color imaging
Failure to dilate with Valsalva manuever[a]
Lack of respiratory phasicity

[a]Applies to femoral vein.

ver can also be used to assess for reflux at the saphenofemoral junction.

Duplex ultrasound is the test of choice for suspected acute DVT (Table 6.5). Normally, a vein should be entirely compressible by the ultrasound probe. The compression test is best performed in the transverse view (vein appears circular). In the longitudinal axis the probe can unintentionally be off the midline, which can falsely lead the examiner to believe the vein is not compressible. Incompressibility of the vein is the principal finding associated with thrombosis. Lack of flow on color-flow mode also suggests an occlusion. Fresh thrombus may be very echolucent, so that its presence in a vein may be difficult to visualize. Over time, thrombus becomes echogenic (white) and chronically may show evidence of recanalization (wall thickening, irregular flow lumen). Central veins, such as the iliac and subclavian veins, are more difficult to directly evaluate with duplex and compression maneuvers, because of their location. Indirect parameters such as phasicity of flow must be examined to assess patency of more central veins. The absence of normal femoral vein dilation with Valsalva maneuver can occur in the presence of iliac vein thrombosis and normal respiratory variation in flow, referred to as phasicity, may also be absent.

ACKNOWLEDGMENTS

We would like to thank David Pendleton, RVT, and Kevin Franklin, RVS, for their expert consultation in formulating this chapter.

SELECTED READING

Bluth EI, Stavros AT, Marich KW, Wetzner SM, Aufrichtig D, and Baker KD. Carotid duplex sonography: a multicenter recommendation for standardized imaging and Doppler criteria. *Radiographics.* 1988;8:487-506.

Moneta GL. Screening for mesenteric vascular insufficiency and follow-up of mesenteric artery bypass procedures. *Semin Vasc Surg.* 2001;14(3):186-192.

Norgren L, Hiatt WR, Dormandy JA, Nehler MR, Harris KA, Fowkes FGR. Inter-society consensus for the management of peripheral arterial disease (TASC II). *J Vasc Surg.* 2007;45(suppl):5-67.

Olin JW, Piedmonte MR, Young JR, et al. The utility of duplex ultrasound scanning of the renal arteries for diagnosing significant renal artery stenosis. *Ann Intern Med.* 1995;122:833-837.

Rose SC. Noninvasive vascular laboratory for evaluation of peripheral arterial occlusive disease. Part I. Hemodynamic principles and tools of the trade. *J Vasc Interv Radiol.* 2000;11:1107-14.

Rose SC. Noninvasive vascular laboratory for evaluation of peripheral arterial occlusive disease. Part II. Clinical applications: chronic, usually atherosclerotic, lower extremity ischemia. *J Vasc Interv Radiol.* 2000;11:1257-1275.

Rose SC. Noninvasive vascular laboratory for evaluation of peripheral arterial occlusive disease. Part III. Clinical applications: nonatherosclerotic lower extremity arterial disease and upper extremity arterial disease. *J Vasc Interv Radiol.* 2001;12:11-18.

Roth SM, Bandyk DM. Duplex imaging of lower extremity bypasses, angioplasties, and stents. *Semin Vasc Surg.* 1999;12(4):272-284.

Rutherford, RB, ed. *Vascular Surgery.* 6th ed. Philadelphia: Elsevier Saunders Publishers, 2005.

Zierler RE. Vascular surgery without arteriography: use of duplex ultrasound. *Cardiovasc Surg.* 1999;7:74-82.

Zweibel WJ. New Doppler parameters for carotid stenosis. *Semin Ultrasound CT MR.* 1997;18:66-71.

Zwolak RM, Fillinger MF, Walsh DB, et al. Mesenteric and celiac duplex scanning: a validation study. *J Vasc Surg.* 1998;27(6):1078-1088.

Identification and Management of Cardiovascular Risk

CHAPTER 7

Risk Factors and Risk Modifications

The aging process can bring multiple health problems. Many of these problems are now well-recognized risk factors for atherosclerosis that have important impact on and increase the risk of coronary artery disease as well as peripheral vascular diseases, such as lower-extremity occlusive disease and cerebrovascular disease (Fig. 7.1). Simply put, the older one gets, the higher the risk of atherosclerosis. When these factors are controlled well, the risk of both vascular disease progression and perioperative events are reduced. However, when these risk factors are not controlled they may work in concert in the development of vascular disease and perioperative events. This chapter focuses broadly on some of these cardiovascular risk factors and on counseling patients about how to minimize cardiovascular events around the time of vascular interventions. Specific pathways that can be used to stratify periprocedural risk once a specific vascular intervention is planned are addressed in Chapter 8.

I. Tobacco abuse. Cigarette smoking has now clearly been identified as an independent predictor of vascular disease and failure of vascular operations or interventions. While smoking has notoriously been associated with coronary artery disease, the cerebrovascular and lower-extremity arteries appear to be more adversely affected by cigarette smoking than the coronary system. Smoking increases the risk of stroke at least twofold and the risk of lower-extremity occlusive disease four- to sixfold (two times that in the coronary arteries). Continued tobacco abuse is responsible for vascular disease progression, while smoking cessation mitigates these effects. Studies have shown that the risk of death, myocardial infarction (MI), amputation, and bypass graft failure are all lower in those who have stopped smoking compared with active smokers. The precise mechanisms of smoking's harmful effects on the heart and blood vessels are not fully understood, due in part to the fact that the chemical milieu produced by the burning of tobacco produces over 8,000 chemical byproducts. It is generally accepted, however, that nicotine is the

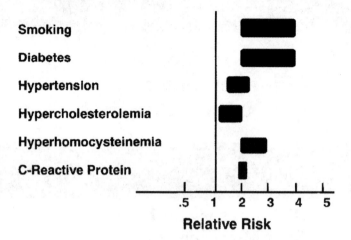

Figure 7.1.   Range of independent impact of each atherosclerotic
risk factor in the development of lower-extremity vascular disease.
Smoking indicates comparison versus former smoking. (From
Hirsch AT, Haskal ZJ, Hertzer NR, et al. for the writing committee.
ACC/AHA 2005 guidelines for the management of patients with
peripheral arterial disease [lower extremity, renal, mesenteric,
and abdominal aortic]: A collaborative report from the AAVS/SVS/
SCAI/SVMB/SIR and the ACC/AHA task force on practice guidelines.
J Am Coll Cardiol. 2005;e1-e192, with permission.)

stimulant and addictive component of tobacco. Despite this
addictive property, nicotine does not appear to participate in
the adverse effects of smoking on the vascular system. In contrast, oxidizing agents in tobacco are known to cause vasoconstriction, hypertension, and endothelial dysfunction, which, in
addition to inhibition of prostacyclin, cause a hypercoagulable
state. The effect of these oxidizing substances in cigarette smoke
lead to augmented lipid deposition, platelet aggregation, and
smooth muscle cell dysfunction. Collectively, these harmful
effects encourage the formation of new atherosclerotic lesions
and cause existing lesions to be less stable and more prone to
thrombosis.

It is no wonder that smoking cessation is critical to improving
cardiovascular outcomes. Convincing smokers to quit is not easy,
as most are affected by chemical addiction. The techniques available to help patients discontinue smoking will not succeed unless
the patient really wants to stop. Those who are convinced that
smoking is related to their vascular disease and have good motivation generally will stop smoking. Unfortunately, these individuals are in the minority and only 40% of men and 30% of women
who quit smoking will remain free of tobacco one year later.

Most studies of smoking cessation pharmacotherapy have
focused on nicotine as the addictive element in tobacco. Nicotine
replacement therapy comes in several forms, including transder-
mal patches, gum, nasal spray, inhalers, and sticks meant to sim-
ulate cigarettes. A newer nicotinic receptor agonist based on the

structure of cytosine, called varenicline (Chantix Pfizer, Inc., New York, NY, U.S.A.) has shown particular effectiveness in helping individuals to quit smoking. The antidepressant bupropion (Wellbutrin and Zyban, GlaxoSmithKline, Brentford, Middlesex, U.K.) has also been used with some success to reduce symptoms of withdrawal and achieve smoking cessation. Combination therapy consisting of bupropion and nicotine replacement has been shown in some studies to improve cessation rates compared to either therapy alone (Fig. 7.2). Interestingly, a new nicotine vaccine is being evaluated that in theory turns the body's immune system against the chemical before it is able to reach the brain and cause its addictive effects. Most studies have found that the effectiveness of any of these medications in assisting with smoking cessation is increased if combined with formal counseling and/or psychotherapy sessions. Regardless of the method used, the best long-term results to date report cessation rates of only 20–25%, although evidence suggests that rates may be higher with the newer nicotine receptor agonists.

II. Hypertension. The management and control of hypertension mitigates the development and progression of peripheral arterial disease and the risk of adverse periprocedural cardiac events defined as stroke, MI, and cardiovascular death. The risk of each of these events is two to four times higher in hypertensive patients compared with patients with normal blood pressure. Traditional guidelines have set a systolic blood pressure of 140 mm Hg or lower and diastolic pressure of 90 mm Hg or lower as "normal" target numbers. More recent information suggests that lower target numbers of 130/80 or lower are beneficial in patients with diabetes, renal insufficiency, and certain forms of heart disease.

Three common categories of antihypertensive medications are **beta-receptor blockers**, **calcium channel blockers,** and medications that alter the renin-angiotensin system, either through **inhibition of the angiotensin-converting enzyme** (**ACE inhibitors**) or through **angiotensin receptor blockade** (**ARBs**). Beta-blockers and ACE inhibitors have both been shown to reduce the incidence of MI and cardiovascular death in

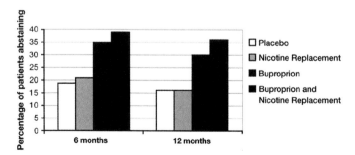

Figure 7.2.   Abstinence from smoking based upon cessation therapy used at 6 and 12 months. (From Jorenby DE, Leischow SJ, Nides MA, et al. A controlled trial of sustained-release bupropion, a nicotine patch or both for smoking cessation. *N Engl J Med.* **1999;340:685-691, with permission.)**

those with coronary disease, and ACE inhibitors have been shown to reduce these same adverse outcomes in patients with peripheral arterial disease. The effectiveness of beta-blocker therapy in reducing periprocedural and long-term cardiac events in those undergoing vascular interventions is so well established that it should be part of every patient's medical management.

In addition to the benefits of reduced blood pressure levels, arterial wall and myocardial cell remodeling are favorably altered by medications that block the renin-angiotensin-aldosterone system. The specifics of these effects remain less well defined and represent an area of active research; however, these medications in particular may modify the cardiovascular system through a mechanism that is independent of their effects on blood pressure levels.

In addition to the categories of antihypertensive medications already mentioned, the central acting medication **clonidine** and the direct vasodilator **hydralazine** are useful in treating more significant hypertension in some individuals. Diuretics such as **hydrochlorothiazide** (often abbreviated HCTZ) and **Lasix** (furosemide) can be used alone or in combination with other antihypertensive agents to successfully treat high blood pressure. Importantly, improvements in blood pressure control can also be realized by healthy lifestyle modifications, such as an improved diet, weight loss, and initiation of an exercise program. If blood pressure measurements remain elevated and refractory despite months of treatment with multiple agents, renal artery occlusive disease (e.g., renovascular hypertension) should be considered as a possible etiology.

III. Hyperlipidemia. Control of high serum lipids may slow the progression of atherosclerosis. In particular, **statin medications** or hydroxymethylglutaryl (HMG) CoA-reductase inhibitors not only control cholesterol but appear to halt atherogenesis and may even lead to plaque regression. They also have helpful effects on the endothelium and vascular smooth muscle and are antithrombotic. Their use has been shown to reduce all types of cardiovascular events. In the **Scandinavian Simvastatin Trial**, drug therapy for hypercholesterolemia was associated with a 38% reduction in the development or worsening of claudication. The **Heart Protection Study** has revealed significant reductions in coronary events, strokes, and peripheral intervention requirements in those with and without diagnosed peripheral vascular diseases using simvastatin (Zocor, Merck & Co., Inc., West Point, PA, U.S.A.) (Fig. 7.3). Retrospective reviews have noted a reduction in carotid endarterectomy restenosis and improved durability in those taking lipid-lowering agents.

In peripheral vascular disease, the **major lipid risk factors** are:

1. Elevated **low-density lipoprotein (LDL)**
2. Elevated **triglyceride levels**
3. Depressed levels **high-density lipoprotein (HDL)**

Normal plasma cholesterol is defined as less than 200 gm/dL/100 mL. However, the risk from serum cholesterol is continuous and increases as the cholesterol level rises. LDL levels greater than 160 mg/dL are considered extraordinarily high and

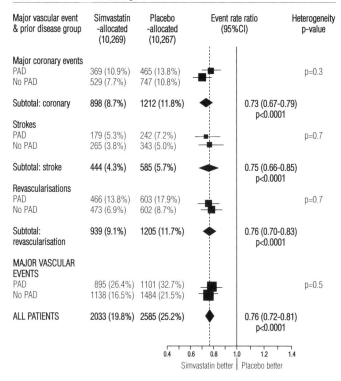

Major vascular event & prior disease group	Simvastatin -allocated (10,269)	Placebo -allocated (10,267)	Event rate ratio (95%CI)	Heterogeneity p-value
Major coronary events				
PAD	369 (10.9%)	465 (13.8%)		p=0.3
No PAD	529 (7.7%)	747 (10.8%)		
Subtotal: coronary	**898 (8.7%)**	**1212 (11.8%)**	0.73 (0.67-0.79) p<0.0001	
Strokes				
PAD	179 (5.3%)	242 (7.2%)		p=0.7
No PAD	265 (3.8%)	343 (5.0%)		
Subtotal: stroke	**444 (4.3%)**	**585 (5.7%)**	0.75 (0.66-0.85) p<0.0001	
Revascularisations				
PAD	466 (13.8%)	603 (17.9%)		p=0.7
No PAD	473 (6.9%)	602 (8.7%)		
Subtotal: revascularisation	**939 (9.1%)**	**1205 (11.7%)**	0.76 (0.70-0.83) p<0.0001	
MAJOR VASCULAR EVENTS				
PAD	895 (26.4%)	1101 (32.7%)		p=0.5
No PAD	1138 (16.5%)	1484 (21.5%)		
ALL PATIENTS	**2033 (19.8%)**	**2585 (25.2%)**	0.76 (0.72-0.81) p<0.0001	

0.4 0.6 0.8 1.0 1.2 1.4
Simvastatin better | Placebo better

Figure 7.3.   The effects of simvistatin use in those with and without peripheral vascular disease on the major cardiovascular endpoints of coronary events, stroke, and revascularization requirements. (From Heart Protection Study Collaborative Group. Randomized trial of the effects of cholesterol-lowering with simvistatin on peripheral vascular and other major vascular outcomes in 20,536 people with peripheral arterial disease and other high-risk conditions. *J Vasc Surg.* 2007;45:645-654, with permission.)

need reduction, ideally to less than 100 mg/dL. In those at highest risk for ischemic events it is recommended to reduce LDL to 70 mg/dL. Triglyceride levels should be below 150 mg/dL, which is usually achieved with fibric and nicotinic acid derivatives such as **gemfibrozil** and **niacin**. Cholesterol may also be lowered by the bile acid–sequestering resins **cholestyramine** and **colestipol** as well as niacin. As a rule, serum measurements of cholesterol and triglycerides should be determined after a 12-hour fast. A low-fat (35% of calories), low-cholesterol (<300 mg daily) diet remains the cornerstone of treatment of hyperlipidemia, and when combined with regular exercise is much more effective. Performance in a regular aerobic exercise program has been shown to be especially effective in increasing levels of the useful form of lipoprotein, HDL. Importantly, alcohol may exacerbate hypertriglyceridemia in some individuals and elimination of alcohol intake should be an initial step in managing hypertriglyceridemia. Although past recommendations called for a 3-month trial of diet management before medications were added, it is now common for statins to be started earlier, particularly as our understanding of the benefits of this class of medications evolves. The side effects of statin therapy are few but include hepatic toxicity and myositis, which can cause significant leg pain or soreness in some individuals. Therefore, patients receiving statins must be evaluated by the prescribing physician and have liver function and creatinine kinase levels monitored during therapy.

IV. Diabetes mellitus. Diabetes has both macrovascular and microvascular effects. It is a strong independent predictor for stroke and lower-extremity occlusive disease. The need for amputation in diabetics with lower-extremity arterial occlusive disease is roughly 10 times that of nondiabetics. While tight glycemic control has been recognized as preventing microvascular events, such as nephropathy, retinopathy, and neuropathy, it remains unclear if this reduces cardiovascular events. It appears likely that in those diabetics with intensive glucose control, claudication, revascularization, and amputation occur less frequently. However, there is no current evidence that good diabetic treatment retards atherosclerosis. Strict control may aid the diabetic in clearing and healing infections and minor skin breakdowns. Collectively, these nuances have led the **American Diabetes Association** to recommend maintaining a **glycosylated hemoglobin (A1C)** of less than 7% in those diabetics with peripheral vascular disease. Meticulous foot care to include appropriate shoes, moisturizing skin care, and daily inspection are critical in order to avoid ulceration, necrosis, infection, and potential sepsis or amputation.

V. Antiplatelet therapy. A significant cardiovascular benefit is realized when patients with peripheral vascular disease take antiplatelet medications. It is important to understand that this benefit is not necessarily related to improved leg symptoms or walking distance, but instead to improved survival over time. Specifically, the **Antithrombotic Trialists' Collaboration** meta-analysis has shown reductions in MI, stroke, and vascular death in those with peripheral vascular disease with the use of antiplatelet therapy. This reduction was between 20% and 30% in those with intermittent claudication, peripheral bypass grafts, or peripheral angioplasty. Antiplatelet therapy also reduces subsequent cardiovascular events in those with asymptomatic cerebrovascular disease and other atherogenic risk factors. Similarly, the use of antiplatelet therapy after previous stroke or prior carotid endarterectomy has been shown to reduce secondary stroke.

Most studies on the effectiveness of antiplatelet therapy have utilized **aspirin**, which competitively inhibits the **cyclooxygenase enzyme** within the platelet. Inhibition of cyclooxygenase blocks the production of **prostaglandin** and **thromboxane A_2 (TXA$_2$)** from arachidonic acid. The detrimental effect of TXA$_2$ comes from its activation of the **GP IIb/IIIa binding site** on the platelet, which allows fibrinogen to bind, which causes platelets to aggregate or begin to clump together. By inhibiting cyclooxygenase and ultimately TXA$_2$, aspirin prevents platelet aggregation. The antiplatelet effect of aspirin lasts for about 72 hours and can be achieved with 81 mg per day, which has a lower bleeding risk than the traditional 325 mg daily dose.

Clopidogrel (Plavix, Sanofi-Aventis/Bristol-Myers Squibb Company, New York, NY, U.S.A.) is another antiplatelet medication (75 mg daily) that works as a noncompetitive inhibitor of the **adenosine diphosphate** (**ADP) receptor** on platelets. The effect of clopidogrel on this receptor is irreversible and lasts the duration of platelet, which is about 7 to 10 days. Binding of ADP to its receptor on the platelet is necessary for activation of the same GP IIb/IIIa receptor triggered by TXA_2. The IIb/IIIa receptor is important as the binding site for fibrinogen, which initiates platelet aggregation. Both low- and high-affinity ADP receptors are present on platelets, and the active metabolite of clopidogrel also inhibits the low-affinity ADP receptor. Through these actions on the ADP binding sites and ultimately the GP IIb/IIIa receptor, clopidogrel provides a more thorough or stronger antiplatelet effect than aspirin in most patients.

Recently, results from the **Clopidogrel versus Aspirin in Patients at Risk of Ischemic Events (CAPRIE)** trial were reported. In individuals with previous MI or stroke, or in those with diagnosed peripheral vascular disease, clopidogrel reduced cardiovascular events by 8.7% (5.32% vs. 5.83% per year) compared with aspirin. In those with peripheral vascular disease, the benefit with clopidogrel was greater, with the risk of vascular death, stroke, or MI reduced by almost 24% (3.71% vs. 4.86% per year) at 3 years. The findings of CAPRIE were statistically significant in favor of clopidogrel, and many who treat those with established peripheral vascular disease use clopidogrel as first-line therapy based on this data. However, the absolute risk reduction with clopidogrel in CAPRIE was small, and aspirin remains an established and less expensive antiplatelet therapy. These facts are especially relevant when considering a medication that will be taken for many years; some providers prefer using aspirin as the initial therapy and use clopidogrel as an effective alternative. Combination therapy with aspirin and clopidogrel is somewhat controversial and no studies to date have shown benefit of dual- versus single-agent treatment. Benefit from dual antiplatelet therapy has been difficult to show in clinical studies because of the increased risk of bleeding associated with the combination of these two agents.

While the question of which antiplatelet medication to use may not have a single answer that applies to all patients, guidelines do exist to assist the provider in this area. Specifically, there is a consensus based on multiple clinical trials that some form of antiplatelet therapy, either aspirin or clopidogrel, is indicated in patients with peripheral vascular disease to reduce the long-term cardiovascular event rate including cardiovascular death (class/level of evidence 1A) (See Table 8.2). Because aspirin has been around the longest, it has the benefit of having demonstrated its effectiveness in more than one randomized controlled study. The use of aspirin is therefore supported by class/level 1A evidence, which denotes the consensus on efficacy (class 1) supported by multiple randomized controlled trials (level A). In contrast, clopidogrel was more recently introduced and has only been shown to be effective in one randomized controlled trial (CAPRIE). Use of clopidogrel in this setting is therefore supported by class/level 1B evidence, indicating the consensus on efficacy (class 1) supported by one randomized controlled trial (level B).

Other medications with differing mechanisms providing antiplatelet effects are also available. These include **picotamide**, a thromboxane synthase inhibitor that directly inhibits the production of TXA_2 and **cilostazol** (Pletal, Otsuka America Pharmaceutical, Inc., Rockville, MD, U.S.A.) and **dipyridamole** (Persantine Boehringer Ingelheim Pharmaceuticals, Gaithersburg, MD, U.S.A.), which inhibit the phosphodiesterase enzyme within platelets. Dipyridamole, which may have a unique role in preventing secondary stroke, also directly stimulates prostacyclin synthesis and potentiates the platelet inhibitory actions of prostacyclin. However, some of these effects may not occur at therapeutic levels of the drug; hence, the mechanism of action of dipyridamole remains somewhat poorly defined.

VI. Hyperhomocysteinemia. It is now understood that high serum levels of the amino acid **homocysteine** are associated with a substantial increase in the risk of arterial occlusive disease. Hyperhomocysteinemia carries an independent two- to threefold increased risk for developing lower-extremity occlusive disease, intermittent claudication, coronary artery disease, and stroke. Increased homocysteine levels are found in 30–50% of those with established cardiovascular disease, and evidence suggests that hyperhomocysteinemia also augments progression of peripheral arterial disease. Even more interesting is the fact that this condition places those with peripheral arterial disease at a three- to fourfold increase in vascular morbidity and mortality compared to those with normal levels of this amino acid.

The causes of hyperhomocysteinemia may include either a genetic alteration in the enzymes responsible for its metabolism, or deficiencies in vitamin B_{12} and folate, which are cofactors in this process. B complex vitamins, cobalamin (B_{12}), pyridoxine (B_6), and folic acid have all been noted to reduce plasma levels of homocysteine and have been targeted as a potentially simple therapy for this risk factor. However, there is as of yet no correlation between reducing amino acid levels and reducing cardiovascular events. In fact, a trend indicating a reciprocal effect has been noted. Trials are ongoing and more information should be available in the coming years.

VII. C-reactive protein and fibrinogen. An association has been noted between elevated plasma levels of the inflammatory markers **C-reactive protein** and **fibrinogen** and vascular disease. Specifically, increased levels of these markers have been identified in patients with lower-extremity occlusive disease, coronary artery disease, and stroke. This relationship is thought to be an association and not causative, meaning that these molecules do not cause vascular disease but are simply markers of the immune-mediated process of atherosclerosis. The role of these molecules in identifying and treating vascular disease is not fully understood and currently no recommendations can be made as to their use in clinical practice.

VIII. Obesity. While obesity may not be in and of itself a risk factor for the development of peripheral vascular disease, it makes treatment difficult. In the setting of extra weight, degenerative joint disease, and respiratory limitations, exercise programs for lower-extremity occlusive disease have very low success rates. Obesity makes endovascular access to the femoral arteries and operative exposure in the groin, abdomen, and retroperitoneum more difficult. Obesity is also a risk factor for periprocedural complications such as pneumonia, venous thrombosis, and pulmonary embolism. In the authors' experience, obesity increases wound complications, specifically those overlying femoral artery exposures in the groin. Consequently, it is the authors' opinion that obese candidates for elective vascular procedures should lose weight prior to the surgery or endovascular therapy, understanding that those with symptomatic or urgent conditions will not have such benefit.

Patients who are 15 to 40 pounds above their ideal weight are considered moderately obese. Morbidly obese patients (100 lbs overweight) seldom can be expected to lose substantial weight before elective surgery. Therefore, the benefits of elective abdominal or extremity vascular reconstruction in excessively obese patients must be weighed carefully against the increased risks of perioperative complications.

Occasionally, providers point out that weight reduction in preoperative patients is difficult to achieve and may be unsafe, and that insistence on weight loss may discourage patients from returning for treatment. This line of reasoning also points out the added cost of dietary consultation and the potential danger of excess weight loss before surgery as obstacles to preoperative weight reduction. In the authors' experience, safe weight reduction can be accomplished in approximately eight of ten moderately obese patients who require an elective procedure. Ideally, the patient's weight should be brought to within 10% of ideal body weight. Furthermore, this effort may serve as a life-altering event in which weight reduction becomes not only necessary for the perioperative time period but is continued throughout the patient's life. If successful, weight reduction improves not only a patient's peripheral vascular health but also their overall well-being. The following guidelines for periprocedural weight reduction are effective.

A. The **importance of preoperative weight reduction** as a means to facilitate operative access and exposure and to decrease complications must be explained to the patient. We emphasize that elective surgery can be safely postponed until weight loss is achieved.

B. A **definite time period** for the diet is proposed and a tentative surgery date is selected. Most moderately obese patients will need to lose 10–30 lbs. To ensure safe, gradual weight reduction, we recommend a weight loss of 1–2 lbs per week. Thus, elective surgery is postponed for 6 to 8 weeks for most patients. Obviously, some patients will need 3 to 6 months of dieting. We also have found it important to recheck patients every 6 to 8 weeks to ensure that they are losing weight and not having any problems with the diet.

C. The diet should be **reduced-calorie** (1,000 to 1,200 calories/day), but balanced. We use a relatively low-fat, low-cholesterol, 1,000-calorie diet. Diets that do not have a balance of carbohydrates, protein, and fat are not safe for older patients with vascular disease and their use may result in catabolism and deficiencies in vitamins, minerals, and trace elements.

D. Although **consultation with a dietician** may be helpful in some cases, a simple explanation of the diet by the physician and office nurse generally will suffice and saves the patient the time and expense of a dietary consultation. In the authors' experience, patients seem to respond best to the firm insistence on and explanation of a diet by the primary surgeon.

E. A specified amount of weight to lose is marked on the front page of the diet. Patients are instructed to take a baseline reading of their weight on a home scale and then attempt to lose the specified weight over the time period of the weight loss program.

F. Alcoholic beverages are a commonly overlooked source of calories. This fact should be emphasized to patients who drink regularly, as they usually must reduce alcohol intake to lose weight.

G. Most patients find it very difficult to lose weight and **stop smoking** at the same time. Consequently, it is recommended to allow some chronic smokers to continue some smoking while they diet. An agreement can be made with the patient that smoking will stop when the patient is hospitalized for elective surgery. Some may question this relatively late discontinuance of smoking, however, in the authors' experience this approach usually results in successful weight reduction and has not led to increased pulmonary morbidity.

IX. Exercise. Regular exercise is important for the patient's overall cardiovascular fitness, pulmonary function, and reduction of excess weight. As mentioned, regular exercise has positive benefits on hypertension, hyperlipidemia, and insulin sensitivity. Regular lower-extremity exercise in the form of a **structured or supervised walking program** is critical in patients with peripheral vascular disease. Walking increases skeletal muscle's metabolic adaptation to ischemia and may enhance collateral blood flow, resulting in stabilization or improvement of claudication. A variety of walking programs can be initiated in patients with peripheral vascular disease; however, a simple program that has helped the majority of the authors' patients emphasizes the following four concepts:

A. Dedicated walking time. Patients set aside a defined period of walking above and beyond that which they perform as part of their normal daily activities. Daily exercise may be too much for older patients; consequently, an every-other-day walking program is ideal, but should be tailored appropriately (e.g., 30–45 minutes, 3 to 5 days per week).

B. Walking instructions. Patients are instructed to walk at a comfortable pace and stop for a brief rest whenever leg pain (e.g., claudication) becomes severe. If patients experience no leg pain, they should continue walking for the 30–45 minutes set aside for the program. In bad weather, patients may use a treadmill or stationary exercise bicycle or walk inside a shopping mall. The walk–rest routine should be continued until the patient has performed at least 30 minutes walking (not including the rest periods). It is helpful to inform patients that as the leg adapts to anaerobic metabolism, the frequency and length of rest stops will decrease.

C. Recording walking time, length, and weight loss. Patients should be encouraged to record their walking program, including time and distance, on a calendar or in a journal. Patients who are obese should combine this record of exercise with daily or weekly weight measurements, as success with walking often goes hand-in-hand with weight loss. Recording their effort holds the patient accountable and offers a means to see successes over time. After 6–8 weeks, most patients can double or triple their comfortable walking distance and may also notice weight loss.

D. Supervision and follow-up. A follow-up visit with a provider or a phone call from one of the patient's vascular team during this period is critical to provide encouragement and supervision of this important endeavor.

SELECTED READING

Bates ER, Babb JD, Casey DE, et al. ACCF/SCAI/SVMB/SIR/ASITN 2007. Clinical expert consensus document on carotid stenting: a report of the American College of Cardiology foundation task force on clinical expert consensus documents. *J Am Coll Cardiol.* 2007;49:126-170.

CAPRIE Steering Committee. A randomized blinded trial of clopidogrel versus aspirin in patients at risk of ischaemic events. *Lancet.* 1996;348:1329-1339.

Hirsch AT, Haskal ZJ, Hertzer NR, et al. ACC/AHA 2005 guidelines for the management of patients with peripheral arterial disease (lower extremity, renal, mesenteric, and abdominal aortic): a collaborative report from the AAVS/SVS/SCAI/SVMB/SIR and the ACC/AHA task force on practice guidelines. *J Am Coll Cardiol.* 2005;e1-e192.

Heart Protection Study Collaborative Group. Randomized trial of the effects of cholesterol-lowering with simvistatin on peripheral vascular and other major vascular outcomes in 20,536 people with peripheral arterial disease and other high-risk conditions. *J Vasc Surg.* 2007;45:645-654.

Norgren L, Hiatt WR, Dormandy JA, et al. Inter-society consensus for the management of peripheral arterial disease (TASC II). *J Vasc Surg.* 2007;45(suppl S):S5-S61.

Smith FCT. The medical management of claudication. In: Hallett, JW, Mills JL, Earnshaw JJ, Reekers JA, eds. *Comprehensive Vascular and Endovascular Surgery.* Edinburgh: Mosby, 2004.

CHAPTER 8

Perioperative Risk Stratification and Clinical Guidelines

Most patients with manifestations of peripheral vascular disease requiring intervention have existing cardiac, pulmonary, and/or kidney diseases that increase their risk of periprocedural morbidity and mortality. Preoperative preparation must include an accurate assessment of the patient's risk related to these vital organ systems, taking into account the indication for the procedure, the type of anesthetic required, and optimization of coexisting medical conditions. This chapter focuses on assessing and reducing periprocedural cardiac risk according to evidence-based guidelines. Additionally, this chapter discusses the significance of coexisting carotid occlusive and chronic kidney disease and optimizing pulmonary function. Finally, new directions in the perioperative management of diabetes mellitus are outlined.

I. Perioperative cardiac risk. A key factor in achieving excellent results from elective vascular surgery, open or endovascular, is accurate assessment of anesthetic risk. Although clinical sense and experience contribute a great deal to an initial impression of anesthetic risk, more objective data also assist with assessment of operative risk. Historically, preoperative physical condition was correlated with anesthetic morbidity and mortality using the American Society of Anesthesiologists (ASA) classification. This grading system refers only to a patient's overall physical condition and does not consider the type of anesthesia, extent of operation, or experience of the surgeon. There are five levels of ASA classification, with 1 indicating a healthy individual and 5 noting extreme coexisting medical conditions. The letter "e" is added to indicate an emergency procedure. In 1977, Goldman developed a more involved scoring system to evaluate perioperative cardiac risk from 1,000 patients having undergone general surgical procedures. When this system was applied prospectively to 99 patients undergoing elective aortic surgery, the **rates of cardiac complications were higher than those in the original study of general surgical procedures**. This finding was among the first reporting the high incidence of significant coronary artery disease (CAD) in patients undergoing vascular procedures.

A. Evidence-based algorithm. MI is the leading cause of death following vascular procedures, occurring in 3–6% of elective cases. Additionally, some degree of myocardial ischemia is present following 20–40% of vascular procedures, depending upon how aggressively the diagnosis is pursued. Hertzer and colleagues of the Cleveland Clinic defined the prevalence of coronary artery disease in vascular patients, demonstrating **that severe but correctable CAD existed in nearly one-third of patients presenting for surgical treatment of peripheral vascular disease** (abdominal aortic aneurysm, 32%; cerebrovascular disease, 26%; arteriosclerosis of the lower limbs, 28%). Severe, correctable CAD was present in about 50% of patients with angina pectoris and 30% with a previous myocardial infarction.

Following this seminal report came more than two decades of study aimed at reducing cardiac morbidity and mortality around the time of peripheral vascular intervention. Much of this effort focused on identifying those with silent but correctable coronary disease prior to the planned procedure; the assumption being that in such individuals, coronary angiography followed by revascularization would reduce perioperative risk and increase survival. While this approach emphasizing coronary revascularization was beneficial in subsets of patients, such as in the **Coronary Artery Surgery study (CASS)**, it is not applicable to all those undergoing vascular procedures. In fact, more recent publication of the **Coronary Artery Revascularization Prophylaxis (CARP)** trial showed that among patients with stable cardiac symptoms, preoperative coronary revascularization does not improve short- or long-term survival. Findings from the CARP study and others like it have resulted in more balanced recommendations that propose a more selective role of preoperative coronary revascularization while emphasizing periprocedural medical therapy (e.g., beta-blockers, statins, and ACE inhibitors). The following paragraphs outline the contemporary guidelines on perioperative cardiac risk assessment.

1. **Eagle and associates identified key clinical markers of increased cardiac risk in patients undergoing vascular operations (Eagle criteria):** (a) angina pectoris, (b) prior MI, (c) congestive heart failure, (d) diabetes mellitus, and (e) age greater than 70 years. The risk for a perioperative cardiac event increases with the number of criteria present (Table 8.1). With three or more, the risk of a perioperative cardiac event is 30%, with 77% of these patients having severe CAD on coronary angiography. Although the Eagle criteria are largely of historical importance, they provide a very good and concise listing of key clinical factors to be considered prior to elective vascular procedures.

2. In 1996 the **American College of Cardiology and American Heart Association published guidelines for preoperative cardiac evaluation.** These guidelines were revised in 2002 and again in 2007 to provide a framework for considering cardiac risk associated with noncardiac surgery. Three prominent themes from the updated 2007 guidelines include:

Preoperative coronary intervention is rarely necessary unless otherwise indicated independent of the planned procedure.

Preoperative evaluation is not performed to "give clearance to operate," but instead should provide an assessment of the patient's medical condition and present a risk profile that can be used to make treatment decisions.

No preoperative testing should be performed unless it is likely to influence patient treatment (e.g., if it will actually change the perioperative management).

Table 8.1.   Eagle criteria

Clinical Criteria	Number of Criteria Present/ % Risk for Cardiac Event
Angina pectoris	
Prior myocardial infarction	0 criteria/2% risk
Congestive heart failure	1 or 2/10% risk
Diabetes mellitus	3 or more/30% risk
Age >70 years	

(From Eagle KA, Coley CM, Newell JB, et al. Combining clinical and thal-
lium data optimizes preoperative assessment of cardiac risk before major
vascular surgery. *Ann Int Med.* 1989;110:859-866, with permission.

Additionally, the 2007 guidelines were converted from tabular
format to listing of recommendations written in sentences to
express more complete thought. Also, a clearer explanation of
the clinical evidence supporting each guideline is provided using
levels of evidence and classification of recommendations
(Table 8.2). Specifically, levels of clinical evidence A, B, or C are
cross-referenced with classification of recommendations (I, IIa,
IIb, and III) to give the provider an estimate of the certainty and
size of each guideline. For example, level A evidence indicates
the strongest estimate of certainty coming from evaluation of
several patient groups with a consistency of direction and magnitude of effect. Level A evidence is supported by more than one
randomized clinical trial or a meta-analysis, while level B evidence stems from a single randomized trial or several nonran-
domized trials. It is important to note that guidelines supported
by level B or C evidence are not necessarily weak. Some clinical
questions are not well suited for clinical trials, or the optimal
time to perform such a trial may have passed. In some cases the
clinical consensus in favor of a test or therapy is so strong that
there is no need for investment to initiate a trial to prove the
point. In such instances **classification of recommendations**
is useful, as it provides a broader perspective than just the published or hard evidence for or against a given test or therapy
(Table 8.2). Armed with this basic understanding of levels of
evidence and classification of recommendations, the provider
can proceed in taking the patient's medical history and perform
a review of systems, focusing on three areas that relate directly
to the cardiac evaluation algorithm in the 2007 guidelines
(Fig. 8.1):

1. Identification of **active cardiac conditions** (Table 8.3)
2. Identification of **clinical risk factors** for cardiovascular
   events (Table 8.3)
3. Evaluation of the patient's **functional capacity** (Table 8.4)

Active cardiac conditions (formerly major predictors in the
2002 guidelines) represent conditions that if present should be
thoroughly evaluated and treated *before* noncardiac surgery,
even if it means a delay in or cancellation of a nonemergent case

Table 8.2.   Levels of clinical evidence and classification of recommendations

Levels

Level A	Evidence from multiple randomized trials or meta-analyses
Level B	Evidence from single randomized trial or nonrandomized studies
Level C	Evidence from retrospective or case studies or from expert opinion

Classification

Class I	Treatment or procedure is useful or effective (i.e., benefit far outweighs the risk and treatment *should* be performed)
Class IIa	Recommendation in favor or treatment or procedure being useful or effective (i.e., benefit outweighs the risk and *it is reasonable* to perform treatment)
Class IIb	Usefulness or effectiveness less well established (i.e., benefit is equal to or greater than the risk and the procedure or treatment may be considered)
Class III	Treatment or procedure is not useful and may be harmful (i.e., risk outweighs the benefits and treatment should not be performed)

(Fig. 8.1). These conditions include unstable coronary syndromes, decompensated heart failure, significant arrhythmias, and severe valvular disease. This guideline represents a class I recommendation supported by level B evidence. The patient should also be evaluated for the presence of one or more of the five **clinical risk factors** (formerly *intermediate predictors*) recognized in the 2007 guidelines. These include history of ischemic heart disease, compensated heart failure, cerebrovascular disease, and diabetes or renal insufficiency (Table 8.3). These factors are used in the final step of the cardiac evaluation and care algorithm in managing patients undergoing a high-risk surgery who have an unknown or poor functional capacity (Fig. 8.1).

Estimation of **functional capacity** is also critical and can be accomplished by simply interviewing the patient about his or her living situation and daily activities. Functional capacity is expressed in **metabolic equivalents (METs)** and has been shown to correlate well with oxygen uptake by formal treadmill testing (Table 8.4). In patients who have moderate or better functionality (>4 METs) without symptoms, preoperative management is unlikely to be changed based on additional cardiac testing. In contrast, cardiac risk is increased in persons who are unable to meet a 4-MET demand, such as performing daily activities, and such persons may benefit from preoperative

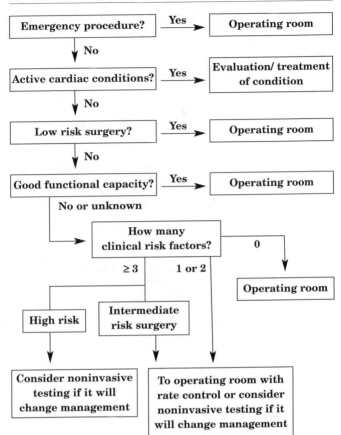

Figure 8.1.   American Heart Association 2007 guidelines for preoperative cardiac evaluation.

cardiac testing depending upon the magnitude of the planned procedure (Fig. 8.1). Once the provider has established the presence or absence of active cardiac conditions and clinical risk factors and assessed the patient's functional status, he or she can move to the **cardiac evaluation and care algorithm** to determine the need for and appropriateness of preoperative cardiac testing. This five-step approach provided as part of the 2007 guidelines, is as follows:

Step 1. *Is the planned procedure an emergency?* If so then the patient should proceed to the operating room (class I recommendation with level C evidence). In these cases the situation does not allow for further cardiac assessment, and recommendations will focus on perioperative optimization with medications and monitoring and surveillance for cardiac events in the postoperative period. If the procedure is not emergent then the provider should proceed to the next step.

Table 8.3.   Clinical assessment of cardiac risk

Active cardiac conditions (should be evaluated and treated before surgery)
Unstable coronary syndromes (myocardial infarction within 30 days, unstable or severe angina)
Decompensated congestive heart failure
Significant arrhythmias (high-grade atrioventricular block, symptomatic ventricular arrhythmias supraventricular arrhythmias with uncontrolled ventricular rate, newly recognized ventricular tachycardia and symptomatic bradycardia)
Severe valvular disease

Clinical risk factors
History of ischemic heart disease
Compensated or prior congestive heart failure
History of cerebrovascular disease
Diabetes mellitus
Renal insufficiency

From the Revised Cardiac Risk Index

Step 2. *Does the patient have active cardiac conditions?* If so then these should be evaluated and treated prior to the planned procedure (class I recommendation with level B evidence). Consideration of proceeding with the operation may be given after these conditions have been evaluated and treated. If the patient does not have any identifiable active cardiac conditions the provider should proceed to the next step.

Step 3. *Is the planned procedure a low-risk operation?* If so then the patient with no active cardiac conditions should proceed to the planned surgery (class I recommendation with level B evidence). A list of procedures considered low, intermediate, and high is provided in Table 8.5. If planned procedure is more than low-risk, the provider should proceed to the next step.

Table 8.4.   Estimated energy requirements for various activities

1 MET
Sitting at rest
Eat, dress, or use the toilet
Walk indoors around the house

4 METs
Light work around the house
Walk a block or two on level ground (at 4 mph pace)
Climb flight of stairs or walk on slight incline
Brisk walk on level ground
Heavy work around the house
Moderate recreational activities (golf, bowling, dancing)

Greater than 10 METs
Strenuous sports (swimming, tennis, jogging)

MET, metabolic equivalent.

Table 8.5.   Estimates of risk for various procedures

Low risk

Diagnostic angiography

Basic extremity endovascular procedures

Intermediate risk

Open carotid endarterectomy

Carotid artery stenting

Endovascular aneurysm repair

Open extremity bypass (femoral-popliteal bypass)

Open extra-anatomic bypass (axillo-bifemoral bypass)

High risk

Open aortic reconstruction for aneurysm disease

Open aortic reconstruction for occlusive disease (aorto-bifemoral bypass)

Other major vascular surgery

Step 4. *Does the patient have moderate or better functional capacity (≥4 METs)?* If so then the patient with no active cardiac conditions and good functional capacity can proceed with the moderate- to high-risk surgery without additional cardiac testing (class I recommendation with level B evidence). If the patient has poor or unknown functional capacity (Table 8.4), the provider should proceed to the final step in the algorithm (Fig. 8.1).

Step 5. *How many of the five clinical risk factors are present?* If the patient has poor or unknown functional capacity or has cardiac symptoms and is undergoing a moderate-to-high–risk procedure, then the **presence and number of clinical risk factors (Table 8.3) determines the need for further evaluation**. If the patient has zero clinical risk factors, then it is appropriate to proceed with the planned procedure with no further evaluation (class I recommendation with level B evidence). If the patient has one or two clinical risk factors, it is reasonable to proceed with the procedure with heart-rate control or consider additional noninvasive cardiac testing if it will change the management (class IIa recommendation with level B evidence) (Fig. 8.1).

Two studies have failed to show a difference in outcome between patients who underwent additional cardiac testing versus those who proceeded to the operating room with optimal medical management in this situation. If the patient has ≥3 clinical risk factors then the magnitude of the planned procedure (Table 8.5) impacts the decision on whether or not to obtain noninvasive cardiac testing. In patients with three or more clinical risk factors who are undergoing *open aortic or other major vascular surgical* procedures, additional cardiac testing should be considered if it will change the patient's management (class IIa recommendation with level B evidence). In patients with three or more clinical risk factors who are to undergo *intermediate procedures* such as carotid endarterectomy, there are insufficient data to determine the best strategy (proceeding with the operation with tight heart-rate control versus further cardiac testing if it will change management).

By definition, if a patient has undergone **previous** coronary revascularization, he or she has a history of ischemic heart disease, which is the first of the five clinical risk factors. In such instances if the revascularization was in the previous 5 years and the patient is asymptomatic with good functional status, then noninvasive cardiac testing is not recommended. If the revascularization is more than 5 years old or if the patient is undergoing a high-risk vascular operation then noninvasive cardiac testing should be considered if it will change the patient's perioperative management.

   B. Noninvasive cardiac testing refers to those methods used to identify areas of myocardium at risk for ischemia and infarction during times of stress. The goal of these tests in relation to vascular patients who may be undergoing an invasive procedure is to recognize those who are asymptomatic and may be at high risk of adverse cardiac outcomes from otherwise undetected coronary disease. Generally, if such tests are positive, patients then undergo invasive coronary angiography to define the anatomy of the coronary arteries, which allows treatment either by percutaneous (**percutaneous translumenal coronary angioplasty**) or open surgical (**coronary artery bypass grafting; CABG**) means. Findings on cardiac testing may also allow for more intensive perioperative monitoring, safer anesthetic techniques, or even changing the operative plan from a high-risk open vascular operation to a less invasive intermediate-risk alternative (e.g., endovascular versus open; or extra-anatomic bypass versus open aortic reconstruction). For simplicity's sake, noninvasive cardiac stress testing can be thought of in three main categories: **exercise stress testing, dobutamine stress echocardiography**, and **radionuclide myocardial perfusion**.

   1. Resting and exercise electrocardiogram (ECG) testing. The resting 12-lead ECG provides good information relating to both perioperative events and long-term morbidity and mortality in patients with known coronary artery disease. An existing Q wave provides an estimate of left ventricular function, perioperative cardiac complications, and long-term mortality. The presence of either left ventricular hypertrophy or ST-segment depression on a preoperative 12-lead ECG has also been shown to predict adverse perioperative events. The 2007 guidelines suggest that preoperative resting 12-lead ECG is reasonable in patients with no clinical risk factors who are undergoing vascular surgical procedures (class IIa recommendation, level B evidence). Generally, the ECG should be obtained within 30 days of the planned procedure.

   The use of a treadmill in combination with the 12-lead ECG (exercise stress ECG) provides much more information about a patient's functional capacity and risk of perioperative coronary events. Exercise ECG was pioneered by **Robert A. Bruce** while at the University of Washington in the early 1960s. Bruce is widely held as the "father of exercise cardiology" and the so-called **Bruce protocol** used during this test bears his name. This protocol has been extensively validated and consists of seven stages, each lasting 3 minutes resulting in 21 minutes of exercise for the complete test. During stage 1, the patient walks at 1.7 mph at a 10% incline; the speed and incline are increased for subsequent stages. There is a modified Bruce protocol that is commonly used in patients whose functional capacity does not allow completion of the full 21 minutes. **The goal during the protocol is for the patient to reach 85% of maximum predicted heart rate, which is roughly 220 (210 for women) minus the patient's age.** In clinical practice patients rarely complete the entire 21-minute protocol, as most are unaccustomed to exercise. However completion of 9–12 minutes of the protocol is adequate, providing the patient reaches the 85% predicted maximum heart rate. The ability of the patient to reach this goal maximum heart rate is in itself a good prognostic sign. **Horizontal or down-sloping ST-segment depression (≥2 mm) is the most reliable indicator of myocardial ischemia during the test.**

The sensitivity of exercise ECG for detecting myocardial ischemia depends upon the extent of coronary occlusive disease. It has been shown that as many as 50% of patients with single vessel coronary disease who have good functional capacity will have a normal exercise ECG. In contrast, the sensitivity and specificity has been shown to be as high as 86% and 53%, respectively, in patients with multivessel disease. Exercise ECG is not appropriate for all patients and should not be performed in those with unstable angina, recent MI, or those with poorly controlled heart failure.

2. Dobutamine stress echocardiography (DSE) combines two-dimensional echocardiography with infusion of the pharmacologic agent dobutamine and has become an important tool to evaluate preoperative cardiac function in patients who are not candidates for exercise ECG. Echocardiography itself is a standard noninvasive ultrasound imaging modality of the heart that is able to assess not only the structural components, such as the chambers and valves, but also the function and contractility of the myocardium (e.g., wall motion). Even the resting or nonstress component of this exam is useful, as resting left ventricular ejection fraction and/or diastolic function have been shown to be important factors in estimating perioperative risk. Infusion of the β_1 receptor agonist dobutamine increases myocardial contractility and heart rate and therefore myocardial stress and oxygen demand. During this "stress" phase of the test, significant coronary artery occlusive lesions can be identified by regional wall abnormalities in the distribution of the affected coronary vessels. Simply put, the myocardium can be visualized as failing in areas where blood flow is restricted during stress. The negative predictive value of DSE has been shown consistently to be above 95%, meaning that patients with a normal exam have extremely low rates of perioperative myocardial events. Increasing experience with DSE has lead to its preference over radionuclide myocardial perfusion imaging in some centers, with studies suggesting that it has twice the sensitivity of other testing modalities. DSE is limited in certain patients in whom echocardiography does not provide good images of the heart. Additionally, dobutamine should not be used as a stressor in patients with serious arrhythmias, severe hypertension, or hypotension.

3. Radionuclide myocardial perfusion imaging is the third main category of preoperative cardiac testing methods. This modality uses nuclear medicine technology to assess the heart at rest and during stress induced by infusion of a pharmacologic agent. During a follow-up image or scan of the heart hours after the baseline and stress images, this technique examines the heart muscle in the "recovered" or post-stress phase. Radionuclide perfusion imaging is accomplished by injection of a radionuclide or tracer into the patient, which is preferentially taken up by the myocardium. The tracer, usually technetium-99 sestamibi or thallium-201, emits small amounts of gamma rays detectable by a gamma camera or imager. Baseline images of the heart are obtained after injection of the tracer, which allows assessment of myocardial perfusion and determination of ejection fraction. A pharmacologic stressor, typically dipyridamole, adenosine, or dobutamine, is then administered to increase cardiac contractility and heart rate. Images are obtained during stress, and areas of myocardium that are malperfused or that fail during stress can be imaged and mapped. Four to six hours following the stress images, a scan is repeated to assess the areas of myocardium where the perfusion defects were visible. If the areas have returned to normal, the ischemia is termed **reversible ischemia** and attributed to a fixed coronary occlusive lesion or stenosis. These areas of myocardium in which reversible ischemia (RI) can be demonstrated are at risk and are felt to be critical during the perioperative period. If the areas remain without perfusion in the delayed imaging phase, the ischemia is termed **irreversible ischemia** and attributed to an area of myocardium destroyed by a previous infarction. Areas of irreversible ischemia are not at risk and are felt to be less important during the acute perioperative period. Radionuclide perfusion imaging with stress has a high sensitivity (90–95%) for detecting patients at risk for perioperative cardiac events. The risk using this modality appears to be directly proportional to the amount of myocardium at risk, as reflected by the extent of reversible ischemia or RI.

To summarize, all three categories of noninvasive cardiac testing are useful in identifying vascular patients at risk for perioperative cardiac events and each has strengths and weaknesses. However, these tests should be used selectively in appropriate patients and only in instances where their findings will result in tangible changes in perioperative management (Fig. 8.1). In general, patients should be considered for coronary angiography only if they have active cardiac conditions or poor functional status, three or more clinical risk factors, and evidence of ischemia during noninvasive cardiac testing. As far as which test to employ, the experience and expertise of an institution's cardiac laboratory in this area plays an important role and may ultimately be as important as the particular type of test ordered.

C. Preoperative coronary revascularization. Following this selective approach only about 5% of patients with peripheral vascular disease will undergo preoperative coronary angiography and some type of coronary revascularization, either open (e.g., CABG) or percutaneous (e.g., percutaneous coronary intervention [PCI]). Although revascularization prior to vascular procedures in patients with coronary disease seems inherently reasonable, the pathophysiology of perioperative cardiac morbidity limits its effectiveness. Specifically, a number of studies have shown that mild, nonobstructive coronary lesions may be just as important in causing myocardial infarction as high-grade stenoses or occlusions seen on coronary angiography. This fact stems from the dynamics of the atherosclerotic plaque, which is often independent of degree of stenosis. Even in sites of milder stenosis, an atherosclerotic plaque may become "unstable" and rupture, causing platelet aggregation and coronary thrombosis. This phenomenon suggests that preoperative revascularization may not reduce perioperative ischemic complications in all patients. This fact combined with the risks associated with coronary angiography and revascularization has resulted in recent studies that support a very selective application of coronary revascularization to certain groups of patients.

An early publication from the Coronary Artery Surgery study (CASS), which looked at outcomes in patients with both peripheral vascular and coronary occlusive disease, demonstrated short- and long-term benefits in those who received CABG prior to vascular intervention. Although favorable from the standpoint of preoperative revascularization, subgroup analysis suggested that the benefits were mostly limited to patients with three-vessel coronary artery disease and were inversely related to ejection fraction. This study and others like it, showing benefit of preoperative revascularization, have mostly been retrospective analyses; not until publication of the **CARP trial** has there been a randomized, prospective study comparing preoperative revascularization (CABG or PCI) versus no revascularization in vascular patients.

In CARP, roughly 500 patients were randomized to either coronary revascularization (n = 258; 141 PCI and 99 CABG) or no revascularization (n = 252). The study enrolled patients undergoing open aortic surgery or open lower-extremity revascularization for severe claudication or critical ischemia. Importantly, the study did not randomize the highest risk patients with left main coronary stenosis (>50%), severe aortic valve stenosis, or depressed ejection fraction (<20%). Conclusions from CARP found that among patients with stable cardiac symptoms, coronary artery revascularization prior to major elective vascular procedures can be done safely (1.7% mortality). However, preoperative revascularization does delay (median time 54 days), and in some cases prevents, the vascular operation (13% of coronary revascularization group did not undergo intended vascular operation). Finally, coronary artery revascularization in stable patients does not provide short-term benefit or improve long-term survival. The lack of benefit of preoperative revascularization today compared to that found in previous studies is undoubtedly due in part to an increase in the use of beta-blockers, antiplatelet agents, ACE inhibitors, and statin medications. Emerging evidence is fairly clear that optimization of such medical therapy in the perioperative and long-term postoperative period decreases cardiovascular morbidity and mortality. It should be noted that despite the excellent findings of the CARP trial, the overall risk of early cardiac morbidity (8.4% early MI) and late mortality (23% mortality at 27 months) was still significant. **Although the clinical evidence relating to coronary revascularization prior to vascular procedures may seem conflicting or even confusing, adherence to the 2007 guidelines offers the clinician the best opportunity to make solid, evidence-based decisions and provide optimal care.**

D. Cardiac conduction abnormalities must also be recognized and defined before any vascular procedure is performed. As was previously noted, the 2007 guidelines suggest that preoperative resting 12-lead ECG is reasonable in patients with no clinical risk factors who are undergoing vascular surgical procedures (class IIa recommendation, level B evidence). Performance of a resting 12-lead ECG within 30 days of the procedure will identify many of these conduction abnormalities. First-degree atrioventricular block, right- or left-bundle branch block, and bifascicular or trifascicular blocks are usually chronic and seldom progress to complete heart block. Thus, temporary pacing is usually not required for these conduction disturbances. In contrast, patients with second-degree, Mobitz type II, or third-degree atrioventricular block should be evaluated for perioperative pacing support, as these disturbances are more serious and prone to progress to complete heart block. Whether such pacing is temporary or permanent largely depends upon the discretion of the cardiology and anesthesia consultants. Permanent pacemakers are usually required for complete heart block or intermittent complete heart block.

Patients with **implanted cardiac pacemakers** present unique challenges during vascular procedures, as electrocautery may adversely affect the pulse generator. To prevent this possibility the rate of the pacemaker can be converted to a fixed-rate prior to the operation. Complexities involving the operation of pacemakers mandate that the vascular specialist consult with a cardiologist familiar with electrophysiology in order to establish a safe yet rational perioperative management plan.

II. Coexisting carotid occlusive disease. This is present in 10% to 20% of patients with vascular disease of the aorta and/or extremities. Most often this disease is asymptomatic and detected by the presence of a cervical bruit. In these instances evaluation with duplex ultrasound is appropriate and has already been performed in many instances. Although the presence of co-existing carotid occlusive disease often raises concerns regarding an increased risk of periprocedural stroke, there is little evidence confirming this correlation, especially in asymptomatic patients. Furthermore, there is no clinical evidence that pre-emptive repair of carotid stenoses decreases the perioperative risk of stroke associated with vascular procedures. Even if the patient is found to have a high-grade asymptomatic carotid stenosis (>80%), the authors' recommended practice is generally to proceed with the planned aortic or extremity procedure. The carotid disease is then managed on its own merit in the weeks and months that follow.

Exceptions to this practice include **symptomatic carotid stenoses**, which should be repaired prior to other planned vascular procedures. Additionally, an asymptomatic high-grade lesion in the setting of a contralateral carotid occlusion may be considered for repair depending upon its appearance on duplex ultrasound and the planned vascular procedure. Finally, bilateral preocclusive lesions are often managed with the same consideration of pre-emptive repair; however, there are limited clinical data to guide the clinician in these cases. In some instances, patients with large or symptomatic aneurysms or limb-threatening ischemia of the leg must have these problems addressed urgently and sometimes accept a small but finite risk of perioperative stroke associated with the carotid disease.

III. Coexisting pulmonary disease. This disease is a leading cause of postoperative morbidity and mortality, with many studies showing that pulmonary complications are at least as common as cardiac complications. Complicating this scenario is the fact that most patients undergoing vascular operation have some degree of chronic lung disease from smoking.

A. The initial **history and physical examination** will identify the patients at highest risk of pulmonary problems. They often are dyspneic at rest or with minimal exertion or exhibit chronic cough and sputum production. Other more advanced findings include a hyperinflated chest with distant breath sounds and use of accessory neck and abdominal muscles to assist with breathing. Patients with a component of reactive airway or bronchospasm may have wheezing. A simple bedside assessment of the degree of airway obstructive disease can be made by having the patient take a deep inspiration and then expire as quickly as possible while the examiner listens with a stethoscope. Normal complete expiratory time is less than 3 seconds; however, for patients with obstructive lung disease, this time is often 4 to 8 seconds. This simple bedside test also can be used to monitor clinical improvement during bronchodilator therapy.

B. A preprocedural **chest x-ray** (anterior-posterior and lateral projections) can provide insight into the chronicity and severity of obstructive lung disease and assess for evidence of lung cancer such as pulmonary nodules or effusions. Chest x-rays also provide a crude estimate of heart size and can be used to follow interstitial lung disease or identify blebs. The authors' practice is to have a new chest x-ray within a month of a procedure performed on active smokers and to insist that one has been performed within the prior 6 months in all others undergoing vascular operation.

C. Pulmonary function testing and measurement of **arterial blood gases** need not be routine but are indicated for patients in whom significant pulmonary disease is suspected. One of the most reliable predictors of high pulmonary risk is the forced expiratory volume at 1 second (FEV_1). Significant postoperative pulmonary complications can be expected in patients with an FEV_1 of less than 15 mL/kg or less than 1 L. If the FEV_1 is less than 70% of that predicted, the spirometry should be repeated after administration of an inhaled bronchodilator. An increase of at least 15% in FEV_1 indicates that preoperative bronchodilator therapy may enhance pulmonary function. This improvement may be especially important for the patient who has marginal lung function and requires elective surgery. Although measurement of arterial blood gases should not be routine, baseline values may help in patients with severe chronic obstructive pulmonary disease (COPD). For example, an elevated P_aCO_2 (>45 mm Hg) is associated with increased perioperative pulmonary risk.

D. Optimizing or improving pulmonary function (Table 8.6) in patients with chronic lung disease before the planned procedure can decrease the incidence of postoperative respiratory complications at least twofold. Preoperative preparation may require that the patient stop smoking, that antibiotics for bronchitis and bronchodilators be administered, and that the patient be instructed in deep breathing.

    1. Smoking cessation for eight weeks before any planned vascular procedure is ideal so that cilia regeneration within the lining of the lungs can occur and chronic cough (e.g., bronchorrhea) can resolve. Complete cessation is often difficult for many patients who are anxious before hospitalization, although most can be convinced to reduce cigarette consumption to some degree, which is also useful. A reasonable request is to reduce smoking to half a pack (ten cigarettes) per day, with a commitment to stop when admitted to the hospital. Often the planned vascular procedure can be used as a reason to initiate a formal smoking cessation

Table 8.6. **Pulmonary risk reduction strategies**

Preoperative
Smoking cessation for at least 8 weeks
Treat airflow obstruction in patients with COPD or asthma (beta-agonist inhalers)
Antibiotic and delay elective surgery if respiratory infection is present
Patient education regarding lung expansion

Intraoperative
Limit duration of surgery to <3 h
Use of epidural anesthesia
Substitute less invasive procedures when possible

Postoperative
Deep-breathing exercises or incentive spirometry
Continuous positive airway pressure if mechanically ventilated
Epidural anesthesia

COPD, chronic obstructive pulmonary disease.
Adapted from Smetana GW. Preoperative pulmonary evaluation. *N Engl J Med.* 1999;340:937-944.

program, which can be of significant help in the perioperative period as well as in the long term for the patient.

2. Respiratory infections in patients with COPD are most often caused by *Streptococcus* or *Haemophilus* species and some type of penicillin antibiotic (e.g., ampicillin or amoxicillin) is effective treatment. Importantly, any respiratory infection must be adequately treated before elective surgery, even if this means delaying the procedure.

3. Bronchodilators remain the cornerstone of therapy for patients with COPD and now are often combined with an inhaled form of steroid. However, we often find that vascular patients with known pulmonary disease are not receiving optimum doses of inhaled bronchodilators or may not be receiving the inhaled steroid component when they are being evaluated for a procedure. If the patient's reactive airway component is known to be significant, the inhaler regimen should be optimized preoperatively, in some instances by use of a nebulizer for a few days. Also, for patients with significant reactive airway disease, a short but high dose of oral steroids may be necessary in the perioperative period to improve (at least temporarily) the patient's pulmonary mechanics.

4. Deep breathing maneuvers with the incentive spirometer have been shown to decrease the incidence of pulmonary complications after open vascular procedures. Furthermore, the effectiveness of this adjunct has been shown to improve if the patient receives preoperative instruction, as opposed to waiting until the postoperative period to teach the method. The practice of sending the spirometer home with the patient days before the procedure is even advocated by some. In these instances the patient can become familiar with the breathing technique and can initiate pulmonary exercises prior to the planned procedure. Avoiding perioperative pulmonary complications is multifactorial and includes nursing instruction, patient motivation, and early postoperative ambulation and adequate pain control.

IV. Coexisting kidney disease. Kidney disease is commonly present in vascular patients and has been shown to be associated with a higher risk of periprocedural cardiac events. The relevance of renal dysfunction in the perioperative period is underscored by its inclusion as one of the five clinical risk factors in the 2007 guidelines (Table 8.3). Pre-existing renal disease (serum creatinine ≥2.0 mg/mL) has also been shown to be a risk factor for postoperative renal dysfunction and increased overall morbidity and mortality. **Estimated creatinine clearance**, which is a more accurate assessment of renal function, provides an approximation of glomerular filtration and has also been used to predict periprocedural morbidity and mortality. This method takes into account patient age and weight as well as serum creatinine levels in the following formula: **Estimated creatinine clearance = (140 – age [yr] × weight [kg]) / (72 × serum creatinine [mg/dL])** *(multiply by 0.85 for women)*. The normal range of estimated creatinine clearance is 55–145 mL/min/1.73 m^2 in men and 50–135 mL/min/1.73 m^2 in women.

A measure of renal function (either serum creatinine or creatinine clearance) should be checked routinely in vascular patients prior to any open or endovascular intervention. The authors' routine includes an assessment of renal function within 30 days of any vascular procedure. Depending upon the degree of renal dysfunction, protective measures may be taken or alterations made in the operative plan to account for this condition. One of the simplest adjuncts in patients with chronic renal disease is preprocedural hydration with crystalloid to establish a urine output of 0.5 to 1 cc/kg. Generally, this requires gentle hydration with 1–2 L of crystalloid in the hours before the planned procedure. Other specific renal protective strategies employed prior to and during endovascular procedures to minimize the harmful effects of contrast agents are discussed in Chapter 10.

V. Diabetes mellitus. This is the most common metabolic condition to occur in vascular patients and its presence should increase suspicion for coronary artery disease. Additionally, perioperative cardiac events have been shown to occur more frequently in those with diabetes and it too has been included as one of the five clinical risk factors in the 2007 guidelines (Table 8.3). Diabetes can be particularly difficult to manage in the perioperative period, when oral intake is varied and physiologic stress is high, resulting in a state of insulin resistance from increased levels of glucagon, epinephrine, and cortisol. Nonetheless, **hyperglycemia has been shown to be an independent risk factor for cardiovascular events and the severity of hyperglycemia has been shown to be directly proportional to mortality during myocardial infarction.** In the perioperative period, blood glucose levels are typically managed with frequent blood sugar measurements and use of adjusted doses or infusions of short-acting insulin. Although blood sugar ranges of 150–250 mg/dL used to be acceptable, more recent evidence strongly supports a more aggressive approach in the perioperative period, using continuous intravenous insulin infusion to maintain blood glucose levels between 100 and 150 mg/dL. Specifically, the **American College of Endocrinology has provided a position statement recommending that preprocedural glucose concentrations should be less than 110 mg/dL, with maximal glucose not to exceed 180 mg/dL in hospitalized patients, and that concentrations should be less than 110 mg/dL in patients in the intensive care unit**. While these strict ranges may not be achievable in all patients, this position statement emphasizes the importance of emerging clinical evidence in this area.

The **preoperative management** of the diabetic patient depends on the timing of the vascular procedure and whether the patient's usual therapy consists of insulin, an oral hypoglycemic, or both. The complicating factor is the fact that patients are kept without food or drink (e.g., nothing per mouth) prior to their procedure predisposing them to hypoglycemia. Patients who are insulin-dependent and scheduled for their procedure early in the day (before 9 A.M.) should not take their insulin dose in the morning. They may be asked to bring their insulin with them if they are a morning admission. The blood sugar level is checked upon arrival and if greater than 100 mg/dL, the patient should receive one-half the usual intermediate-acting insulin dose. If the blood sugar is less than 100 mg/dL, the patient should receive a dextrose-containing solution once an intravenous line is established. Insulin-dependent patients who are scheduled for a procedure later in the day should be asked to take one-half the usual dose of intermediate-acting insulin instead of the full dose in the morning with whatever is allowed to be taken by mouth. Patients taking oral hypoglycemic agents should be advised not to take the oral agents on the morning of the vascular procedure.

The so-called brittle diabetic can have wide variations in blood sugar levels despite frequent glucose monitoring; in these patients levels are optimally controlled with a continuous intravenous insulin drip. An infusion of 1 to 4 units of regular insulin per hour generally results in good control. In the acute postoperative period, various sliding scales of intravenous infusion rates (units/hour) exist that allow the infusion of insulin to change according to blood glucose levels. **However, rare, severe, and sustained hypoglycemia can cause significant neurologic damage and is a particular risk related to the use of continuous insulin infusions.** To avoid inadvertent rapid insulin infusion we recommend mixing only 10 units of regular insulin in 250 mL of D5W or D5NS and infusing at a rate of 25 to 100 mL/h (1 to 4 units) using an infusion pump. One should also infuse a dextrose containing solution when using an insulin drip and have an ampule of high concentration dextrose nearby for use should the patient become hypoglycemic.

SELECTED READING

Beattie WS, Abdelnaem E, Wijeysundera DN, Buckley DN. A meta-analysis comparison of preoperative stress echocardiography and nuclear scintigraphy imaging. *Anesth Analg.* 2006;102:8-16.

Clinical factors associated with long-term mortality following vascular surgery: outcomes from the coronary artery revascularization prophylaxis (CARP) trail. *J Vasc Surg.* 2007;46:694-700.

Eagle KA, Rihal CS, Mickel MC, Holmes DR, Foster ED, Gersh BJ. Cardiac risk of non-cardiac surgery: influence of coronary disease and type of surgery in 3368 operations. CASS investigators and University of Michigan Heart Care Program. Coronary artery surgery study. *Circulation.* 1997;96:1882-1887.

Fleisher LA, Beckman JA, Brown KA, et al. ACC/AHA 2007 guidelines on perioperative cardiovascular evaluation and care for noncardiac surgery. *J Am Coll Cardiol.* 2007;50:e159-241.

Garber AJ, Moghissi ES, Bransome EDJ, et al. American College of Endocrinology position statement on inpatient diabetes and metabolic control. *Endocr Pract.* 2004;10:77-82.

McFalls E, Ward H, Moritz T, et al. Coronary artery revascularization before elective major vascular surgery. *N Engl J Med.* 2004;351: 2795-2804.

O'Neil-Callahan K, Katsimalis G, Tepper M, et al. Statins decrease perioperative cardiac complications in patients undergoing noncardiac vascular surgery. The statins for risk reduction in surgery (StaRRS) study. *J Am Coll Cardiol.* 2005;45:336-342.

Poldermans D, Bax J, Schouten O, et al. Should major vascular surgery be delayed because of preoperative cardiac testing in intermediate-risk patients receiving beta-blocker therapy with tight heart rate control? *J Am Coll Cardiol.* 2006;48:964-969.

Rihal CS, Eagle KA, Mickel MC, Foster ED, Sopko G, Gersh BJ. Surgical therapy for coronary artery disease among patients with combined coronary artery and peripheral vascular disease. Coronary Artery Surgery study (CASS) registry. *Circ*. 1995;91: 46-53.

CHAPTER 9

Perioperative Planning and Care of the Vascular Patient

Optimal care of the vascular patient in the operating room or endovascular suite requires a keen understanding and awareness of details related to **monitoring, patient preparation and positioning**, and **anesthesia**. The improved awareness of the vascular provider in each of these areas ensures the best chance for a safe, technically successful procedure with the lowest possible risk of morbidity and mortality. Each vascular procedure, whether it is an open aneurysm repair in the operating room or a percutaneous lower-extremity arteriogram and stent in the imaging suite, requires a well thought-out and communicated plan in regard to these topics. Optimal patient preparation and positioning may be accomplished through a "final time out" or **operating room or endovascular suite briefing** and are imperative to ensure that the correct procedure is performed on the correct patient at the correct surgical sight. The monitoring and anesthesia plans are especially relevant in transition to care of the patient in the post-procedure setting, which can be the recovery room, post-anesthesia care unit (PACU), inpatient ward, or intensive care unit (ICU). This chapter emphasizes the principles of basic cardiac and respiratory monitoring, patient preparation and positioning, and anesthesia. An understanding of these should be of particular value to surgical house staff, nurses, and other vascular providers who are often the first into the operating room or endovascular suite and the first to recognize and treat problems during the postoperative period.

OPERATIVE PLAN AND ANESTHESIA

Improved anesthetic management has been a key factor in the reduction of perioperative morbidity and mortality in vascular and endovascular surgery. The preoperative assessment of the patient and his or her comorbidities form the basis for selecting the most appropriate anesthetic. The anesthesia team must be aware of the planned procedure and the procedural conduct—much more than simply reading the name from the operating room list of the day. The type and depth of anesthetic varies widely among the range of vascular and endovascular procedures to be performed. Therefore, for the smooth conduct of any vascular or endovascular operation, regardless of level of complexity, communication between the vascular and anesthesia providers must begin before the start of the case and continue throughout.

Clinical examples that emphasize the need for communication include the **requirement for patients undergoing certain endovascular procedures to remain fully awake and directable** during the procedure. In these instances patients may need to remain still, hold their breath, or have neurologic evaluation during the procedure (e.g., during carotid arteriography or stenting). Any conscious sedation at all in such cases may be too much and result in an overly sedated, noncooperative patient and a suboptimal procedure. The **effectiveness of regional anesthesia for certain extremity procedures** also needs to be discussed well before the procedure to avoid placement of a peripheral nerve block or regional anesthetic that does not fully anesthetize the planned area of operation (e.g., nerve block that anesthetizes the forearm and hand when the planned operation is the upper arm and axilla). And finally, the **anesthesia team must be aware of specific aspects of the procedure, open or endovascular, that are most stressful to cardiac, cerebral, respiratory, and renal function** in order to manage the patient effectively. This chapter provides an overview of physiologic monitoring that applies to the operating room or endovascular suite and focuses on perioperative care for carotid, aortic, and lower-extremity procedures.

I. Perioperative physiologic monitoring provides clinical data critical to assessment and maintenance of cardiac, respiratory, neurologic, and renal function during and after any open or endovascular procedure. The magnitude of the procedure and the patient's medical condition determine the extent of monitoring, and it should be recognized that in some instances the information gathered may be misleading or imprecise and may not influence the overall outcome of the patient. It is important to understand the limitations of monitoring and use only techniques and devices that will provide useful or actionable information.

    A. Basic intravenous access and monitoring. All patients should have at least one sizable (14- or 16-gauge) intravenous line and electrocardiographic (ECG), temperature, and blood pressure monitoring. A urinary catheter and collection system to measure urine output is needed for operations that last longer than a few hours or endovascular interventions that may require the patient to remain supine for several hours following the procedure.

    B. Pulse oximeters, which attach to a finger or toe, are used to continuously measure arterial oxygen saturation of hemoglobin. Pulse oximetry functions by positioning a pulsating arterial vascular bed between a two-wavelength light source and a detector. A familiar plethysmograph waveform results. Because the detected pulsatile waveform is produced from arterial blood, the amplitude of each wavelength is related to reduced versus oxidized or oxyhemoglobin and allows continuous beat-to-beat calculation of oxygen saturation. The instrument's ability to accurately calculate saturation can be impaired by hypothermia, hypotension, and vasopressor medications. The placement of an additional pulse oximeter probe on another site in these instances is recommended (at the alternate extremity or a more central location such as ear or nose).

    C. Arterial and central venous access. More significant open vascular cases or cases in which the patient's blood pressure can be expected to be labile may require an indwelling radial artery line and, occasionally, a central venous catheter. The arterial line allows easier blood sampling for measurements of arterial blood gas, hematocrit, electrolytes, and glucose, as well as continuous blood pressure tracings. The central venous line allows measurements of central venous pressure

(CVP) and infusion of resuscitative fluids and medications at a more brisk rate, depending upon the size of the catheter or sheath.

D. Pulmonary capillary wedge pressure measured with a **Swan-Ganz pulmonary artery (PA) catheter** is a reliable guide to left-sided (left atrium and left ventricle) filling pressures and even left ventricular function. The PA catheter also allows the measurement of cardiac output and mixed venous oxygen saturations (SvO_2) as an indicator of oxygen delivery and end-organ extraction. Although some anesthesia providers prefer a PA catheter in all major open vascular cases, its routine use is controversial, as some studies have shown that is does not improve overall patient outcome. **Therefore, use of PA catheters on a selective basis in patients with ventricular dysfunction, unstable angina, or recent myocardial infarction who require open vascular surgery on an urgent or compelling basis is recommended.** If there is question about the need for a PA catheter, the surgeon and anesthesia provider should discuss the indications in the context of the overall operative plan. If it remains unclear whether or not a PA catheter will be needed, an introducer can be placed in a central vein at the start of the operation allowing for the catheter to be placed later if necessary. Figure 9.1 illustrates the pressure tracings as the Swan-Ganz catheter is floated through the right heart to a wedge position in a pulmonary artery. Although there are complications related to the use of a PA catheters, most of the risks are incurred in the process of obtaining central venous access.

Oximetric PA catheters allow continuous monitoring of SvO_2, which is an early indicator of change in the patient's physiologic well-being. SvO_2 may be used to assess the effectiveness of a specific intervention, with a decrease in saturation indicating worsening oxygen delivery (e.g., myocardial infarction) or increased end-organ extraction (e.g., sepsis). An SvO_2 of less than 60% indicates physiologic compromise and

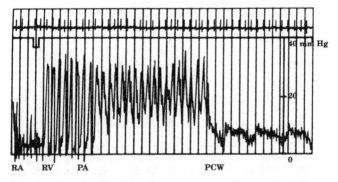

Figure 9.1. Swan-Ganz pulmonary catheter tracings as the catheter is advanced from the right atrium (RA) through the right ventricle (RV) and pulmonary artery (PA) to a wedged position in a pulmonary artery (PCW). The pressures shown are within normal limits. Abnormal values are discussed in the text.

should prompt a reevaluation of the patient, to find the source or explanation. The Svo_2 can then be followed as an early measure of treatment success such as the response to administration of an inotropic agent. Oximetric pulmonary artery catheters are more expensive than the standard PA catheters and should only be placed in cases where such physiologic detail will be used. **Despite the physiologic information that this technology provides, the value of the Swan-Ganz catheter is debatable, as some prospective studies have shown its routine use does not improve mortality.** **E. Transesophageal echocardiography (TEE)** is another option for monitoring cardiac function in the operating room, but it is less commonly used outside of the operating room in the postoperative setting. TEE is a sensitive method to detect myocardial ischemia manifest by the development of **myocardial wall motion abnormalities** and can accurately assess left ventricular filling and function (e.g., ejection fraction).
F. Core temperature monitoring is critical for all open aortic or extremity vascular cases that last for more than two to three hours. Hypothermia ($<35°C$) is associated with risk for cardiac events, including ventricular tachycardia related to elevated levels of circulating catecholamines. In addition, hypothermia contributes to coagulopathy by adversely effecting the enzymes that participate in the clotting cascade. Esophageal, intravenous, or bladder thermistor monitoring are all generally accurate. Warming the operating room to 75°F before the patient enters and using warm air plastic drapes (Bair Hugger, Augustine Medical, Inc., Eden Prairie, MN, U.S.A.) are helpful in maintaining the core temperature of the patient.
II. Patient positioning and operating room briefing. Positioning the patient on the operating or endovascular table is critical and should occur as part of the **final time out** or **operating room briefing program**. This preparatory step assures that the members of the team know each other as well as the patient and the planned procedure, including its stepwise conduct. The surgical site and procedure are reviewed and critical steps and necessary equipment are anticipated among the four key players in the room: **surgeon or endovascular specialist, surgical assistant, circulating nurse,** and **anesthesia provider.** Optimally, this briefing is led by the surgeon or endovascular specialist and occurs with all present at the same time. The operating room briefing program has been shown to serve in conjunction with the more basic and familiar "time out" to reduce wrong patient and wrong site procedures and to improve overall patient safety and procedural efficiency in the operating room and endovascular suite.
Once the final time out or operating room briefing has occurred, final patient positioning and setup can take place. Special attention should be paid to whether or not to tuck the patient's arms next to his or her side on the table and where any fluoroscopic imaging will take place during the procedure. Again, anticipation and planning before the final sterile preparation and draping is critical for a safe, effective, and efficient procedure.
In addition to positioning for proper retraction and/or fluoroscopic imaging, patient positioning has been shown to be critical

in avoiding pressure-related injuries to the skin and peripheral nerves in certain susceptible areas. The most common pressure-related problems in the authors' experience have been lateral heel and malleolus ulcers. These ulcers are multifactorial and often occur in patients with lower-extremity ischemia who undergo longer duration procedures. Pressure-related heel ulcers can be prevented by elevating the legs on soft towels so that the heels do not rest directly on the operating table or by placing soft egg-crate padding under the heels themselves. Another potential problem occurs when the upper extremities are tucked along the sides of the patient and pressure from the edge of the operating table compresses the ulnar nerve, causing a neuropraxia. This bothersome problem can be prevented by gently wrapping the elbow region with a soft egg-crate pad to keep pressure off of the ulnar nerve.

Positioning of the head, eyes, ears, and neck should also be performed with care. Patients with carotid disease or musculoskeletal conditions such as arthritis may be particularly susceptible to injury secondary to poor positioning. Gentle positioning of the neck in the neutral position is best when possible and the eyelids should be gently taped closed to avoid corneal abrasions. Limitations of range of motion involving the neck or extremities should be noted before patient positioning, and movement after induction of anesthesia should not involve motion beyond these limits. The risk of injury to the skin can be minimized by accounting for the ECG leads, catheter connectors, or three-way stopcocks and jewelry that may be in contact with the skin of the patient. In addition, the patient's skin should not be directly exposed to metal.

III. Anesthetic plan for aortic surgery. The determinants of safe anesthesia for aortic surgery (endovascular or open) include careful control of the patient's blood pressure, intravascular volume, and myocardial performance within context of the patient's baseline cardiac risk. As these patients commonly have coronary artery disease, tachycardia, anemia, or extremes of blood pressure can result in myocardial ischemia and perioperative myocardial infarction. Therefore, the anesthesia team must be aware of the stages of the operation and their hemodynamic consequences. The surgeon must be aware of specific organ system performance during the operation (e.g., tachycardia or oliguria), as this provides insight into the management of these systems in the postoperative period. Some of the most useful information regarding the patient's physiologic responses can be obtained during the operation. Furthermore, the surgeon must understand how the anesthesia team manages the patient during critical parts of the operation and be willing to contribute information that he or she deems important.

Anesthesia for aortic surgery may consist of a **regional technique (e.g., epidural or spinal), a mixed regional and general technique, or a general anesthetic technique**. The selection of anesthetic is of course influenced by type of aortic surgery—open or endovascular. All open aortic cases require a general anesthetic, which can be performed as the sole method or augmented by addition an epidural. Endovascular aneurysm repair (EVAR) can be performed under an epidural anesthetic alone, although some surgeons prefer general anesthesia in these cases to allow for more direct control of the patients respiratory status. Local anesthesia and conscious sedation is used for percutaneous aortic interventions and has even been described as feasible for certain EVARs in patients in whom the risk of general and regional anesthetic was prohibitive.

The mixed technique is most common with open aortic cases and consists of continuous epidural anesthesia with a mixture of local anesthetics (e.g., bupivacaine) and narcotics (e.g., fentanyl) supplemented with general anesthesia and intubation. Epidural catheters are safe in vascular patients and can be used even in patients who will be heparinized as part of the procedure but only after the epidural catheter has been placed. In these cases, the heparin is held for several hours before and after the time of catheter removal to reduce the incidence of epidural or subdural hematomas. These complications are rare, especially in instances where an atraumatic puncture and placement of the catheter were made at the initiation of the anesthetic.

It is important to remember that epidural anesthesia with local anesthetics may cause peripheral vasodilation and reduced blood pressure, requiring volume or even vasopressors in rare instances. The use of a mix of narcotics and local anesthetics or just narcotics for the epidural in such cases usually alleviates this sometimes challenging response. The authors have also found that a continuous epidural narcotic infusion is a safe and effective method of controlling postoperative pain for 48 to 72 hours after open abdominal or lower-extremity operations. General endotracheal anesthesia may offer the greatest control of the hemodynamics and respiratory system for patients with significant pulmonary and cardiac disease. Although balanced general anesthesia with nitrous oxide, narcotics, relaxants, and barbiturates provides excellent operative conditions, a small amount of an inhalation agent or an intravenous vasodilator frequently is required to manage hypertension.

A. Unexplained hypotension during aortic surgery (open or endovascular) must be met with a calm but rapid assessment of the patient for possible causes.

    1. Palpation of the aorta or transduction of femoral sheath pressures should be performed to confirm what the anesthesia monitors indicate. If there is a strong aortic pulse or normal pressures transduced through the femoral access sheaths, attention should be focused on the monitoring systems (e.g., compression or occlusion of the arterial line).

    2. Bleeding from endovascular access vessel can occur during placement of device sheaths through the iliac vessels and even the aortic bifurcation. The diagnosis of iliac or aortic perforation can be accomplished by performing flush aortography or retrograde angiography through the femoral sheaths. If there is a high suspicion that perforation of an access vessel is responsible for hypotension, a large compliant balloon and covered stent should be quickly readied on the back table as the diagnostic maneuvers are performed.

    3. Myocardial infarction or arrhythmia should be indicated by findings on ECG or TEE.

    4. Tension pneumothorax resulting from preoperative central venous line placement will be accompanied by distended neck veins and high airway pressures.

5. **Cardiac tamponade** from right atrial injury during preoperative line placement will also be accompanied by distended neck veins but more normal airway pressures initially.

6. **Malignant hyperthermia** is a rare but serious complication accompanied by increases in end-tidal CO_2 and in the patient's core temperature.

7. **Manipulation or withdrawal of the intestines** from the abdomen during open aortic surgery may also cause hypotension, which usually can be corrected with a fluid bolus or a one-time dose of ephedrine or a phenylephrine.

8. **Blood pressure may also decrease when the inferior vena cava is compressed or retracted** secondary to decreased venous return to the heart (preload); the surgeon should inform the anesthesia team prior to performing this maneuver.

B. **One of the most stressful steps for the myocardium** during open aortic operations is placement of the **aortic cross-clamp**, which acutely increases after load. Blood pressure and pulmonary capillary wedge pressures also increase and ST-segment changes or ventricular irritability may be seen on the ECG monitor. The healthy heart can tolerate these changes fairly well; however, the impaired heart is at a higher risk. In the case of a severely impaired heart, the blood pressure and cardiac output may actually decrease with placement of the aortic cross clamp. In such cases and in an apparent paradoxical step, titration of peripheral vasodilators is necessary to reduce after load acutely. Inotropic support should also be added if necessary to stabilize the hemodynamics in these instances. For these reasons, it is imperative that the surgeon and anesthesia team communicate regarding timing and position of the aortic cross-clamp and its release.

With placement of the aortic cross-clamp, renal cortical blood flow and urine output may decrease even if the clamp is below the renal arteries. This effect can usually be prevented by establishing a diuresis before the cross-clamp with hydration and mannitol (12.5 to 25.0 g intravenously). The preoperative central venous or pulmonary wedge pressure and left ventricular function must confirm that the patient is adequately hydrated prior to initiating a diuresis. If mannitol is not effective, 10 to 20 mg of furosemide (Lasix, Hoechst Marion Roussel, Kansas City, MO, U.S.A.) may also be given, although this decision should be well communicated between the surgical and anesthesia teams. During any diuresis, potassium must be carefully monitored and supplemented to prevent serious arrhythmias that result from hypokalemia.

C. **Blood loss**

1. **Significant blood loss** may occur during open aortic operations when the aneurysm sac is opened, as back-bleeding from lumbar arteries and the inferior mesenteric artery can be brisk. Here again, the anesthesia team should made aware of this operative maneuver so they may anticipate the need for increased volume resuscitation while these vessels are oversewn.

2. **Blood loss can be substantial** enough during open aortic cases to require transfusion. The alternative to

banked blood transfusion is **autotransfusion**, which can be accomplished by use of the cell saver device set up at the beginning of the case. Dilutional coagulopathy may occur after 4–6 units of blood are transfused and platelets and clotting factors must be given to the patient in this scenario. The use of the **thromboelastogram (TEG)** can also provide a qualitative analysis of the ability of the blood to clot, which can be used to guide specific factor replacement. Empiric transfusion of blood products in anticipation of aortic clamp removal can be performed but should be carefully considered. Fresh plasma and platelets may be especially important when the graft is opened, as any coagulopathy may result in problematic anastomotic or retroperitoneal bleeding. The threshold hemoglobin level to begin transfusion should be determined on a patient-by-patient basis depending upon the severity of underlying disease and type of operation performed. **The surgeon and anesthesia team should communicate openly about the transfusion of blood and blood products.**

D. Fluid replacement. Throughout the aortic procedure, adequate amounts of fluid, usually crystalloids such as normal saline or Ringer's lactate, must be given continuously. Fluid replacement should be guided by indices of ventricular filling, maintenance of a good cardiac index, and adequate urine output (at least 0.5 cc/kg/h). It is not uncommon for crystalloid to be administered at rates up to 750 to 1,000 mL/h during open aortic procedures due to evaporative fluid loss from exposed bowel and associated blood loss. Because patients are prone to becoming hypothermic during long open operations, crystalloids and blood products should be warmed as they are infused. In addition, we attempt to prevent hypothermia during such cases by using an upper-body heating tent (Bair Hugger) and by warming the operating room.

E. One of the most critical times of an open aortic operation is release of the aortic clamp. This maneuver decreases after load and profound hypotension can occur. The surgeon should prepare the anesthesia team several minutes before unclamping and the clamp should be released slowly while the surgeon views the arterial blood pressure tracing. If significant hypotension occurs, the clamp can be partially or completely reapplied while resuscitation is achieved. Hypotension can be minimized by intravascular volume loading, avoidance of myocardial depressants, and vasodilators, as well as inhalation agents prior to clamp release. Occasionally, small amounts of sodium bicarbonate will be beneficial; the authors generally give intravenous calcium chloride, which increases myocardial contractility and blood pressure. **If one reverses heparin with protamine at the end of the operation, it must be administered slowly (e.g., use an initial test dose), as it can cause hypotension or bradycardia.** In rare cases, protamine may lead to severe bronchospasm and hemodynamic instability.

IV. Carotid artery surgery. Anesthesia for carotid artery interventions (open or endovascular) must be administered carefully to avoid swings in blood pressure and cerebral perfusion. Additionally, it is necessary to avoid oversedation in cases where patients need to be awake for neurologic assessment. In addition to **general anesthesia** for carotid interventions, options include **cervical block** for awake, open carotid operations and simple **local anesthetic with mild sedation** for carotid artery stenting (CAS).

The common clinical concern during any carotid intervention is cerebral perfusion and neurologic evaluation in the cases where the patient may be awake. During both awake, open carotid operations and CAS, it is important for the patient to be communicative and directable to assess neurologic status as a marker of adequate cerebral perfusion. Too much sedation during these cases can result in the inability to determine whether the patient's decreased neurologic status is due to the anesthetic or the carotid intervention. During carotid interventions, the surgeon must understand basic control mechanisms for cerebral blood flow, methods of monitoring cerebral perfusion, and the effects of different anesthetic agents on cerebral metabolism.

A. Cerebral blood flow. There are four major determinants of cerebral blood flow in the normal brain.

    1. Local metabolic factors. Accumulation of local metabolic products causes vasodilation of blood vessels as part of normal autoregulation and increased local intracerebral flow.

    2. Arterial oxygen tension (P_aO_2). Within wide limits, P_aO_2 does not significantly influence cerebral blood flow.

    3. Arterial carbon dioxide tension (P_aCO_2) affects cerebral blood flow throughout its physiologic range. As P_aCO_2 is decreased, cerebral blood flow decreases, and vice versa.

    4. Cerebral perfusion pressure (mean arterial pressure minus intracranial pressure or venous pressure). Within wide ranges of perfusion pressure, cerebral blood flow is maintained in a steady state by autoregulation.

    In diseased states, these control mechanisms are altered. Autoregulation is altered so that the acceptable mean arterial pressure is different and the point at which autoregulation becomes lost is also altered. Blood vessels in an ischemic brain are maximally vasodilated and therefore blood flow becomes a direct function of perfusion pressure (i.e., mean arterial pressure). During carotid clamping, normotension to slight hypertension should optimize cerebral perfusion via collateral routes including the contralateral carotid and vertebral arteries.

B. Monitoring. There are at least three methods to assess adequate cerebral perfusion during carotid cross-clamping or occlusion:

1. Awake patient who has no neurologic changes with carotid occlusion
2. Normal electroencephalogram (EEG) that does not change with carotid occlusion
3. Measurement of carotid artery stump pressures as a reflection of cerebral perfusion

These methods as well as the indications for use of a temporary vascular shunt during open carotid endarterectomy are described in greater detail in Chapter 11.

C. Types of anesthesia and anesthetic agents. The goals of anesthesia for carotid surgery include maintenance of a consistent blood pressure, regulation of the patient's P_aCO_2 to maximize blood flow to ischemic brain, and rapid emergence from general anesthesia for neurologic examination in the operating room. **General anesthesia** during open carotid operations is preferred by some surgeons and may afford more direct control of the patient's blood pressure and the patient's airway and therefore ventilatory status. General anesthesia is also advocated by some in a teaching setting, where the length of the case may be slightly increased and instructional comments are made more openly. One of the most common general anesthetic techniques for carotid surgery is **balanced anesthesia** of barbiturates, nitrous oxide, narcotics, and muscle relaxants. Volatile agents and barbiturates may offer some protection against ischemia because cerebral oxygen demand is reduced.

In contrast, many surgeons prefer **local or regional anesthesia** for awake, open carotid operations as a safe technique that allows immediate detection of neurologic change when the carotid artery is clamped. This technique avoids the potential cardiodepressant effects of general anesthesia and may afford patients a quicker recovery. Regardless of whether one prefers general or regional anesthesia, safe results can be achieved. In the authors' opinion, the choice lies with the experience and judgment of the surgeon and the anesthesia team.

Volatile anesthetics are generally considered cerebral vasodilators, with halothane being the most potent and isoflurane the least. In contrast, most of the intravenous anesthetic agents are cerebral vasoconstrictors. The effects that these agents have on the abnormal cerebral vasculature is variable and, as a result, the impact of one anesthetic choice versus another is less important than a normal to slightly elevated **blood pressure** in maintaining cerebral perfusion. The ability of either volatile or intravenous agents to suppress metabolism and provide cerebral protection occurs only at anesthetic depths that could impair hemodynamic stability. Halothane can cause hypotension and myocardial depression. Deep anesthesia with a volatile agent such as halothane may also increase intracranial pressure and promote intracerebral blood flow steal from ischemic areas. Prevention of ischemia with direct augmentation of cerebral perfusion either by supporting the mean arterial pressure or placement of a temporary vascular shunt is almost certainly more beneficial than any attempt with anesthetics to prolong the brain's tolerance to ischemia.

V. Lower-extremity arterial reconstructions. Lower-extremity arterial reconstructions can be performed using either **general anesthesia** or **regional anesthesia** alone, or **mixed general and regional anesthesia**. Simple **local anesthesia with sedation** may also be used for percutaneous lower-extremity interventions. The choice depends upon on whether the case is open or endovascular, patient comorbidities, and anesthesia and surgeon experience and preference. In our experience, continuous epidural anesthesia is an excellent method for open femoral popliteal bypass grafting, including instances of a concomitant retrograde iliac stent placement (i.e., hybrid open and endovascular procedure). In the early postoperative period, the epidural catheter is left in place for additional pain relief or for reoperation if early graft thrombosis occurs. In addition to excellent pain relief, the fact that epidurals infused with local anesthetic cause lower-extremity vasodilation is proposed by some to provide additional circulatory benefits in these cases.

The indication and appropriateness of a regional technique should be decided by the anesthesia team in consultation with the vascular providers. The surgeon should give appropriate input on the choice of a regional anesthetic and any potential ramifications, and patient acceptance of a regional anesthetic as well as its safety must be considered. Many factors may reduce the advisability of a regional technique, such as dementia, risk of pulmonary aspiration, or previous back or spine injury. Prolonged sedation is often required in many of these lower-extremity arterial reconstructions. In addition, some patients may have cardiovascular conditions that may disqualify them for regional anesthesia because of venous and arterial dilation (e.g., hypertrophic cardiomyopathy or severe aortic stenosis).

The use of regional anesthesia in patients requiring anticoagulation or antiplatelet therapy remains controversial, and decisions are often made on an individual patient basis. Although most studies reveal very low complication rates of epidural anesthesia placed in association with antiplatelet therapy or low molecular weight heparin, the risk is not zero. Because bleeding complications in this setting are so significant, the authors defer to their anesthesia colleagues on a case-by-case basis as to which patients are candidates for epidural anesthesia. Furthermore, once the epidural catheter is in place, this same expertise is necessary with regard to the need to hold these same medications (antiplatelet and/or heparin) before and around the time of catheter removal.

Anesthesia for acute lower-extremity ischemia, such as in the instance of an arterial embolism, is often complicated, as these cases tend to occur in critically ill patients at high risk for general anesthesia. If necessary, exposure of the femoral artery and performance of a thromboembolectomy can be accomplished using local anesthesia. However, general anesthesia is preferred for most cases of acute lower-extremity ischemia because they invariably take a longer time period than anticipated. This is especially the case because operative arteriograms, arterial bypasses, or fasciotomies are frequently necessary as part of operating on acute lower extremity ischemia.

VI. Lower-extremity venous procedures. Lower-extremity venous cases may be performed using a general, regional, or simple local anesthesia, depending upon the planned procedure. Local anesthesia with or without an oral or intravenous anxiolytic such as diazepam is all that is necessary to perform basic endovenous ablation of the saphenous vein with laser or radiofrequency. In the authors' experience, even most open venous operations, such as stab phlebectomy and high ligation and removal of the saphenous vein, can be accomplished with local anesthesia and intravenous conscious sedation. Here again, communication is essential with the anesthesia provider, who is able to optimally time the dose of pain and amnestic medications with the removal or "stripping" of the vein. Careful consideration and performance of the procedure can avoid the need and therefore the small risk associated with epidural or spinal anesthesia in many of these cases. Certainly patient, surgeon, and anesthesia experience and preference play a large part in the decision as to which anesthetic type is optimal in these situations.

SELECTED READING

Brewster DC, O'Hara PJ, Darling RC, et al. Relationship of intraoperative EEG monitoring and stump pressure measurements during carotid endarterectomy. *Circulation.* 1980;62(Suppl 1):I4-I7.

Bush HL Jr, Hydo LJ, Fischer E, et al. Hypothermia during elective abdominal aortic aneurysm repair: the high price of avoidable morbidity. *J Vasc Surg.* 1995;21:392-402.

Clagett GP, Valentine RJ, Jackson MR, et al. A randomized trial of intraoperative autotransfusion during aortic surgery. *J Vasc Surg.* 1999;29:22-31.

Cullen ML, Staren ML, el-Ganzouri A, et al. Continuous epidural infusion for analgesia after major abdominal operations: a randomized, prospective, double blind study. *Surgery.* 1985;98: 718-728.

Ereth MH, Oliver WC Jr, Santrach PJ. Perioperative interventions to decrease transfusion of allogeneic blood products. *Mayo Clin Proc.* 1994;69:575-586.

Frank SM, Fleisher LA, Breslow MJ, et al. Perioperative maintenance of normothermia reduces the incidence of morbid cardiac events. A randomized clinical trial. *JAMA.* 1997;277:1127-1134.

Makary MA, Mukherjee BA, Sexton JB, et al. Operating room briefings and wrong-site surgery. *J Am Col Surg.* 2007;204(2):236-243.

Mangano DT, Layug EL, Wallace A, et al. Effect of Atenolol on mortality and cardiovascular morbidity after noncardiac surgery. *N Engl J Med.* 1996;335:1713-1720.

Mannucci PM. Hemostatic drugs. *N Engl J Med.* 1998;339:245-253.

Valentine RJ, Duke ML, Inman MH, et al. Effectiveness of pulmonary artery catheters in aortic surgery: a randomized trial. *J Vasc Surg.* 1998;27:203-212.

Wiklund RA, Rosenbaum SH. Anesthesiology. First of two parts. *N Engl J Med.* 1997;337:1132-1141.

Wiklund RA, Rosenbaum SH. Anesthesiology. Second of two parts. *N Engl J Med.* 1997;337:1215-1219.

Youngberg JA, Lake CL, Roizen MF, et al., eds. *Cardiac, Vascular and Tthoracic Anesthesia.* Philadelphia: Churchill Livingstone, 2000.

Catheter-Based and Endovascular Concepts

CHAPTER 10

Indications and Preparation for Angiography

Angiography is the direct intravascular administration of radiographically visible dye in order to gain anatomic information about a particular blood vessel or group of blood vessels. **Arteriography** is defined as angiography of the arterial system, and **venography** is angiographic imaging of the veins. Historically, angiography has mostly served a diagnostic purpose, providing a road map to guide appropriate surgical intervention. The past two decades, however, have witnessed considerable growth in minimally invasive techniques to treat disease and injury from within the vessel lumen—the so-called **endovascular procedures**. As many of these procedures are performed using small wires and catheters, another commonly used term is **catheter-based procedures**. Common endovascular procedures are angioplasty, stenting, stent-graft repair of aneurysms, embolization, and catheter-directed thrombolysis. A number of vascular specialists are trained in angiography and endovascular procedures, from the disciplines of interventional radiology, cardiology, and vascular surgery. Perhaps a more encompassing term for a physician performing endovascular procedures is the "**vascular interventionalist**" or "**endovascular specialist.**"

I. Indications. Nearly every vessel in the human body can be imaged with angiography by a motivated and skilled vascular interventionalist. However, the indications for angiography are just as important as the skills required to perform it. Even the simplest angiographic procedures carry risk to the vessel(s) being imaged and to the patient as a whole. Therefore *angiography should not be undertaken without clear and appropriate indications*. History, physical exam, and noninvasive tests are nearly always sufficient to make the diagnosis of peripheral arterial disease (PAD). The specific indications for lower-extremity, cerebrovascular, and renal and mesenteric arteriography are discussed in detail in their respective chapters. In general, angiography should only be employed **when the additional anatomic information will clearly affect the sound clinical management of the patient.**

Informed consent for angiography includes an explanation of the indications, alternative methods of diagnosis, and potential complications. Patients should understand that angiography can be either diagnostic or therapeutic and that, in general, solely diagnostic angiograms are becoming less common given the imaging capability of noninvasive modalities (duplex, computed tomography angiogram [CTA], and **magnetic resonance arteriography** [MRA]). Additionally, endovascular treatments are often possible in the same setting as the diagnostic angiogram following the diagnostic phase. The vascular interventionalist may plan a solely diagnostic angiogram under certain circumstances, such as determining suitability for complex endovascular interventions such as carotid stenting or aortic endografting. Angiography is the best test for the rapid diagnosis of some specific vascular emergencies, such as acute mesenteric or limb ischemia and can also help solve certain diagnostic dilemmas—for example, vasospastic disorders versus occlusive disease of the hands, Buerger's disease, temporal arteritis, and periarteritis nodosa.

The objective and potential outcomes of the angiogram should be understood from the outset and explained to the patient. The patient should understand that attempts at diagnosing and/or treating the condition with noninvasive modalities have been exhausted and that angiography is necessary for clinical decision making. We inform patients undergoing a lower-extremity arteriogram for chronic limb ischemia of three possible outcomes of the procedure:

1. Diagnostic information leading to an endovascular therapy at that setting or at a later date
2. Diagnostic information leading to an open treatment at a later date
3. Diagnostic information leading to no intervention due to disease pattern or severity

The decision to proceed with endovascular or surgical treatment depends on the patient's anatomy, medical comorbidities, and clinical presentation. In many cases, either endovascular or open surgical therapy may be appropriate. It is important that the patient be presented with **balanced and realistic expectations** about any procedure, its durability, the need for future interventions, and potential complications.

Endovascular procedures are attractive to both patients and clinicians. As an example, endovascular aortic aneurysm repair has reduced mortality and morbidity compared with open aneurysm repair, and has allowed treatment in patients who would not be suitable for open repair (Chapter 15). However, the dizzying angiographic success and rapid recovery that patients often experience with endovascular procedures should be viewed in the context of evidence supporting longer term outcomes both of the procedure and the patient (i.e., will they last and will the patient have good mid- to long-term survival?). Vascular specialists should be cautious not to lower the threshold for the treatment of vascular diseases simply because of the availability of endovascular techniques. The potential benefits of intervention should be tempered with an understanding of the natural history of the disease and life expectancy of the patient. The majority of patients with claudication, for example, can be treated medically and will experience no worsening in their disease.

Treatment, whether endovascular or surgical, should be limited to the minority of patients with progressive, lifestyle-limiting claudication.

II. Preparation.

A. Prior to angiography, the endovascular specialist should **review the patient's history, lab work, and indications for the procedure**. The informed consent forms are also reviewed and the patient should have the opportunity to ask "last minute" questions.

B. An **abbreviated physical exam** should be performed just prior to the procedure to confirm previous findings and assure no interval change.

1. An evaluation of the planned **access vessel** is critical in the pre-procedure holding area. The absence of or change in a pulse should prompt reconsideration of the access site except in cases of access distal to known disease that is the target of intervention (e.g., femoral access distal to iliac disease that is target of intervention).

2. Distal pulses or Doppler signals should be confirmed prior to lower-extremity angiography and ABIs recorded if an intervention is likely. The absence of a pulse or Doppler signal after intervention implies embolization, vessel dissection, or poor technical result. Ankle-brachial indices should be recorded after any lower-extremity endovascular intervention and compared with pre-procedure values.

3. Newly recognized or poorly treated medical conditions such as severe hypertension, arrhythmia, or renal insufficiency generally contraindicate angiography.

4. Patients with foot ulcers or gangrene should have their wounds reassessed, as they may benefit from debridement prior to or just following the endovascular procedure.

C. Previous open surgical or endovascular procedures are particularly relevant and should be reviewed as part of this pre-procedure routine. Vessels that have been accessed multiple times in the past or the presence of an extremity bypass may affect the location and method of access for angiography. For example, previous aortobifemoral bypass will present specific challenges related to scar and number of patent lumens at the femoral level (e.g., prosthetic bypass limb and native femoral/iliac lumen). In this same scenario the bypass graft presents a narrow bifurcation at the aortic position that generally prevents placement of a sheath into the contralateral limb of the graft. The locations of prior endovascular interventions, along with balloon and/or stent sizes, and complications from prior procedures should be recorded, noting access problems.

D. Allergy to iodinated contrast material should be ascertained and can occur in 2–5% of patients. These reactions are usually mild, with itching and urticaria. Rarely, more severe anaphylactic reactions occur, manifested by wheezing, bradycardia, and hypotension. Patients with prior contrast reactions are at higher risk for recurrent allergic complications with repeat angiography. Although the benefits of some type of pretreatment in this high-risk group are controversial, it is generally recommend that a "prep" consisting of steroids and diphenhydramine (Benadryl, Johnson and Johnson, New Brunswick, NJ, U.S.A.) be administered prior to the angiogram. One such regimen includes 50 mg of prednisone by mouth 13, 7, and then 1 hour prior to the procedure. A single dose of 25 to 50 mg of diphenhydramine may also be given 1 hour prior to the administration of contrast. When an urgent angiogram or CTA is obtained, an emergency prep can be administered with 50 mg diphenhydramine intravenously and 100 mg hydrocortisone intravenously.

E. The patient should be questioned as to his or her **current medications.**

1. Care must be exercised in the use of iodinated contrast in patients taking **metformin** (Glucophage, Bristol-Myers Squibb, New York, NY, U.S.A.). This oral agent used to treat non–insulin-dependent diabetes mellitus can cause a severe lactic acidosis that can be precipitated by contrast agents. The risk is especially high in patients with renal dysfunction. In general, patients should not take metformin for 48 to 72 hours after the use of iodinated contrast agents. This is especially true in patients who have a baseline creatinine of greater than 1.5 mg/dL.

2. Anticoagulants such as warfarin should be stopped before procedures that involve arterial access. This usually means stopping warfarin for 2 to 4 days and allowing the international normalized ratio to fall below 1.5. Of course, the indications for anticoagulation must be noted because some patients, such as those with mechanical heart valves or known pulmonary emboli, should not be off of anticoagulation. A heparin "window" can be used in patients at high risk for stopping anticoagulation. The patient is kept fully anticoagulated on intravenous unfractionated heparin (UFH) while the warfarin is held. UFH has a short half-life (90 minutes) compared to warfarin (36 hours), so that it can be held for several hours prior to and after the angiogram. The development of low molecular weight heparins now allows a number of patients at moderate risk for holding anticoagulation to "bridge" at home with subcutaneous injections. **Antiplatelet agents** such as aspirin and/or clopidogrel (Plavix) are commonly taken by patients with peripheral vascular disease. Some interventionalists insist these drugs are held prior to angiography, while others do not. Prior to some interventions such as carotid or renal stenting, many physicians ensure that antiplatelet agents are "on board" or even administer high doses on the day of the procedure. There is no consensus on the use of antiplatelet agents and angiography. At present, each case must be assessed individually, balancing the risk of bleeding with thrombosis. Patients with a personal or family history of **bleeding problems** should be carefully evaluated with a platelet count and coagulation studies (prothrombin time and partial prothrombin time). A hematology consultation should be sought if heritable bleeding disorder is suspected.

F. Renal function is assessed by measuring serum creatinine and blood urea nitrogen. Contrast material can be nephrotoxic, especially in the elderly, patients who are dehydrated, those with diabetes, and in patients with renal insufficiency. **Adequate urine output** (0.5 mL/kg/h) should be established in these patients prior to contrast angiography by intravenous hydration, and the administration of bicarbonate may reduce the risk of contrast nephropathy. For those patients with a creatinine greater than 1.5, the authors administer a mixture of three ampules of **sodium bicarbonate** (8.4%, 50 mL) added to dextrose 5% in water at a rate of 3 cc/kg/hr for the hour prior to the angiogram and 1 cc/kg/hr during and for 6 hours after the procedure. The use of **acetylcysteine** (Mucomyst, Bristol-Myers Squibb, New York, NY, U.S.A.) to prevent contrast nephropathy has been extensively studied. Although consistent evidence of its benefit is lacking, acetylcysteine's use is relatively innocuous when prescribed as an oral regimen of 600 mg orally twice daily for the day prior to and of the procedure.

G. Skin preparation of the access or puncture site should include cleansing with an antiseptic soap such as chlorhexidine or povidone-iodine. In the case of femoral access, both groins should be prepped.

H. Pre-procedural antibiotics are not necessary for routine angiography. However, antibiotics may be beneficial prior to implanting a permanent intravascular stent or if the access site must be a prosthetic graft.

III. Risks. The main risks of angiography are hemorrhage from the access site; allergic reactions to the contrast material; thrombosis of the punctured vessel; and embolization of a clot from the catheter, air, or atheromatous material. In experienced hands, these complications occur in about 1% of all cases. Mortality is less frequent (0.05%) but is a definite risk that the patient must understand.

IV. Selection of access vessel. Every endovascular procedure begins with intravascular access. Although percutaneous vascular access is usually straightforward, this most basic technique can also be quite foreboding. The most frequent complications of angiography occur at the access site (2–4%) and include hematoma, pseudoaneurysm, and arteriovenous fistula. Careful selection of the access vessel is critical to the safety and success of the angiogram. The most commonly selected vessels for arteriography are the femoral and brachial arteries.

A. The common femoral artery is accessible and large enough to accommodate sizeable sheaths. The primary disadvantage of femoral access includes the risk of retroperitoneal hemorrhage, which can occur with an inadvertent high puncture and access into the external iliac artery. In contrast, low puncture or access into the superficial femoral artery increases the risk of pseudoaneurysm, vessel dissection, and thrombosis.

The technique of femoral artery access requires careful attention to specific anatomic landmarks, including those on the patient's skin and one key landmark identified by fluoroscopy. The optimal site for access into the common femoral artery is just below the inguinal ligament at the level of the femoral head. At this level the **femoral artery courses over the medial one-third of the femoral head** (Fig. 10.1) and access at this location improves the effectiveness of manual compression of the vessel when the access sheath is removed following the procedure. Fluoroscopic confirmation of

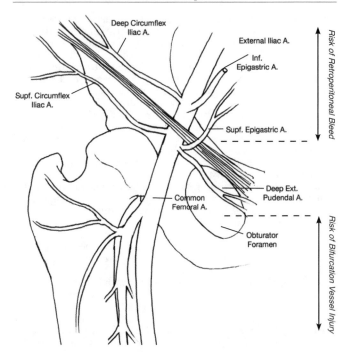

Figure 10.1. Bony landmarks are useful for identifying the level of the common femoral artery. The inguinal ligament runs between the pubic tubercle and the anterior superior iliac spine, marking the top of the common femoral artery. High puncture or laceration of the inferior epigastric artery can lead to serious retroperitoneal bleeding. Puncture at or below the femoral bifurcation is also to be avoided.

this location is simple and important to avoid misadventures associated with punctures based solely on the inguinal skin crease, which is often misleading. A line between the anterior superior iliac spine and the pubic tubercle marks the inguinal ligament, and by using a hemostat placed at the planned puncture site and fluoroscopy, one can confirm that the access is over the femoral head. This technique is particularly helpful in obese patients in whom the skin landmarks are distorted as well as in patients with diminished pulses.

B. Arterial access can be accomplished in a **retrograde** or **antegrade** manner and consideration of these options should be made prior to attempting to enter the vessel. **Retrograde arterial puncture** refers to the needle being placed opposite the direction of blood flow. For lower-extremity arterial disease, the femoral artery opposite the more symptomatic leg is often selected for retrograde puncture. This allows for a full aortogram and runoff or imaging of the most symptomatic lower extremity without interference from the femoral access sheath.

Access via the contralateral femoral artery also offers working room if needed, to treat the symptomatic leg by going "up and over" the aortic bifurcation. An **antegrade stick of the femoral artery** is placed heading with the direction of blood flow down the lower extremity and allows for a focused unilateral arteriogram. The antegrade approach provides a more supportive platform when treating severe disease or total occlusions of the distal femoral, popliteal, and infrapopliteal arterial segments. Antegrade access generally requires more precision to allow access of the femoral artery in its most proximal segment away from the femoral bifurcation and profunda femorus artery. Even with accurate access, directing the wire into the superficial but not the deep femoral artery can be challenging, because of limited working room between the entry site and the femoral bifurcation. Because of these technical challenges, antegrade femoral access has a slightly higher risk of access site complications compared with the more standard retrograde access.

C. Brachial artery access may be selected in patients with poor femoral pulses or with other compelling reasons to avoid access in the groin, such as the presence of a bypass graft. Additionally, downward-sloping vessels such as those of the mesentery are often easier to catheterize with selecting wires brought from above, a configuration which is afforded by brachial access. The portion of the brachial artery just above the antecubital crease is superficial and suitable for access. **Access through the left brachial artery is preferable to the right** because it avoids traversing the origins of the common carotid arteries with wires and possibly sheaths. Right-sided brachial access requires crossing both common carotids with these devices and therefore harbors a small risk of stroke from embolization of atheromatous plaque or debris. The smaller size of the brachial artery makes access more technically challenging, and accurate entry into the brachial artery may be facilitated with an ultrasound guided puncture. The brachial artery can rarely accommodate larger than a 6 Fr sheath, which may curtail procedures requiring larger devices unless an open exposure of the artery is performed to allow direct repair after removal of a larger sheath. Lower-extremity interventions cannot usually be performed from a brachial approach due to the limited length of commercially available endovascular devices. The location of the brachial artery and its proximity to the median nerve in a small fixed space or sheath in the arm necessitates good hemostasis following access sheath removal. In contrast to femoral access hematomas, which are most often managed without surgery, even a small hematoma over the brachial artery can result in median nerve compression, requiring operative intervention.

V. Methods.

A. Pain or discomfort associated with angiography is usually minimal and transient. Such discomfort is related to vessel puncture, sheath placement, and contrast injection. Occasionally, the use of balloon angioplasty and/or stents may result in visceral pain if the vessel wall is stretched significantly. Pain accompanying contrast injection has been markedly reduced with the use of **iso-osmolar or only**

slightly hyperosmolar contrast agents. If an older hyper-   AQ4
osmolar contrast agent is used, the patient may experience an
intense hot or burning pain that lasts seconds but is remark-
ably uncomfortable. In general, the authors manage the
patient's pain and anxiety with the oral administration of a
short-acting benzodiazepine or use of an intravenous dose of a
short-acting narcotic such as fentanyl and rarely resort to an
intravenous sedative such as propofol (Diprivan, AstraZeneca,
Wilmington, DE, U.S.A.). Local anesthetic is used around
the puncture site and in most cases is all that is required.
Transient visceral pain with balloon angioplasty or stenting is
mediated by adventitial receptors and indicates vessel stretch;
severe or persistent pain suggests rupture or impending perforation of the vessel.

B. A variety of **nonionic contrast agents** are used today,
which are much improved over older ionic contrast agents.
Many of these nonionic agents are iso-osmolar or only slightly
hyperosmolar, which represents the greatest improvement
over older agents, which were extremely hyperosmolar and
painful during injection. Excreted by the kidneys, contrast
agents can induce acute renal dysfunction in patients with or
without pre-existing renal insufficiency. However, individuals
with known renal failure, proteinuria, diabetes mellitus, and
dehydration are at higher risk. Postangiographic renal dysfunction peaks at 48 hours and can be minimized by intravenous hydration, limited contrast loads, and, rarely, mannitol
infusion. Contrast-induced nephropathy is usually transient
and improves within a week's time.

C. The modified Seldinger technique is used to obtain
access to the vessel (Fig. 10.2) and entails puncture of the
anterior wall of the vessel with a hollow, beveled needle. Once
pulsatile flow is confirmed, a guidewire (e.g., floppy J-wire) is
advanced into the artery. The needle is withdrawn while manual pressure is held over the entry site to prevent bleeding. A
sheath that contains a soft, tapered inner dilator is then
placed over the wire into the lumen and the inner dilator
removed. **The sheath acts as a working port within the
vessel, through which catheter and wire exchanges can
be made with minimal bleeding or trauma to the vessel
wall**. The smallest sheath that can effectively accomplish the
goals of the angiogram should be selected to minimize access
site complications. If initial passage of the wire into of the
artery is impeded, the needle may not be completely within
the lumen, in a side branch of the artery, or up against a piece
of plaque. Advancing the wire under these circumstances can
cause damage, and any resistance to wire advancement should
lead to examination under fluoroscopy to avoid coiling of the
wire, which can be seen with extraluminal placement or dissection. In these cases, the wire is removed and the arterial
back-bleeding again confirmed. The endovascular specialist
may try to angle the bevel of the needle in a different direction
or withdraw the tip slightly, in an effort to enter the true
lumen and then reinsert the wire under fluoroscopic guidance,
looking for resistance free placement. In instances where
blood flows freely from the needle but the wire will not pass, a
small contrast injection under fluoroscopy may help identify

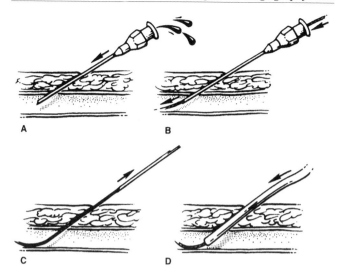

Figure 10.2.   Modified Seldinger technique for percutaneous angiography. (A) Introductory needle is passed into femoral or brachial artery. **(B)** Smaller flexible guidewire is passed through the introductory needle into the artery. **(C)** Introductory needle is withdrawn over the guidewire, which is left in the artery. **(D)** Larger flexible angiographic sheath or catheter is passed over the smaller guidewire into the artery.

the problem. Failure of these simple maneuvers should prompt withdrawal of the needle, manual pressure, and a new puncture.

The classic Seldinger technique is worth mentioning and involves not only puncture of the anterior vessel wall but also the back wall of the artery as well (**double puncture technique**). With this technique the needle is withdrawn until a flash of pulsatile blood confirms intraluminal placement. The double puncture technique is best avoided by those with limited experience, as it is technically more challenging and bleeding from the posterior wall puncture into the femoral sheath or even retroperitoneum can be a problem.

Difficult arterial access may also be due to poor pulsation or large body habitus. In these situations, bony landmarks in relation to the chosen access location are especially helpful and should be evaluated using fluoroscopy. In more difficult cases, the endovascular specialist may wear a lead glove and attempt to access the artery under real time fluoroscopy. Doppler or duplex ultrasound can also be used as an adjunct to locate the vessels (e.g., ultrasound-guided access). The SmartNeedle (Escalon Medical Corp, Wayne, Pennsylvania, U.S.A.) has a built-in Doppler probe and can also be used for difficult access scenarios. Calcium deposits in the femoral and iliac arteries may actually form a cast of the vessel that can also be used as a guide to the vessel using fluoroscopy. If a catheter-based intervention mandates femoral access, one last option is to perform a preliminary or marking arteriogram via the brachial artery in order to identify the position of the femoral arteries in groin to guide the puncture location.

VI. Venography.

A. Diagnostic venography of the extremities typically consists of two parts, **ascending and descending**, and may also be referred to as **phlebography**. This two-staged exam allows for study of venous anatomy and patency by injecting contrast from venous access distal in the extremity to proximal in the direction of venous flow (i.e., ascending). Typically, the descending venogram is performed from a remote venous access site to allow injection of contrast down the extremity against the flow of venous blood to assess competence of the venous valves. Traditionally, ascending and descending venography is performed on a tilt table to allow gravity-induced changes in venous flow during different stages of the exam. While duplex has nearly replaced venography in the diagnosis of deep vein thrombosis (DVT) and in identifying venous reflux, there has been a resurgence of venography performed in conjunction with catheter-directed thrombolytic treatment for acute venous thrombosis. Venography is also useful in complicated venous cases to define lower-extremity anatomy for patients needing deep venous valve reconstruction or venous bypass.

B. Patient preparation and risk. Steps in preparation for and the risk of venography are nearly the same as those discussed for arteriography and include recognition of contrast allergies, renal insufficiency, and need for a suitable puncture or access site. About 3% of venographic studies will be complicated by minor allergic reactions, **contrast-induced thrombophlebitis** or thrombosis, or contrast extravasation at the puncture site.

C. Methods. The quality and safety of leg venography can be optimized by paying attention to the two previously mentioned aspects of the technique.

    1. Ascending venography is performed by injecting contrast into a vein on the distal extremity in a direction away from the foot. The patient should be positioned at 30° to 45° reverse Trendelenburg on a tilt table, with no weight bearing on the affected limb. Weight bearing causes the gastrocnemius and soleus muscles to contract, preventing adequate filling of some deep veins. For general diagnostic purposes, a vein on the dorsum of the foot is punctured with a 21-gauge needle. Rarely, a cutdown exposure of the great saphenous vein at the ankle is necessary. Diluted nonionic contrast in a volume of 60–90 mL per extremity is usually suitable and may reduce the risk of contrast-related phlebitis. Views of the superficial and deep veins can be obtained without a tourniquet unless leg swelling is severe and causes increased compartment pressures. In this situation an ankle tourniquet to occlude the superficial system is used to promote better filling of the deep veins. Images of the leg are made with external and internal rotation of the foot and the same views are obtained over the knee and thigh. Finally, the pelvic film is exposed after the table is returned horizontal and the leg elevated. The venous system is flushed with 60 mL of normal saline at the completion. **Ultrasound-guided popliteal vein access** with the patient in the prone position is often chosen for catheter-directed thrombolytic treatment of acute DVT involving the proximal femoral and/or iliac veins. A form of ascending venography, this approach provides excellent support for crossing acute venous thrombus with wires and catheters and provides optimal imaging of the proximal femoral, iliac, and even caval circulations.

2. The normal ascending venogram is able to image the lower extremity up to and including the inferior vena cava. During normal ascending venography, the deep and superficial veins are opacified, except for the profunda femorus vein, which is rarely filled. Deep venous trunks in the calf are paired, the smallest being the anterior tibial veins. These deep leg veins have smooth, straight walls except where the valves are positioned and then a beadlike appearance of the vein can be appreciated. Venous sinuses within the muscle of the leg are large and fusiform in the young but appear smaller with advancing age. The popliteal and femoral veins are usually single but may be paired in some individuals. Normally, contrast should flow quickly up the deep system after leg elevation, allowing for visualization of the proximal femoral, iliac, and even caval circulations. For more complete opacification of these proximal venous segments and depending upon the size and location of the distal access vein in the leg it may be necessary to place a sheath to allow placement of a catheter near or into the proximal venous segment of interest. Injection of contrast into a catheter placed more proximally allows more full and complete filling and imaging of these venous segments. Alternatively, the proximal venous segments may be imaged as part of the descending venogram.

3. Descending venography of the lower extremity is performed by accessing the contralateral femoral vein and crossing over the bifurcation of the inferior vena cava with a wire and catheter. This allows placement of a catheter above the venous segment of interest for injection of contrast to assess the valvular reflux. Once the catheter is placed above the segment of interest the patient is positioned in a steep reverse Trendelenburg position (i.e., head up), while contrast boluses are injected through the catheter and images recorded. The patient may perform a **Valsalva maneuver**, which increases intra-abdominal pressure and transiently halts venous emptying from the legs to increase the sensitivity of descending venography. In the setting of normal valvular function, the contrast will only descend as far as the next set of competent valves, which prevent flow down the venous segment. Conversely, in the setting of valvular incompetence, contrast will flow down the venous segment of the leg until a competent set of valves intervenes.

4. Acute lower-extremity deep venous thrombosis is confirmed by filling defects in the deep veins on more than one view. The contrast column will end abruptly when the thrombosis obstructs the vein. Deep veins also may be nonopacified because of external compression from muscle swelling in the fascial compartments. Chronic changes from **post-thrombotic syndrome** reveal well-developed collaterals and partial recanalization with intraluminal webs or synechiae. Chronic venous insufficiency as a result of primary valvular degeneration or post-thrombotic syndrome is evident by the degree of contrast reflux visualized on descending venography.

5. Upper-extremity venography can accurately diagnose and potentially treat central venous stenosis or thrombosis. Although duplex is the initial test of choice in this situation, the intrathoracic position of the central veins makes them difficult to exam directly with ultrasound. The use of chronic central venous catheters for parenteral nutrition, chemotherapy, and dialysis predisposes the subclavian and innominate veins to stenosis and/or thrombosis, which may require central venous angiography to diagnose. In such cases an often distended superficial arm vein may serve as a site for access and injection of diluted contrast. **Ultrasound-guided basilic vein access** allows placement of a venous sheath and therefore a wire and catheter into more proximal venous segments for imaging and potential treatment. The presence of a dialysis fistula or graft in the arm provides an obvious site for venous access and intervention in select cases. In the case of acute **axillo-subclavian venous thrombosis, also referred to as Paget-Schroetter syndrome,** distended antecubital veins may facilitate venous access. Venography in this scenario is often combined with catheter-directed thrombolysis to treat the acute DVT, which often forms as a result of thoracic outlet syndrome. In the absence of acute axillo-subclavian venous thrombosis but suspected thoracic outlet syndrome, diagnostic venography should include provocative maneuvers (abduction and external rotation or the arm), which may provide the diagnosis.

SELECTED READING

Barrett BJ, Parfrey PS. Preventing nephropathy induced by contrast medium. *N Engl J Med.* 2006;354:379-386.

Criado FJ. Percutaneous arterial puncture and endoluminal access techniques for peripheral intervention. *J Invasive Cardiol.* 1999;11:450-456.

Garrett PD, Eckart RE, Bauch TD, et al. Fluoroscopic localization of the femoral head as a landmark for common femoral artery cannulation. *Catheter Cardiovasc Interv.* 2005;65:205-207.

Hodgson KJ, Mattos MA, Sumner DA. Access to the vascular system for endovascular procedures: techniques and indications for percutaneous and open arteriotomy approaches. *Semin Vasc Surg.* 1997;10:206-221.

Lasser EC, Berry CC, Talner LB, et al. Pre-treatment with corticosteroids to alleviate reactions to intravenous contrast material. *N Engl J Med.* 1987;317:845-849.

Merten GJ, Burgess WP, Gray LV, et al. Prevention of contrast-induced nephropathy with sodium bicarbonate: a randomized controlled trial. *JAMA.* 2004;291:2328-2334.

Rupp SB, Vogelzang RL, Nemcek AA, et al. Relationship of the inguinal ligament to pelvic radiographic landmarks. *J Vasc Interv Radiol.* 1993;4:409-413.

CHAPTER 11

Catheter-Based Technology and Devices

In order to participate in a meaningful discussion of endovascular therapies or to take part in endovascular procedures, the provider or trainee needs a fundamental understanding of equipment and techniques. This chapter is designed to prepare the reader with that basic familiarity and understanding and includes sections on catheter-based technologies and thrombolytic therapy. Additionally, this chapter provides a brief discussion of post-angiogram care and complications specific to endovascular procedures. As a starter and because the use of catheters in these cases is ubiquitous, the term ***catheter-based*** should be thought of as synonymous with **endovascular** procedures.

I. Basic equipment. The exponential growth of endovascular procedures to treat vascular disease and certain patterns of vascular injury has driven the development of catheter-based technology. Competition in the industry to "build the better mousetrap" has led to a seemingly countless number of endovascular tools, some of which are interchangeable. The wide array of endovascular technologies can seem at first overwhelming. However, a basic understanding of certain core elements is all that is necessary for most basic endovascular procedures. The following section describes these core tools that that are used as part of nearly all endovascular procedures: **sheaths, wires**, and **catheters (Table 11.1)**. Categories of therapeutic technologies, including **balloons, stents, covered stents or stent grafts**, and **intravascular ultrasound** are described followed by a discussion of concepts related to **catheter-directed thrombolysis.** Finally, a summary of post-catheterization care and complications unique to endovascular procedures is provided.

The nuances of different device brands are not discussed here, as the purpose of this chapter is to provide a broad overview of each class of equipment. Where brand names are mentioned, these may imply a frequent practice of the authors but are not intended to profess superiority of a particular device. In many cases, the obvious utility of catheter-based interventions has led to widespread usage prior to FDA approval for such applications. For example, bare metal stents were originally FDA-approved only for use in the biliary tree, and covered stents for the tracheobronchial tree. **The following discussion includes some off-label use of catheter-based technology and the reader is advised to consult the individual manufacturer's guidelines for every endovascular device prior to usage**.

A. Sheaths. The primary function of **sheaths** is to maintain hemostatic access to the inside of the vessel once entry has been accomplished by the modified **Seldinger technique**. Sheaths act as ports through which wires, catheters, and other devices can be exchanged without causing trauma to the vessel or significant blood loss. The hemostatic valve at the end of

Table 11.1.   Categories of catheter-based tools

Access needles
  18-gauge
  21-gauge micro-puncture kit
Sheaths—4 Fr and greater
  Short straight (10-12 cm and 22-25 cm lengths)
  Long straight (90 cm)
  Preshaped crossover sheaths (45-60 cm)
Wires— 0.014 to 0.035 inches diameter (regular and exchange-length)
  Hydrophilic (e.g., glide wire)
  Nonhydrophilic (i.e., working wires)
  Starter (e.g., starter J-wire or Bentson wire)
  Stiff (e.g., Amplatz, Cook, Inc., Bloomington, IN)
Catheters
  Nonselective flush (e.g., straight, pigtail, Omni)
  Selective/end hole (e.g., angled glide, Bernstein, Cobra, Simmons)
  Infusion (e.g., multiside hole thrombolytic)
Guide Catheters
Balloons
  Compliant
  Noncompliant
  Cutting
  Cryo-balloons
Stents
  Balloon-expandable
  Self-expanding
  Covered (i.e., stent grafts)
Intravascular ultrasound (IVUS)
Mechanical thrombolysis (e.g., Angiojet, Possis Medical, Minneapolis, MN)
Access or puncture site closure devices

the sheath through which these devices are passed from outside of the patient to inside the blood vessel is often referred to as the diaphragm. A side port, also toward the end of the sheath, allows it to be flushed proximal to the diaphragm or transduced to measure the pressure within the vessel. **Sheaths are sized based on their inner diameter with 1 Fr unit equaling 0.33 mm**. This is important to keep in mind, understanding that a 5 Fr sheath has a 1.65 mm inner diameter but an outer diameter that creates a slightly larger opening in the vessel. The majority of diagnostic procedures are performed through sheaths 10–12 cm long, with longer sheaths (e.g., 45 and 90 cm) available to provide a platform for endovascular procedures at distances farther from the access site. Sheaths that are shaped with preformed curves are also available, such as the popular "crossover" sheath that has a wide U shape for optimal positioning over the aortic bifurcation into the contralateral iliac or femoral artery. Using this longer preformed sheath, arteriograms and catheter-based interventions can be performed on the leg contralateral to the femoral access site

The smallest sheath suitable for the task at hand should be used in order to minimize the size of the hole in the vessel and lessen the risk of access site complications. The most common sheath sizes used range from 4 Fr to 10 Fr. Very large diameter sheaths up to 25 Fr are necessary to accommodate certain devices for endovascular aneurysm repair.

B. Wires. Catheter-based interventions are initiated with placement of a wire maneuvered into a desired location using fluoroscopic guidance. Once the wire is in the desired location, the endovascular tool needed to accomplish the next step (e.g., catheter, balloon, or stent) may be placed over a wire though the sheath, with the wire acting as a rail on which the device travels. Once a wire has been positioned to its desired location, it should not be advanced or withdrawn until the given intervention is complete. Meticulous **wire control** or **wire management** is important to avoid injury to vessels or structures beyond the desired location and critical once placed beyond a stenosis targeted for therapy. Should the wire be inadvertently pulled back proximal to such a lesion, regaining wire access can be difficult; multiple wire passes can cause adverse events such as embolization or dissection.

Wires are sized based on their diameters and lengths. The most common wire diameters are 0.035, 0.018, and 0.014 inches. Because they are the largest, 0.035" wires are most easily handled and can be used for the majority of basic diagnostic and large vessel interventions. Because of their small size, 0.014-inch wires are more difficult for the less experienced endovascular specialist to handle and maneuver. The 0.014-inch wires were originally designed for use in the coronary arteries and are therefore compatible with smaller profile balloons, stents, and other endovascular devices. A benefit unique to the 0.014-inch wire pertains to **monorail catheter technology**. The monorail mechanism allows the wire to exit from an opening of a device (e.g., catheter, balloon, or stent) much closer to the forward tip of the device instead of out of the back or rear of the device (Fig. 11.1). This technique allows for more rapid exchanges over a shorter length of wire, reducing manipulation and making the exchange easier for one individual to accomplish. The 0.014-inch wire system is most often used in small vessels (e.g., carotids or tibials) or when wire movement must be kept to a minimum (e.g., renals). The "working wires" for the endovascular specialist include **standard lengths** (145–180 cm) and **exchange lengths** (240–300 cm). Exchange-length wires are necessary when performing over-the-wire interventions so that catheter or balloon exchanges can be made without losing wire access. **The length of wire needed for a given procedure can be estimated using the following formula: distance from the access site to the target lesion location + length of the catheter + 10 cm.**

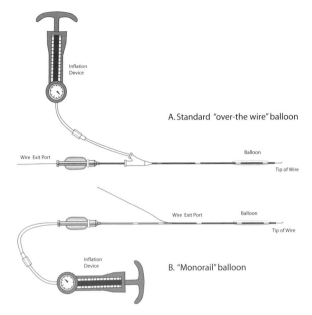

Figure 11.1. (**A**) "Over-the-wire" balloons typically go over a 0.035- or 0.018-inch wire, which exits at the end of the balloon. (**B**) Monorail technology utilizes a 0.014-inch wire that exits via a side port in the balloon.

Wire properties also vary with respect to their **steerability**, **trackability**, and **stiffness**. Starter wires are used at the onset of vascular access to facilitate sheath and initial catheter placement. A typical starter wire has a low degree of stiffness and a floppy, straight, angled, or J-shaped tip that makes initial intravascular passage atraumatic. Wires with an angled tip are steerable in that the interventionalist can turn the tip in a desired direction as the wire is advanced, allowing it to navigate circuitous turns. Wires with a hydrophilic coating are useful for negotiating tortuous vessels and tight stenoses and for selecting or entering the orifice of target vessels. **Hydrophilic wires** are frictionless or slick when kept wet, which is a necessary step to maintain their handling and trackability. Because these wires are often too slick to manipulate with the user's fingers alone, tools referred to as **torque devices** that grip the wire may be used to effectively steer or spin the tip of the wire. Care must be taken with hydrophilic wires, as they are prone to enter the subintimal plane. This can be advantageous if a subintimal angioplasty is desired, but can also create unwanted dissections or even vessel perforations. The stiffness of a wire's body depends on its diameter and composition, although the segment at the leading edge is typically floppy.

Once the starter and hydrophilic wires have accomplished access to the desired intravascular location, an exchange to a more **stiff wire** is often performed to allow endovascular work over a rail with more substance. Specifically, stiff wires are often necessary to negotiate a sheath into position at a distance far from the access site without losing wire position. Stiff wires also tend to straighten tortuous vessels and provide appropriate support for the deployment of larger endovascular devices, such as endografts for aortic aneurysm repair. Examples of more stiff wires in order of increasing rigidity include the **Rosen, Wholey, Meier, Amplatz,** and **Lunderquist** wires. Finally, specially designed **pressure wires** are now available that can be placed to measure intravascular pressure waveforms at their distal segments or tips. These recently developed wires are useful to directly transduce intravascular pressure and to determine the presence or absence of a pressure gradient across a vascular stenosis.

C. Catheters and guiding catheters. Catheters are long, flexible tubes with hollow lumens that are placed over and used to direct wires through vessels or across stenoses or occlusions. Once the wire has been removed from the catheter, contrast may be injected through the lumen for performance of angiography (Fig. 11.2). Catheters are sized based on their outer diameter and come in two broad categories, **nonselective flush catheters** and **selective end-hole catheters**. Nonselective angiography is performed through flush catheters, which have multiple side holes near the tip and can accommodate high pressure (400–600 psi), high flow injections without causing catheter motion (i.e., catheter whip) within the vessel during injection. Flush catheters are designed to image larger, high-flow vessels such as the aorta and vena cava and come in various lengths and shapes, including the straight flush catheter, the pigtail flush catheter and the Omni SOS catheter (AngioDynamics, Queensbury, NY, U.S.A). A wide assortment of selective or end-hole catheters is available to permit the endovascular selection or cannulation of all types of blood vessels. The choice of a particular catheter depends on the diameter and tortuosity of the main access vessel and the angle of takeoff of the branch vessel targeted for cannulation. Most often, several different catheters may be suitable for

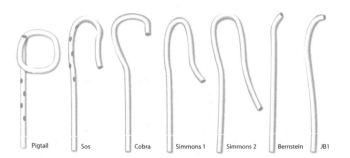

Pigtail   Sos   Cobra   Simmons 1   Simmons 2   Bernstein   JB1

Figure 11.2.   **A sampling of commonly used catheter shapes. Catheters with a complex curve must be reformed to their preformed shape in vivo (e.g., Vitek, Simmons).**

engaging a given vessel, such that the interventionalist's preference and familiarity with the catheter is a major factor in its success. Once the catheter is engaged in the orifice of the desired vessel, the wire may be removed and a selective angiogram performed or advancement of the catheter over the wire can continue into a more distal position. Catheters with a single curve such as the **angled glide**, **visceral selective (VS)**, or **cobra catheters (C1-3)** are advanced by simply pushing them forward over the wire. Catheters with a complex curve must be reformed within the vessel once the wire is withdrawn. Paradoxically, some complex catheters must be withdrawn by the endovascular specialist in order to allow them to advance into the vessel. Examples of complex curve catheters are the **Simmons** and **Vitek catheters**.

Guiding catheters, sometimes simply called guides, are essentially larger catheters through which other devices such as balloons and stents may be passed. **Like catheters (and unlike sheaths), guides are measured according to their outer diameter**. Therefore, an 8 Fr guide that has a 2.66 mm outer diameter will fit through an 8 Fr sheath that has the same inner diameter. The inner diameter of the guide is of course smaller and determines what size devices may pass through. Also, like catheters, guides come in a variety of preformed shapes, which facilitates their placement in angled orifices such as the renal and mesenteric arteries. Although guides can be positioned directly over a wire into a vessel's orifice, unlike sheaths they typically do not come with a tapered inner dilator. Therefore, there is an increased risk of atheromatous embolization with this maneuver because of the step-off (i.e., size mismatch) between the wire and the opening at the end of the guide. An alternative technique involves telescoping the guide over a catheter and wire. The catheter is then withdrawn, leaving the guide in position to conduct interventions. A **Tuohy-Borst** adapter may be placed over the wire and attached to the external end of the guide to prevent backbleeding. This device allows injection of contrast through its side port into the guide to facilitate angiography while the wire remains in place, exiting out the back end of the Tuohy-Borst.

D. Unfractionated heparin (UFH) is used during many peripheral interventions in order to prevent thrombus formation, however, consistent recommendations for its use are lacking. Higher doses of UFH (75–100 mg/kg) are often used for carotid interventions and femoral or tibial angioplasty in which the catheters or wires may be near-occlusive or when prolonged or complex interventions are anticipated. Lower doses (50 mg/kg) may be suitable for more straightforward cases such as limited iliac angioplasty. The authors also suggest lower doses of systemic heparin when working through larger femoral sheaths (7 Fr or more) or via brachial artery access. Heparin may be directly reversed with the use of **protamine** at the end of the procedure or simply allowed to wear off over a period of 1–2 hours prior to removal of the access sheath. Protamine binds to heparin at a ratio of 1 mg protamine: 100 U heparin, induces histamine release, and can cause hypotension and (rarely) anaphylaxis. Accordingly, 50 mg of protamine would neutralize 5,000 units of heparin;

however, the time since the heparin dose should also be considered. The half-life of unfractionated heparin varies (30 minutes to 2 hours), depending on the dose.

E. Vasodilators can be used in select cases to alleviate distal vessel spasm related to catheter or wire manipulation. **Nitroglycerine** can be delivered through the sheath or catheter directly into the blood vessel in increments of 50–100 mcg. The main side effect of nitroglycerin is headache related to vasodilation. When the hemodynamic significance of a mild or moderate stenosis visualized on arteriography is in question, pressures should be transduced proximal and distal to the stenosis. This can be accomplished by transducing the end of the catheter when it is proximal to the stenosis and then slowly withdrawing the catheter across the stenosis distally. A pressure wire can also be used to measure the pressure proximal and distal to the identified stenosis. A **resting mean arterial pressure gradient** of greater than 5 mm Hg or **systolic pressure gradient** greater than 10–15 mm Hg across a stenosis is considered hemodynamically significant. If there is no resting gradient identified across a moderate stenosis, **intra-arterial papaverine** (10–30 mg) can be administered in attempt to unmask the gradient. Papaverine causes distal vasodilation, thereby increasing the velocity across any proximal stenosis mimicking the effects of walking or exertion. A mean arterial pressure gradient of greater than 10 mm Hg or more than 15% following administration of papaverine is significant.

II. Catheter-based therapeutic technologies can be used in cases of acute or chronic occlusive disease, aneurysms, and even in select patterns of vascular injury. Once the endovascular specialist has decided to proceed with a catheter-based intervention, the tools for that intervention need to be selected. If a diagnostic angiogram has already been performed, the basic equipment for the case can be decided upon in advance and set aside. When the intervention is done at the same sitting as the diagnostic angiogram, the interventionalist should take a few minutes to mentally plan an approach to the lesion. The plan should then be discussed with personnel in the catheterization laboratory or operating room. The staff's understanding of the "game plan" encourages active involvement and anticipation of the methods and tools to facilitate the treatment goal.

A. Indications for angioplasty. Since its revival in the late 1970s, angioplasty has been used successfully to dilate or recanalize arteries or grafts in every anatomic region. Catheter-based interventions generally have lower morbidity and mortality than open surgical approaches and in some cases are less expensive since the length of hospitalization is shorter. Patient recovery is excellent, with ambulation occurring on the same or following day. However, endovascular therapies are generally less durable than operative revascularization. The specific indications and options for intervention depend upon the anatomic area being treated and are discussed in detail in the chapters on specific diseases. Guidelines such as the **Trans-Atlantic Inter-Society Consensus (TASC)** provide recommendations for catheter-based versus surgical treatment of lower-extremity occlusive disease (see Chapter 14). For example, a short common iliac stenosis is best treated by endovascular revascularization, whereas open surgery (aortobifemoral bypass) is more fitting for diffuse aortoiliac disease. Nonetheless, the decision for or against a catheter-based intervention should be carefully considered in the context of the anatomy, patient comorbidities, and the skill set of the interventionalist. The authors also feel that success of a given intervention must be documented by improvement of both symptoms and hemodynamic measurement (ankle brachial indices, Doppler wave forms, pulse volume recordings, or transcutaneous oxygen measurements).

B. Percutaneous transluminal angioplasty (PTA) is the most fundamental and popular technique used for treating vascular occlusive disease and generally uses polyethylene catheters that have an inflatable balloon near the tip. Balloon angioplasty represents a variation of the original translumi-nal arterial dilatation described by **Dotter and Judkins**. The Dotter technique used a relatively large 12 Fr Teflon catheter introduced over an inner 8 Fr catheter and passed through the stenosis to dilate it. No balloon was involved. **Gruntzig** popu-larized balloon catheters in the late 1970s, and their use now is common practice.

The first step in PTA is to cross the lesion with the selected wire as described in the previous section. An angled hydrophilic or glide wire is particularly effective in this maneuver and can be steered into and beyond the stenosis. An angled catheter can also be used to direct or steer a straight hydrophilic wire to the appropriate position to navigate across the lesion. Alternatively, the endovascular specialist can enter a subintimal plane when crossing total occlusions (e.g., **subintimal angioplasty**) (Fig. 11.3). With this technique, the wire is directed into an eccentric plane at the start of the lesion forming a loop in the subintimal plane. A catheter can then be used to follow the wire until it re-enters into the true lumen beyond the stenosis or occlusion. A characteristic "give-way" sensation followed by smooth pas-sage of the wire and catheter signals the interventionalist that

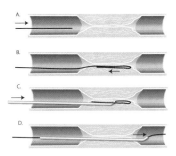

Figure 11.3. Subintimal angioplasty. A steerable wire is used to enter the occlusion in an eccentric plane. The wire begins to loop once in the subintimal plane. A catheter is advanced over the wire into the subintimal plane. After the wire is felt to re-enter the lumen, contrast is injected into the catheter to confirm intraluminal place-ment. The wire is replaced and the catheter is removed. The wire is maintained past the lesion for the duration of the intervention.

the true lumen has been re-entered. Contrast must be injected into the catheter once the lesion has been crossed to confirm re-entry or positioning into the true lumen of the vessel on the other side of the target lesion. Once the wire and catheter have crossed the lesion, a wire exchange can be performed through the catheter to allow placement of a more substantive working wire over which the balloon angioplasty catheter can be placed. Both transluminal and subintimal angioplasty are successful for treating aortoiliac and infrainguinal disease.

The mechanisms by which PTA dilates a stenotic vessel are complex. **First, balloon dilatation causes a focal dissection**, disrupting the plaque and the artery wall. With rupture of the plaque and partial separation from the media there is stretching of the adventitia to increase the cross-sectional area of the lumen (Fig. 11.4). **Second, the intimal plaque protrudes into the lumen**, accounting for the angiographic appearance of local flaps and dissection channels visualized in some cases. **Third, remodeling occurs** by adherence of the intimal flaps with little change in plaque volume. Thus, long-term patency depends on sufficient stretching of the vessel and an adequately remodeled lumen. Restenosis may occur because of insufficient dilatation (compliance), from extension of dissection channels into nondilated segments and from **myointimal hyperplasia**.

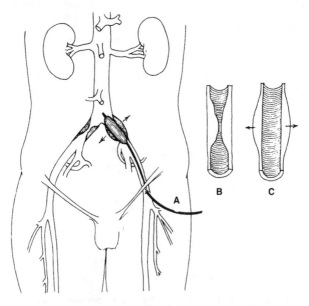

Figure 11.4. Percutaneous transluminal angioplasty (PTA). (**A**) By the Seldinger technique, a catheter with an internal flexible guidewire is passed into and gently insinuated through the area of arterial stenosis. (**B, C**) The balloon is inflated to several atmospheres of pressure. When the PTA is complete, the arterial lumen is larger and the local artery is stretched.

The selection of a balloon for angioplasty is based on the diameter of the vessel (oversized by 1.1 times) and length of the lesion. A variety of techniques can be used to measure or estimate the normal diameter of the target vessel so that the appropriate diameter balloon may be selected. These include marking tapes and catheters with radiopaque markers at known distances from one another and use of the known sheath tip size. Intravascular ultrasound (IVUS) is a newer technology that allows more accurate measurement of vessel diameter from within and can also be used to estimate balloon size. Balloon sizes commonly used for peripheral interventions range from 2.5–10 mm in diameter and 20–100 mm in length. Often, for peripheral interventions, a simple over-the-wire approach is taken with the balloon. When minimal wire movement is important, and for smaller vessels, the **monorail balloon catheter** compatible with a 0.014-inch wire may be chosen (Fig. 11.1). Just like the monorail catheters described previously, the monorail balloon devices have a side port for exit of the wire so that only the initial 20–30 cm of the catheter are involved with each exchange.

Once the balloon is positioned within the target lesion an inflation device is used to expand it to a desired pressure. Every balloon has a **nominal pressure** at which its full or prescribed diameter is reached. The **rated burst pressure** is the pressure below which the balloon is guaranteed not to rupture with 95% confidence. Typical nominal and burst pressures are 6–8 and 12–16 atmospheres, respectively, and are affected by the balloon's compliance or degree of softness. **Highly compliant balloons** are softer and track easily due to their composition but will also expand beyond their designated diameter and length at higher pressures. For this reason more compliant balloons are generally not effective for angioplasty of inflexible calcified stenoses. In fact, very large compliant balloons such as the CODA (Cook, Inc., Bloomington, IN, U.S.A) and Reliant (Medtronic, Inc., Minneapolis, MN, U.S.A) balloons are useful for gently expanding stent-grafts after endovascular aneurysm repair and can also be used to temporarily occlude the aorta or other bleeding or injured arteries. **Noncompliant balloons** are stiffer and are better and more effective for angioplasty of tight stenoses, as they expand to their predetermined diameter without elongating. Very rigid or resistant stenoses can occur in some native arterial lesions as well as with in-stent or recurrent stenosis due to neointimal hyperplasia. These types of rigid or recalcitrant stenoses may be seen at the venous anastomosis of hemodialysis grafts and may have elastic recoil that does not respond to traditional angioplasty. Such lesions can be treated with ultra–high-pressure, noncompliant balloons with rated burst pressures from 20–30 mm Hg. Alternatively, **cutting balloons** have several microblades circumferentially positioned on a balloon, such that longitudinal incisions are made in the plaque with balloon inflation. This technology can also be helpful to overcome the rigidity of very fibrous lesions.

C. Stents are tubes composed of a wire latticework that can be deployed within a vessel in order to overcome elastic recoil and expand the vessel's lumen. Stents are broadly categorized as either **balloon expandable** or **self-expanding** and either **covered** or **bare metal**. Most stents today are composed of either stainless steal or the metal alloy referred to as nitinol. Placement of endovascular stents falls into one of two strategies: **selective stenting** or **primary stenting**. Selective stenting refers to the practice of stent placement only in response to an inadequate technical result seen on completion angiography following PTA. The usual criteria for selective stenting are a residual stenosis or dissection from the angioplasty that compromises 30% or more of the lumen. The presence of a residual pressure gradient also indicates a technically imperfect result and may be an indication for stent placement. In some cases, the original intent is to **primarily stent** the target lesion. The carotid and renal arteries are common targets for primary stenting, due to its superiority versus PTA alone in these locations. With improved balloon and stent technologies and the demonstrated effectiveness of primary stenting, this practice has become more common in recent years. In some cases the target lesion may need to be **pre-dilated** with an undersized balloon to create a small channel within the stenosis in order to position the stent. In these cases the term primary stenting still applies.

Similar to balloons, stents are available in a variety of lengths and diameters. Typically, the stent is oversized slightly for the diameter of the vessel and should nearly match the length of the lesion so that normal segments of vessel are not stented. In cases of selective stenting, a device that has a 1–2 mm greater diameter than the angioplasty balloon is generally selected. It is important to recognize the different properties and applications of balloon-expandable and self-expanding stents (Table 11.2).

Balloon-expandable stent technology originated with the Palmaz design. Today these devices are typically made of stainless steel and are premounted on a less compliant balloon that matches the diameter and length of the stent. When this balloon is inflated the stent expands simultaneously and is deployed at the time of angioplasty. Balloon-expandable stents can be precisely positioned by the operator, which is critical in certain locations such as the renal and mesenteric arteries and aortic arch vessels. Precision and control of placement is an advantage that balloon-expandable devices have over their self-expanding counterparts. Balloon-expandable stents can also be expanded beyond their set diameter (i.e., **overexpansion**) by inflating a balloon with a diameter 1–2 mm larger than the stent once it is initially deployed. Overexpansion will result in some **foreshortening** of the stent as the lattices withdraw from the ends as the diameter goes beyond the designed measurement. These stents are vulnerable to deformation or compression from external forces, and placement of balloon-expandable devices in locations where they could be crushed or fractured, such as an extremity, should be avoided.

Self-expanding stent technology stemmed from the original **Wall stent** design and most stents today are made of nitinol, a metal that assumes its preformed shape when warmed to body temperature. Although the initial **radial force** or **hoop strength** of self-expanding stents is not as great as the

Table 11.2   Bare metal stents are either balloon-expandable or self-expandable. Different properties influence their selection for use.

Property	Balloon-expandable	Self-expandable
Precision of deployment	Excellent	Fair
Radial force	Very strong	Moderately strong
Trackability in tortuous anatomy	Poor	Fair to good
Crushable with external compression	Significantly	Minimally
Continuous self-expanding properties	No	Yes
Can be enlarged beyond set diameter	Yes[a]	No
Conformability to the vessel	Absent	Excellent[a]
Flexibility	Poor	Fair to good

[a] Balloon-expandable stents can be further enlarged by using a larger balloon. Self-expanding stents will conform to a smaller portion of the vessel if a size discrepancy exists. However, an undersized self-expandable stent cannot be further expanded and is vulnerable to migration.

balloon-expandable devices, the self-expanding component of the design works to assume the prescribed diameter and shape over time. In contrast, the balloon-expandable stents, which have greater initial radial force, do not increase in size after placement. Self-expanding stents are generally more flexible than balloon-expandable devices and therefore are better suited for tortuous anatomy. Common locations for self-expanding stents include the carotid arteries, arteries of the extremities, and iliac veins. Intuitively, certain anatomic areas contain flexion or compression points, and may not be well suited for stenting. Examples of such locations are the thoracic outlet, common femoral artery, and popliteal artery. There are concerns for stent fracture and early stenosis that must be balanced with the risks of alternative treatment such as surgery. Some interventions can be performed as **hybrid, open-endo procedures** in which one portion of the procedure is open surgical and the other endovascular. An example of this tactic is a retrograde iliac artery stent before or after an open femoral artery endarterectomy.

Covered stents are made of a wire exoskeleton covered by plastic (polytetrafluoroethylene) or fabric (Dacron). Covered stents are often referred to as stent-grafts and can be used to reline or to exclude a portion of an artery from the circulation. One such application is the treatment of a **pseudoaneurysm**. A pseudoaneurysm is a localized outpouching or area of bleeding from a disrupted artery or artery-graft anastomosis that is contained by only the adventitia or surrounding tissues. Traumatic pseudoaneurysms or arterial disruptions from penetrating or blunt trauma or from iatrogenic injury (post-catheterization) are often suitable for catheter-based treatment. In these cases a covered stent can be deployed across the pseudoaneurysm to exclude it so that it thromboses, while maintaining axial flow through the main vessel. Similarly, an **arteriovenous fistula** from penetrating injury can be successfully treated by placement of a covered stent on the arterial side, effectively sealing the fistula. Of course, surgical treatment can also be undertaken for more complex patterns or clinical scenarios involving these problems. The choice for catheter-based or surgical therapy is often influenced by the location of the lesion. **Endovascular aneurysm repair** is based on the principle of aneurysm sac exclusion with modular stent-graft components (see Chapter 15). Along the same lines, covered stents (Viabahn, W.L. Gore and Associates, Flagstaff, AZ, U.S.A.) have been used as an alternative to surgery in patients with popliteal artery aneurysms, with promising early results. The use of covered stents has recently been extended to occlusive disease, specifically in the superficial femoral artery. A theoretical disadvantage of covered stents in the treatment of occlusive disease is the coverage of potentially important collateral or side-branch vessels, although relining of the diseased segment is intuitively appealing. A randomized prospective study is underway to determine whether covered stents have any advantage over bare metal stents in treating occlusive disease in the superficial femoral artery.

D. Miscellaneous catheter-based technologies also have a niche in the treatment of vascular occlusive disease and in some cases may act as an adjunct to the more established use of stents. Some innovative strategies target neointimal hyperplasia, the principal cause of mid-term angioplasty failures, while others focus on removing or vaporizing plaque burden within the vessel. **Cryoplasty** is one technology that uses a combination of angioplasty with freezing in order to enact both a physical and a biological response (apoptosis) in attempts to decrease rates of intimal hyperplasia and restenosis. Randomized data comparing cryoplasty with standard PTA/stenting is not yet available. **Brachytherapy** or radiation in the superficial femoral artery has shown some benefit in the short-term prevention of restenosis, but data demonstrating its advantage over the long-term are lacking. **Drug-eluting stents** release antiproliferative agents (**sirolimus, paclitaxel**) and have been shown to reduce the short-term risk of restenosis in the coronary arteries. However, drug-eluting stents have not yet been shown to be superior to bare metal stents in the iliac or superficial femoral arteries.

"**Debulking**" technologies such as **laser therapy** and **atherectomy** that vaporize or excise atheromatous plaques are intuitively appealing. A prospective randomized evaluation of the excimer laser in the superficial femoral artery (SFA) failed to show superiority when compared with PTA with selective stenting, although the need for stenting in the laser arm was reduced. Additional randomized studies comparing debulking therapies to PTA/stenting need to be performed before their widespread use can be advocated. Locations considered unfavorable for stenting, such as the popliteal artery or bifurcation vessels, may benefit from technology that reduces the need for stent placement.

IVUS allows for internal imaging and measurement of vessels and has a multitude of clinical applications. Because IVUS images are in cross section, they can provide additional information not seen on two-dimensional angiography. Technical results after angioplasty can be assessed using IVUS to determine if significant residual stenosis or dissection exists and stent apposition can be assessed for completeness. IVUS is useful for verifying measurements of length and diameter for stent-graft repairs of aortic aneurysms. In these instances the origin of the renal arteries can be identified and the exact neck diameter can be measured from inside of the aorta and the presence of plaque or thrombus can also be identified. IVUS can also be used following catheter-directed thrombolysis of deep vein thromboses (DVTs) to assess completeness of the therapy and to identify external compression that may elude venography (e.g., May-Thurner syndrome).

III. Catheter-directed thrombolytic therapy. Despite widespread interest in thrombolytic drugs, their role in peripheral arterial and venous disease remains relatively selective. Enthusiastic reports in the early 1980s have been balanced by more critical analyses from more recent clinical trials. Although the authors have used thrombolytic agents in a variety of clinical settings, it is most often for indications that have been supported by these randomized trials. Currently, the most commonly used thrombolytics are **urokinase, recombinant tissue plasminogen activator (rt-PA), and t-PA mutants (e.g., reteplase)**. Urokinase was withdrawn by the FDA from the market in 1998, but was reintroduced in 2002. It is currently approved for treatment of pulmonary embolism, although off-label use in the arterial and venous circulation is widespread. The use of any of these agents must be undertaken with careful consideration of their pharmacokinetics, indications, and possible complications. The main complication of pharmacologic thrombolysis is bleeding. The emergence of mechanical thrombectomy devices provides an alternative treatment with less risk of bleeding and may be used in combination with pharmacologic thrombolysis or alone.

    A. Pharmacokinetics. Thrombolytics are plasminogen activators that lead to clot lysis by enhancing the fibrinolytic system via conversion of plasminogen to its active form, plasmin. These agents not only act on plasminogen within a clot but also on plasminogen throughout the circulation, and systemic fibrinolysis may result. **Streptokinase** must first form an activated complex with plasminogen, which completes the conversion of excess plasminogen to plasmin. This agent is seldom used anymore, primarily because of high antigenicity and allergic response with repeated exposure. **Urokinase** acts by directly cleaving plasminogen to plasmin, with a greater affinity for fibrin-bound plasminogen than streptokinase. **rt-PA** is currently the most commonly used agent in catheter-directed thrombolysis and is very specific for plasminogen bound to fibrin clot. Although systemic fibrinolysis can occur with t-PA; it happens to a lesser degree than that observed with streptokinase. This advantage reduces bleeding complications. **Reteplase,** a third-generation t-PA mutant, has improved clot penetration, longer half-life, and faster initiation of thrombolysis compared with rt-PA.

The half-life for most thrombolytic drugs is short: streptokinase, 10 to 12 min; urokinase, 11 to 16 minutes; t-PA, 4 to 6 minutes; and reteplase, 15 minutes. Consequently, the effect of the drug dissipates rapidly, although depleted fibrinogen levels may take at least 24 hours to normalize. In the authors' experience, the need to use ε-aminocaproic acid (Amicar; Xanodyne Pharmaceuticals, Inc., Newport, KY, U.S.A.) or fibrinogen concentrates to reverse the thrombolysis rarely occurs.

B. Indications. Selective use of catheter-directed thrombolysis in cases of severe proximal DVTs actively reduces if not eliminates thrombus burden, thereby preserving venous endothelial and valvular function. Subsequently, in select cases, with the appropriate application of catheter-directed thrombolysis, the severity of post-thrombotic syndrome can be reduced. Although initial concerns regarding bleeding complications limited widespread use of thrombolysis, recent data suggests that serious bleeding mishaps are rare. Furthermore, the recent and effective use of **mechanical thrombectomy devices** (**Angiojet,** Possis Medical, Minneapolis, MN, U.S.A.) can reduce the amount and duration of catheter-directed thrombolysis, further decreasing the risk of bleeding. This therapy is also effective in treating acute axillo-subclavian vein thrombosis associated with central venous catheters, effort thrombosis, or thoracic outlet syndrome. In summary, catheter-directed thrombolysis for the treatment of acute DVT should be considered in all symptomatic patients with proximal extremity DVTs, not only for symptomatic relief but also to reduce long-term morbidity associated with post-phlebitic syndrome.

The benefits of thrombolytic therapy for arterial thrombosis are controversial. The **Surgery versus Thrombolysis for Ischemia of the Lower Extremity (STILE) trial** suggested that patients with **acute limb ischemia** (0 to 14 days) who were treated with thrombolysis had improved amputation-free survival and shorter hospital stays. Surgical revascularization was more effective and safer than thrombolysis for patients with **chronic ischemia** (>14 days). There was no difference in efficacy or safety between urokinase and rt-PA. Subgroup analysis demonstrated that patients treated with thrombolytics for acute bypass graft occlusions had a higher rate of long-term limb salvage than those with native artery occlusions. Surgical revascularization fared better for native artery occlusions. Also of importance, failure of optimal catheter placement occurred in 28% of patients who were randomized to lysis in the STILE trial.

The **Thrombolysis or Peripheral Arterial Surgery (TOPAS) trial** examined patients with acute arterial occlusions with a duration of less than 14 days. Although amputation-free survival between thrombolysis and surgery was not significantly different, two secondary outcomes were interesting. First, patients undergoing thrombolysis had a decreased need for open surgical procedures, a benefit that extended into the follow-up period. Second, thrombolytic results again appeared superior in patients with bypass graft occlusions compared with those with native artery thrombosis.

Other uses of thrombolysis for acute arterial occlusion are situations for which surgery has traditionally poor results, or for which high operative mortality makes a nonoperative approach attractive. Acutely thrombosed popliteal aneurysms with tibial artery thrombosis, thrombosis of autogenous vein grafts, and lower-extremity arterial embolism associated with myocardial infarction are examples, although the authors' experience with thrombolysis in these situations has not been uniformly successful.

C. Methods. In the setting of arterial or venous occlusion, catheter-directed thrombolysis occurs as the drugs are delivered via continuous infusion through a multi-side hole catheter directly into the thrombus. The infusion catheter is placed within the thrombus over a selecting wire via standard endovascular techniques and comes with variable infusion lengths (10–40 cm). Several different regimens of treatment are effective and the choice is at the discretion of the endovascular specialist. Urokinase can be given intra-arterially as per the STILE trial protocol as a 250,000-IU bolus followed by 4,000 IU/min for 4 hours and then 2,000 IU/min for 36 hours. A lower dose of urokinase at 30,000–60,000 IU/hr may also be effective. Rt-PA can be effective at relatively low doses (0.05 mg/kg/h for 12 hours). This dose is lower than that tried initially in the STILE trial (0.1 mg/kg/h), where higher doses were associated with more bleeding from puncture sites. Another reasonable regimen administers even lower doses: 2 mg the first hour, followed by 1 mg/hr, which further minimizes bleeding complications. For reteplase, a clot-lacing dose of 5 units is recommended and followed by 0.5 to 2.0 units/h. (**Note that rt-PA doses are in mg, and reteplase doses are units**.) The use of thrombolytics intraoperatively has been described as an adjunctive technique for eliminating distal thrombus after surgical thromboembolectomy. A single bolus of urokinase 250,000 IU can be infused directly to the site of residual thrombus.

Mechanical thrombolysis is a relatively new tool that has been popularized for the treatment of acute arterial and venous thrombosis, either alone or in combination with pharmacologic thrombolysis. The indications are similar to those for pharmacologic thrombolysis. However, these devices may be used in patients with contraindications to pharmacologic agents, such as bleeding diathesis or recent surgery. When used as an adjunct, these devices may hasten the process of clot lysis by mechanically debulking a large amount of the thrombus. The Angiojet is one such device that works by instilling a high-velocity saline jet into the thrombus, resulting in a vacuum effect, such that the macerated clot can be aspirated into the catheter. There is a risk of distal embolization (2–10%) that may be reduced by adjunctive period of pharmacologic thrombolysis. Early technical success and limb salvage with mechanical thrombolysis is promising and comparable with pharmacologic thrombolysis alone. The **Trellis system** (Bacchus Vascular, Santa Clara, CA, U.S.A.) has proximal and distal balloons that can be inflated to exclude the segment of vessel to be treated. The thrombolytic agent is instilled into this segment and a rotating wire macerates the thrombus, which is then aspirated. The potential advantages of this device are the isolation of the thrombolytic drugs and reduced risk of embolization. Prospective data comparing mechanical thrombolysis with surgery is not yet available.

Two important laboratory tests to document a lytic state are measurement of **thrombin time** and **fibrinogen level**. When clot lysis occurs, **fibrin split products** also generally rise. However, changes in the constituents of the fibrinolytic system do not consistently correlate with bleeding complications. Lower fibrinogen levels and higher partial prothrombin time (PTT) levels have been linked to bleeding. Hemorrhagic problems usually occur at the arterial puncture site and are related to catheter size and manipulation.

When a thrombolytic drug is administered, heparin is usually administered concomitantly in order to prevent clot accumulation around the infusion catheters and improve the completeness of thrombolysis. However, heparin may increase the risk of hemorrhage at the catheter infusion site. The authors generally start heparin through the sheath at the onset of regional lytic therapy to avoid **pericatheter thrombus formation.** Low doses from 300–700 units per hour are typical, and PTT levels can be followed to ensure levels are not supratherapeutic.

D. Complications. Catheter-directed or regional thrombolytic therapy is complicated by bleeding, thrombosis, or embolism in 10% to 15% of patients. In the authors' experience, bleeding at the vessel access site has been the most common problem. Distal emboli are often small and sometimes can be resolved with continued thrombolytic administration. Nonetheless, about 5% to 10% of patients will require surgical intervention to manage these complications. Unfortunately, regional low-dose infusions have not eliminated these problems. The most devastating bleeding complications associated with catheter-directed thrombolysis are those related to **intracranial hemorrhage**. Although this complication is rare (<1%), it can occur as a result of too high of doses of thrombolytic drug over too long a period of time and is particularly prone to occur in the elderly and those with underlying hypertension or previous history of stroke. The rare occurrence of intracranial hemorrhage as a complication emphasizes the extreme care that must be taken when evaluating potential patients for this therapy and the attention to detail that must occur among all providers once the therapy is initiated.

IV. Postangiogram care. Any patient who has undergone angiography should be monitored hourly for at least 4 to 6 hours. Most early complications become evident during this time. Nursing personnel can perform most routine checks, but a physician or physician assistant/nurse practitioner should also examine the patient during the recuperative period, as they are on-call for complications arising outside the hospital after patient discharge. The baseline post-procedure exam is helpful if problems occur after discharge and should include: **(a) evaluation of the patient's general appearance and mental status (especially after cerebral studies), (b) heart rate, (c) blood pressure, (d) inspection of puncture sites, (e) palpation of**

extremity pulses, and (f) hematocrit if any signs of hemorrhage exist.

In addition, adequate hydration must be maintained for 12 to 24 hours, since contrast material causes a diuresis and can lead to dehydration. The combination of diuresis and the nephrotoxicity from the contrast material can cause renal deterioration, especially in patients with diabetes mellitus or chronic renal insufficiency. The authors maintain an intravenous infusion for 4 to 6 hours after the angiogram, with alkaline fluids if renal insufficiency is present. Oral fluids are encouraged for 24 hours after the procedure to maintain hydration in all patients.

At the completion of a catheter-based procedure, the final step is access **sheath removal**. If systemic heparin has been given during the procedure, time should be allowed for the anticoagulant effect to wear off or protamine may be given to more quickly reverse the heparin. The primary goal of sheath removal is to achieve hemostasis at the puncture site, without compromise of the vessel lumen. Numerous commercial devices, called **closure devices**, are available for safe and hemostatic sheath removal from the common femoral artery. Suture-mediated closure devices, such as the **Perclose ProGlide** (Abbott Medical, Redwood City, CA, U.S.A.), place a pre-tied knot at the site of the puncture. The **Angio-Seal** (St. Jude Medical, St. Paul, MN, U.S.A.) is a collagen plug that is cinched against the vessel wall and absorbs within 90 days. The **Duett Pro system** (Vascular Solutions, Minneapolis, MN, U.S.A.) achieves hemostasis by the delivery of a procoagulant thrombin and microfibrillar collagen mixture into the tract outside of the artery. Rare instances of distal embolization, femoral artery occlusion, or even early infection of the suture material with these devices have hampered their routine usage by many providers. The overall complication rate associated with closure devices is 2–3% and appears to be decreasing as experience with them increases. Although these devices reduce time and energy expenditure, they do add to the overall cost of the endovascular case. For these reasons, some endovascular specialists prefer the use of manual pressure, held to the artery for 15–20 minutes after sheath removal. External pressure devices, such as the **FemoStop** (Radi Medical Systems, Wilmington, MA, U.S.A.), may also be used as an adjunct to sheath removal and are especially helpful in some instances in which long periods of pressure are indicated. The danger of such devices is that they tend to apply more diffuse and not focal pressure, which is less effective at achieving hemostasis and can lead to a false sense of security among the attending team.

If manual pressure is used to achieve hemostasis following sheath removal, the patient should lie flat with the head slightly elevated for 4–6 hours afterward. In the authors' experience, patients dislike this portion of the procedure because they find it difficult to lay flat for a prolonged time. Following this period, they are allowed to ambulate under close observation and most patients can be discharged shortly thereafter. Closure devices allow the patient to return to ambulation within a couple hours, much sooner than with manual pressure.

V. Complications.

    A. Neurologic deficits. Aortic arch and selective cervical arteriography can rarely result in transient or permanent neurologic deficits that may be delayed, or occur minutes to hours after the angiogram. Neurologic deficits that happen during the study are most likely embolic from dislodged atheroma or catheter thrombus. Meticulous care must also be taken during arch and carotid angiography to assure that no air is injected through the imaging catheter, as air embolization is a recognized cause of neurologic complication during these procedures. Delayed neurologic deficits may also be secondary to hypoperfusion or thrombosis associated with contrast-induced diuresis and dehydration. Urgent carotid endarterectomy should be considered in the event of an immediate neurologic deficit on the side of a tight carotid stenosis, especially if a post-procedure duplex scan or arteriogram confirms that the internal carotid artery has occluded suddenly.

Sometimes the neurologic change is subtle, such as confusion, mild facial paresis, dysarthria, or dysphagia. If the neurologic deficit is not recognized for several hours (>4 hours) and is not resolving, the patient probably has suffered a stroke. Emergency endarterectomy may not be advised in such cases, since it may worsen neurologic deficits by changing an ischemic infarct to a hemorrhagic infarct. A CT scan or MRI should be done in 12 to 24 hours to define infarct areas, intracranial hemorrhage, and edema. Patients with transient neurologic deficits should be given antiplatelet agents (aspirin or clopidogrel) and a duplex ultrasound to rule out carotid thrombosis.

If a cerebrovascular accident has occurred, several measures can help minimize cerebral edema and stroke progression. Intravenous fluids should be limited to maintenance levels (1 mL/kg/h) so that cerebral edema is not worsened by excessive hydration. Systemic anticoagulation to prevent distal internal carotid clot propagation should be considered if there are no signs of intracerebral hemorrhage.

B. Hemorrhage. Small hematomas and ecchymosis at the access site are not uncommon; however, expanding hematomas indicate continued bleeding into the perivascular spaces. The first treatment for a hematoma should be the reapplication of manual pressure for 15–30 minutes. Significant hypertension or coagulopathy should be corrected, as these both contribute to bleeding from the puncture site. Expanding or pulsatile hematomas should be evaluated immediately by ultrasound. Often, an active pseudoaneurysm can be closed by ultrasound-guided compression or ultrasound-guided thrombin injection. In some patients an acute arteriovenous fistula may also resolve with ultrasound-guided compression. **After brachial puncture, any hematoma that compresses the brachial plexus, causing pain or other neurologic change, should be decompressed in the operating room.** Significant retroperitoneal hemorrhage can also occur after angiography, particularly with a high femoral or external iliac artery access. Early indications of such bleeding may be persistent back pain, tachycardia, hypotension, and anemia. Flank ecchymosis is a delayed finding. Abdominal CT scan will demonstrate a periaortic or psoas muscle hematoma, and treatment is initially supportive: correction of coagulopathy, transfusion, and bedrest. Most episodes of retroperitoneal bleeding will have resolved by the time they are discovered. Ongoing bleeding or instability indicates a significant femoral or iliac injury and indicates immediate angiography or surgery. Repeat arteriography and placement of a covered stent can sometimes be used to seal the leaking vessel.

C. Diminished or absent pulses (compared with baseline) following the angiogram suggest partial or complete arterial occlusion. Although arterial spasm may occur, it is rarely the cause of diminished pulses that persist beyond 30 to 60 minutes. **The most common causes of compromised extremity blood flow after angiography are: (a) arterial injury (intimal flap), (b) a clot stripped off the catheter, (c) arterial occlusion associated with a misplaced percutaneous arterial closure device, and (d) compression by a hematoma in the arterial wall or extrinsic to it.** Stent thrombosis can rarely occur in the early post-intervention period and is usually secondary to a technical defect, poor inflow or runoff, or failure to administer antiplatelet therapy. Antiplatelet therapy with at least aspirin is recommended after angioplasty and/or stent placement to reduce the thrombotic risk on a freshly injured endothelial surface. **Clopidogrel** (Plavix) is often prescribed in addition to aspirin after catheter-based interventions at a dose of 75 mg daily. Loading doses of 300 mg are administered in some cases, when the patient is not already on steady-state dose. The added benefit of clopidogrel in preventing thrombosis after intervention is not known, but warrants further investigation. Clopidogrel is often prescribed for locations where stent thrombosis would be disastrous, such as the carotid artery.

The acutely ischemic extremity that is painful, pallid, and pulseless requires emergent revascularization. In contrast, an intimal flap may diminish but not obstruct arterial flow. The extremity will be asymptomatic, but pulses and Doppler pressures (ankle-brachial index) will be diminished compared with those prior to the angiogram. Such asymptomatic cases with mild pressure reduction (10 to 20 mm Hg) can initially be managed nonoperatively. Angiogram or duplex ultrasound should be performed to confirm the diagnosis. Small intimal flaps usually will adhere to the arterial wall and resolve in several days to a few weeks. Systemic heparinization for 24 to 48 hours followed by antiplatelet drugs for 4 to 6 weeks has been a successful regimen in our experience. Ankle-brachial indices at rest and after exercise can be followed to document improvement or deterioration. However, we emphasize that the presence of any ischemic symptoms and the absence of previously palpable pulses require emergent intervention to restore normal extremity circulation.

D. A **pulsatile mass** at the access site represents either a hematoma transmitting a pulse from the artery underneath or a **false aneurysm** (pseudoaneurysm). This is a difficult distinction to make in the early post-procedural period and a duplex ultrasound is diagnostic. In some situations, small (<3–4 cm) acute hematomas can be eliminated by **ultrasound-guided compression**. Although this process may take more than an hour and can be uncomfortable for the patient, the success rate is over 90%. Small pseudoaneurysms frequently resolve with time and should be reimaged with ultrasound at a month. Pseudoaneurysms that are initially missed and then noted at a later examination should be repaired about 6 to 8 weeks after the arteriogram. By this time, local inflammation generally has resolved and dissection and repair may be easier. Chronic pseudoaneurysms have a developed capsule that is not likely to resolve with ultrasound-guided compression. If the pseudoaneurysm has a narrow neck, as many do, **ultrasound-guided injection of thrombin** (0.1 cc at a time of diluted 5,000 IU in 5 cc) is often a very effective means of treatment, as flow in the pseudoaneurysm will cease with administration of a small amount of thrombin. Any postarteriogram hematoma that suddenly causes pain and local subcutaneous hemorrhage is a ruptured pseudoaneurysm and usually requires urgent surgical evacuation and repair of the artery. Pseudoaneurysm rupture is most likely to occur within 7 to 10 days of the initial angiogram. For this reason, it is the authors' suggestion that all patients with local hematomas remain close to a surgical facility during this time

E. Infection. Local access site infection is unusual with meticulous sterile technique. Such technique should include (a) cleansing the site with a surgical scrub soap before the study, (b) standard sterile preparation at the time of the study, and (c) standard surgical attire for members of the angiogram team. If present, superficial pustules at the skin puncture site should be incised, drained, and cultured. If cellulitis extends around this site, oral or parenteral antibiotics should be started. Most local infections will be secondary to hospital-acquired *Staphylococcus aureus* or Streptococcus. Abscesses should be incised and drained in the operating room, since hemorrhage from an infected artery may occur and require repair or ligation. **Any elective synthetic bypass, especially aortofemoral grafting, should be postponed until local groin infections are resolved completely.**

SELECTED READING

Ahn SS, Obrand DI, Moore WS. Transluminal balloon angioplasty, stents, and atherectomy. *Semin Vasc Surg.* 1997;10:286-296.

Bjarnason H, Kruse JR, Asinger DA, et al. Iliofemoral deep venous thrombosis: safety and efficacy outcome during 5 years of catheter-directed thrombolytic therapy. *J Vasc Interv Radiol.* 1997;8:405-418

Clair DG. Critical limb ischemia: Will atherectomy and laser-directed therapy be the answer? *Semin Vasc Surg.* 2006;19:96-101.

Comerota AJ, Gravett MH. Iliofemoral venous thrombosis. *J Vasc Surg.* 2007;46:1065-1076

Comerota AJ, Weaver AJ, Hosking JD, et al. Results of a prospective, randomized trial of surgery versus thrombolysis for occluded lower extremity bypass grafts. *Am J Surg.* 1996;172:105-112.

Curi MA, Geraghty PJ, Merino OA, et al. Mid-term outcomes of endovascular popliteal artery aneurysm repair. *J Vasc Surg.* 2007;45:505-510.

Diehm N, Silvestro A, Do DD, et al. Endovascular brachytherapy after femoropopliteal balloon angioplasty fails to show robust clinical benefit over time. *J Endovasc Ther.* 2005;12:723-730.

Kasirajan K, Haskal ZL, Ouriel K. The use of mechanical thrombec-tomy devices in the management of acute peripheral arterial occlusive disease. *J Vasc Interv Radiol*. 2001;12:405-411.

Koreny M, Riedmuller E, Nikfardjam M, et al. Arterial puncture clos-ing devices compared with manual standard compression after cardiac catheterization: systemic review and meta-analysis. *JAMA*. 2004;291:350-357.

Laird J, Jaff MR, Biamino G, et al. Cryoplasty for the treatment of femoropopliteal arterial disease: results of a prospective, multi-center registry. *J Vasc Interv Radiol*. 2005;16:1067-1073.

Nadal LL, Cynamon J, Lipsitz, et. al. Subintimal angioplasty for chronic total occlusions. *Tech Vasc Interv Radiol*. 2004;7:16-22.

Ouriel K, Veith FJ, Sasahara AA. A comparison of recombinant urokinase with vascular surgery as initial treatment for acute arterial occlusion of the legs. *N Engl J Med*. 1998;338:1105-1111.

Powell RJ, Fillinger M, Bettmann M, et al. The durability of endovas-cular treatment of multisegment iliac occlusive disease. *J Vasc Surg*. 2000;31:1178-1184.

Scott EC, Biuckians A, Light RE, et al. Subintimal angioplasty for the treatment of claudication and critical limb ischemia: 3-year results. *J Vasc Surg*. 2007;46:959-964.

Sohail MR, Khan AH, Holmes DR, et al. Infectious complications of percutaneous vascular closure devices. *Mayo Clin Proc*. 2005;80: 1011-1015.

Tepe G. Drug-eluting stents for infrainguinal occlusive disease: progress and challenges. *Semin Vasc Surg*. 2006;19:102-108.

The STILE Investigators. Results of a prospective randomized trial evaluating surgery versus thrombolysis for ischemia of the lower extremity: the STILE trial. *Ann Surg*. 1994;220:251.

Van de Ven PJ, Kaatee R, Beutler JJ, et al. Arterial stenting and bal-loon angioplasty in ostial atherosclerotic renovascular disease: a randomised trial. *Lancet*. 1999;23:282-286.

CHAPTER 12

Basic Fluoroscopic Concepts and Applied Radiation Safety

Most vascular patients who require an intervention for the severity or refractory nature of their disease will eventually undergo some type of angiographic procedure in the endovascular suite or operating room. **Fluoroscopy, which refers to the digital or photographic formation of images using electromagnetic radiation, is the main principle behind angiography, which pertains specifically to imaging of the blood vessels.** With the aid of devices and contrast material within the vessel lumen (i.e., endovascular), fluoroscopy becomes angiography and allows the provider to see the contour of the vasculature to diagnose, quantify, and even treat disease. Simply put, electromagnetic radiation applied with the techniques of angiography allows the provider to have x-ray vision of the patient's vascular system. While angiography has led to remarkable advances in the treatment of vascular disease, its expanded use must be viewed in balance, with recognition of the potentially harmful effects of radiation to both the patient and provider.

This point is relevant given that much of the recent enthusiasm for angiographic procedures has outpaced provider awareness of basic radiation terminology and radiation safety. In contrast to even a decade ago, when most angiographers had formal instruction in radiology and were dedicated to interventional fluoroscopic procedures, today's endovascular specialist has a more diverse training and practice background. Although well versed in the natural history of vascular disease and the range of management options, today's vascular specialist may not have had dedicated schooling in radiation science. In lieu of such formal training, basic concepts are often passed down to trainees by mentors who may not stress a basic understanding of a few key radiologic principles. While practical, this method may not be ideal in a time when the number and complexity of endovascular procedures is increasing along with the diversity of providers enlisting to perform them.

The intent of this chapter is to recognize this important aspect of vascular care and to present basic radiation terms and concepts including the effects of radiation on patients and providers. Basic steps toward radiation safety are presented, including steps to minimize radiation risk. To cover the entire field of interventional fluoroscopy is beyond the capacity of this chapter and therefore the reader is encouraged to use this as a primer to familiarize and to stimulate additional reading.

I. **Basic radiation concepts.**
   A. **X-rays are a form of electromagnetic radiation.** The main characteristics of x-rays are similar to those of visible light and radiation is frequently quantified in a unit called a photon. **A single photon is a quantum of electromagnetic radiation containing a defined amount of energy, in this instance defined in terms of electron volts (eV)**

Table 12.1.   Basic radiation terminology

Term	Definition	Unit of Measure
Electromagnetic radiation	A form of energy emitted from a source	Photons or electron volts
Radiation dose	Amount of energy absorbed from the radiation source at a point divided by the mass of the tissue at that point	Gray
Quantity dose equivalent	A quantity defined for radiation protection purposes that expresses on a common scale for all types of radiation the irradiation incurred by exposed persons	Sievert
Exposure	A measure of the quantity of radiation present at a particular location and formally determined by air ionization	KERMA

KERMA, kinetic energy released per unit mass of air.

(Table 12.1). The stronger the radiation source, the more photons per second can be produced. It takes thousands of x-ray photons per square millimeter to form a single fluoroscopic frame that is thousands of times greater than the energy contained in a photon of visible light. X-ray photons used for imaging have energies that range from 10,000 to 150,000 eVs. The source of radiation or x-ray tube converts electrical energy into electromagnetic quanta and heat is generated as a side product. Radiation is the transport of this energy away from the x-ray tube by these electromagnetic quanta. **It is important to remember that the intensity of an x-ray beam decreases inversely as the square of the distance between the source and the measuring point (e.g., the greater the distance, the less the beam intensity).**
B. Radiation units and quantities are found in the International System (SI) of Units and include the important unit of radiation dose, referred to as the gray (Gy). Radiation dose is the amount of energy absorbed from the radiation source at a point divided by the mass of tissue at that point (Table 12.1). Surprisingly a very small amount of energy is actually absorbed by or deposited into tissue during medical procedures. In fact, the amount of energy absorbed by tissue is similar to the amount of radiation energy absorbed by the surrounding air. **1 gray (Gy) = 1 joule of energy absorbed per kilogram of material.** A gray is a large unit of radiation. In relation, radiation therapy doses are in the 1–2 gray range meaning that 1–2 joules of energy are delivered per kilogram of radiated tissue. In contrast, a standard chest x-ray delivers a dose of approximately 100 μGy.

Table 12.2.   Maximum permissible doses

Occupational Exposures	
Whole body exposures: effective dose limits	20–50 mSv/yr
Partial body exposure: equivalent dose annual limits for tissues and organs	
Lens of the Eye	150 mSv/yr
Hands	500 mSv/yr

mSv, millisievert or 1/1,000[th] of 1 sievert.
(From the United States National Commission on Radiation Protection and Measurements and the International Commission on Radiation Protection)

Taking into account all forms of radiation, including natural, industrial, nuclear, and others, different types of radiation produce vastly different biological effects for the same number of Gy or dose. So **the quantity dose equivalent (H)** was developed to account for this range for radiation protection purposes and is expressed in units called **sieverts (Sv)**. The dose equivalent expresses on a common scale for all forms of radiation the amount of irradiation incurred by exposed persons and was established by means of an experimentally defined quality factor. While quality factors for some forms of radiation are as high as 20, conveniently the quality factor for medical x-ray energies is 1: 1 Sv = 1 Gy × quality factor.

Finally, the term *exposure* refers to the strength or quantity of the radiation field at a given point (Table 12.1). Most SI measurements of exposure are actually measurements of air dose, which, as was previously noted, has very similar absorption properties to human tissue. Therefore, our standard measures of "exposure"are actually measures of the x-ray beam's ability to ionize air caused by the small amount of absorbed energy. The working unit of exposure is the **kinetic energy released per unit mass of air** acronym (KERMA), which is a measure of the energy extracted from the x-ray beam by air. The unit of measurement for exposure is also the gray. Note that the unit measure of exposure was formally referred to as the Roentgen (R) which was the measure of ionization produced per one gram of air. An air-KERMA of 1Gy corresponds to an exposure of 114 R.

C. Radiation measuring device. A radiation measuring device called a **dosimeter is necessary to determine the dose of radiation emitted by any given source at a particular location**. Dosimeters come in different forms, depending upon the type and amount of radiation that will be monitored or measured. Some basic instruments directly measure the ionization produced in a defined volume of air (i.e., KERMA) within a cylindrical instrument called an ionization chamber. The Geiger counter is another type of radiation detection device, which uses a Geiger tube and associated electrical display components. While these devices provide an accurate representation of soft tissue dose, they are not designed to monitor lesser amounts of exposure to patients or providers on a routine basis.

The more familiar and clinically practical dosimeters are available on clips to be worn by providers and or patients in the endovascular suite or operating room. These devices are often thermoluminescent, which means that the amount of radiation exposure to that point on the dosimeter is determined by the degree of color change in the device (i.e., the greater the radiation exposure the greater the change in color). These dosimeters, sometimes referred to as radiation badges, are used to sample radiation levels at various locations on the provider and should be recorded or logged each month. Typically, these dosimeters are worn in three locations on the provider to assess exposure and to assure effectiveness of the lead shielding. Specifically, they should be worn on the collar outside of the thyroid shield of the neck, at the waist outside of the lead apron, and at the waist underneath the lead apron. These dosimeters report their dose in sieverts and most have a minimal detectible level of 0.01 millisievert (mSv). The safety dose limits for occupational exposure with respect to different body areas (e.g., neck, body, and hands) recommended by the **United States National Commission on Radiation Protection and Measurements** and the **International Commission on Radiation Protection** are provided in Table 12.2 and are defined using mSv per year.

D. Components of basic imaging and the fluoroscopic device. It is important for the provider to have an understanding of the components of a fluoroscopic system in order to be effective in the endovascular imaging suite while minimizing radiation exposure to all persons in the room. **The basic setup of a fluoroscopic system is diagrammed in Figure 12.1 and includes a generator and controls, an x-ray tube, a collimator, and an image receptor or image intensifier**. The purpose of the generator and its controls are to convert available electrical power into the exact form needed to operate the x-ray tube, which is typically underneath the patient (Fig. 12.1).

The **x-ray tube is a lead-shielded device with an exit port positioned toward the patient that converts the electrical energy from the generator into x-rays**. This process is very inefficient, with less than 1% of the applied electrical energy converted to x-rays and the remaining 99% converted into heat. Although x-ray tubes are designed to handle this heat byproduct they can "overheat,"especially during longer endovascular procedures, which results in an aggravating system shutdown. Several maneuvers can be implemented by the endovascular specialist to minimize heat production. These same maneuvers reduce the amount of radiation used during a given case, which makes their judicious use even more appealing. **Specifically, the use of "pulse," instead of the continuous mode of imaging, and reducing the frames per second reduces the amount of heat produced by the x-ray tube**. Also, moving the patient as close as possible to the image intensifier automatically decreases the strength of the x-ray beam and therefore the amount of heat generated. While the first two of these simple maneuvers may reduce the quality of the image, they are suitable for certain, less complex aspects of the endovascular procedure.

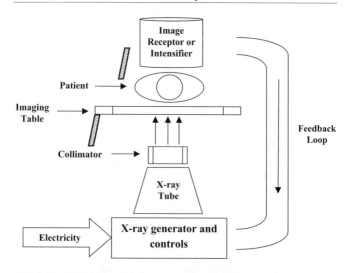

Figure 12.1. Basic components of a fluoroscopic system including x-ray generator and controls, x-ray tube, and image receptor or intensifier. The dark hatched objects represent lead shields that accompany most imaging units and tables.

Moving the patient close to the image receptor or intensifier actually widens the field of imaging and slightly improves its clarity. Finally, high level fluoroscopy uses an even higher intensity of energy to generate more detail and should be used very rarely and only when such degree of image detail is necessary.

The x-ray beam collimators control and minimize the size of the x-ray beam, and when used effectively will decrease radiation dose and scatter during an endovascular procedure. These tools are important because x-rays are emitted uniformly from the generator and are designed to radiate the entirety of the image intensifier, sometimes irradiating a field larger than the image receptor. By focusing or collimating down to only the area of clinical interest, the radiation field and scatter are reduced while subject contrast is improved and the image quality enhanced. **Radiation scatter is the secondary radiation that arises after the x-ray beam contacts the patient**. These photons of electromagnetic radiation are less intense than the primary x-ray beam but still constitute a radiation risk. Scatter is always more intense on the side where the x-ray beam contacts the patient. This side of the imaging setup is referred to as the *zone of high intensity scatter*, which is often underneath the imaging table (Fig. 12.2). The area between the patient and the image receiver constitutes the *zone of low intensity scatter*. Understanding these zones will help the provider and assistants effectively position and shield themselves in the endovascular suite or operating room to minimize radiation exposure.

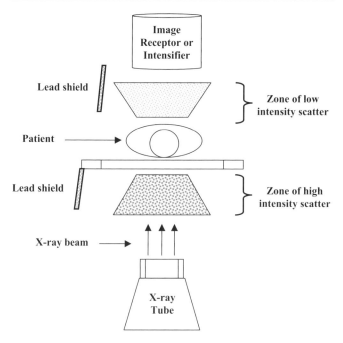

Figure 12.2. Zones of high- and low-intensity radiation scatter in relation to the x-ray beam and patient position. Note the zone of high intensity scatter is on the side where the radiation strikes the patient, which is under the imaging table in this figure.

The **image intensifier,** also referred to as the image receptor, is an electro-optical device that captures and converts an x-ray image into a visible form. The size of the image intensifier has steadily increased with technology, which permits clearer and more comprehensive imaging of the abdominal, thoracic, and peripheral vessels. However, with such large image intensifiers—most are now at least 12 to 15 inches in width—use of collimators becomes even more important in order to focus the radiation field to clinically relevant areas. **Moving the patient toward the image intensifier will broaden the image field and reduce intensity of the radiation beam and the amount of scatter** (Fig. 12.1).

The endovascular specialist should develop a checklist in his or her mind pertaining to these simple components of the fluoroscopic system for optimization of images and reduction of radiation exposure. A review of the following points prior to any imaging series will serve the provider, the patient, and others in the room well during endovascular procedures:

1. Collimator position
2. X-ray beam setting (i.e., continuous versus pulsed)
3. Frames per second
4. Position of the patient in relation to the image intensifier
5. Use of appropriate lead shielding

II. Radiation biology, including genetic and carcinogenic effects of radiation.

A. Radiation effects on human tissue are referred to as either deterministic or stochastic. Deterministic effects have a radiation threshold below which there is no probability of harmful radiation. However, once the threshold has been reached there is a direct relationship between further radiation dose and the adverse biological effect. In contrast, the stochastic effect is related more to chance than to a known effect of an increased dose up to and beyond a threshold. An example of this is a mutation occurring from a single or random dose of radiation that results in a mutation leading to malignancy.

B. Direct and indirect ionization. Absorption of radiation by living cells can result in an interaction with an important target molecule in one of two ways, direct or indirect. **Direct ionization means that the energy from the x-ray is directly absorbed by the target molecule. Indirect ionization refers to x-ray absorption and damage to the water around the molecule**. The indirect radiation and breakdown of water within living cells and tissue is called radiolysis, which results in the formation of damaging ions called free radicals. Studies have shown that radiation damage to living tissue occurs mostly (about 80%) from indirect radiation, while the minority (about 20%) occurs as a result of direct radiation effects.

C. A variety of molecules or cellular structures can be affected by radiation, although DNA appears to be the main target. DNA, which exists in the form of a double helix structure within the nucleus of the cell, contains the operation plans for cellular life as well as the genetic code for reproduction. Direct or indirect radiation damage can break the structure of DNA so it is unable to program these activities. While most cells can repair minor or single strand breaks in the DNA, more significant injury to both strands of the double helix often results in permanent damage.

The effect of radiation on cells is influenced by how rapidly they are proliferating and the sensitivity of specific cell types to radiation. In general, rapidly dividing cell types such as skin cells are more sensitive to radiation than cell types that are less active. Other organ types that are known to be sensitive to radiation exposure are the thyroid, the breast, the lens of the eye, the lung, and the bone and bone marrow. **Two modes of cellular death can occur after exposure to radiation: reproductive death and apoptosis**. Reproductive death refers to proliferative cells that have sustained various levels of DNA injury—some of which may be repaired initially—that ultimately results in failure to proliferate and cell death. Apoptosis is programmed cell death, which is a more uniform and active process in which organized cellular events take the cell down a definite path of demise.

D. Radiation biology is the study of how living cells and organisms react to radiation. At the cellular level, one can conceptualize one of four outcomes that can occur following radiation exposure or damage.

    1. If the damage is to **critical cellular components,** or is too great, the cell can no longer function and dies.

2. Some radiation damage may be repaired fully by the cell with **no identifiable adverse effects**.

3. The damage may be repaired and the cell survives, but with **decreased function or capacity**.

4. Damage may be partially or incorrectly repaired resulting in a **mutation**. In this last group of radiation induced cellular injury, a malignancy or cancer can develop years later. **Genetic mutations can occur in cells that are damaged by radiation but do not die or repair themselves correctly following exposure**. A gene mutation from radiation occurs due to a nonlethal, nonrepaired flaw in the DNA, which results in a failure to produce a protein that is necessary to support or control cell proliferation. In instances where the mutation results in failure to control or shut off a cell line these cells will proliferate unchecked, resulting in malignancy or cancer. Although the understanding of the link between radiation exposure and cancer is relatively limited, there are specific types of cancers known to be related to radiation exposure.

It is important for the vascular provider to realize that the levels of radiation exposure associated with cancer are generally much higher than those encountered during medical fluoroscopy. However, they are worth noting if for no other reason than to underscore the seriousness of radiation exposure and the importance of protective measures. The thyroid gland may be the most radiation-sensitive tissue and is known to be associated with radiation-induced malignancy. The first human cancer to be linked to radiation exposure was skin cancer, which continues to receive considerable attention given its prevalence and relation to sun exposure. Other forms of cancer that have a recognized association with radiation exposure include bone cancer, lung cancer, and leukemia (i.e., bone marrow).

E. Radiation injury with the use of medical fluoroscopy occurs most commonly in the skin and the lens of the eye. This is because radiation exposure to providers and patients occurs at the surface where radiation first makes contact. Skin injury from radiation is particularly prone to occur in those with underlying collagen vascular diseases such as lupus erythematosus and scleroderma and those with diabetes mellitus. Skin injury can range from mild erythema and hair loss, which result from as little as 2–3 Gy, to dermal atrophy, induration, and even necrosis, which can occur with doses in the 10–15 Gy range.

Cells that make up the lens of the eye are also prone to radiation injury, which causes them to lose their clarity or lucency. **Because these cells are continually produced and form layers on the lens over time, if a significant number are adversely affected an opacity, or cataract, can form.** A cataract may or may not impair vision and generally requires radiation doses in excess of 1Gy delivered at one time in an otherwise healthy lens. The threshold for induction of cataracts is greater when the radiation exposure is in lower doses over extended periods. The time between radiation exposure and diagnosis is delayed, often more than five and 10 years for cataracts caused by lesser doses received over extended periods.

III. Practical radiation safety. With the above concepts of fluoroscopic imaging systems and radiation biology in mind, the goal in the interventional suite is to facilitate indicated patient care while minimizing the risk of radiation exposure. Understanding the risk of radiation exposure underscores points made throughout this book that indications for angiographic procedures must be sound and that noninvasive alternatives should be explored. Assuming that the endovascular procedure is indicated or must be performed to provide optimal care for the vascular patient **providers should expect or be willing to accept a risk of radiation exposure that is as low as reasonably achievable (ALARA).**

Regulatory authorities define a maximum permissible dose of radiation per year (Table 12.2). These levels are an *absolute maximum*, which no individual provider should come close to on an annual basis. Establishing the lowest level (i.e., ALARA) is somewhat arbitrary, but should be a number that careful providers know and strive for in their practice. For example, in well-designed endovascular rooms providers usually have total body doses of 0.5–15 mSv per year. For providers to consistently meet an established ALARA goal requires some amount of discipline and good endovascular habits, some of which have been mentioned briefly in previous sections. The five main operational factors to reduce radiation dose that each provider should consider prior to any endovascular procedure are: **distance, time, shielding, beam management, and situational awareness** (Table 12.3).

A. Beam management by the primary operator includes stepping on the pedal and producing x-rays only when necessary. The temptation to stay on the pedal or to inadvertently step on the pedal when no provider is looking at the image screen should be eliminated. This often requires a team effort and a willingness to remind the primary operator to stay "off of the x-ray" when this occurs. Collimating the x-ray beam to tightly image only the necessary anatomy reduces the intensity of stray radiation and increases the quality of the image. Use of low-dose or pulsed imaging is also a useful beam management tool that reduces radiation dose during the initial or final parts of some procedures.

B. Situational awareness includes providers and supporting staff knowing when the fluoroscopic unit is active. This is typically keyed by a light and a characteristic noise, but the primary operator should also state that he or she is ready to begin the imaging so that everyone in the room is aware. Typically there is a light on the outside of the endovascular room to alert those who may consider coming

Table 12.3.   Elements of practical radiation safety

Beam management

Situational awareness

Distance

Time

Shielding (structural and wearable)

into the room that imaging is taking place. The primary operator needs to be aware of the position of his or her technicians and other assistants in the room so that imaging does not occur while a nurse is tending to the patient in direct line or in close proximity of the x-ray beam.

C. Distance from the radiation source should be maximized understanding that doubling the distance from the source of radiation decreases the intensity fourfold. For example, increasing one's distance from the emitting beam from 1 to 2 meters decreases the intensity from 100 mGy/hr to 25 mGy/hr. Patient proximity to the image receiver or imaging intensifier is also important to consider. An increase in the distance between the patient and the image intensifier increases the required x-ray beam output and scatter. Positioning the patient close to the image intensifier (Fig. 12.1) is a easy way to reduce radiation requirements and exposure risk.

D. Time of radiation use is also a key component to operational safety and is closely related to beam management. Time in this context relates both to the operators' initiation of the x-ray beam and time that assisting staff are in areas of higher radiation risk. Familiarity with the system is important in order to maximize tools such as last image hold, replay, and adjuncts that can accentuate certain aspects of the previously taken and stored image. Use of these adjuncts maximizes clinical decision making with the fewest number of fluoroscopic images and radiation time. Finally, the alarm that sounds with each 5-minute interval of time should serve as a reminder for the primary operator that judicious use of fluoroscopic time is an important part of operational safety.

E. Shielding comes in all shapes and sizes, including fixed shields that come from above to rest between the primary operator and the patient and those that hang from the imaging table itself (Fig. 12.1). Shields should also be available for assisting staff members to stand behind during the imaging. Ideally, most team members should be able to provide their assistance (e.g., record the case log) outside of the imaging room. These individuals can enter the room to provide supplies or patient adjustments when the beam is off.

The lead apron, the mainstay of wearable shielding, is at least 0.5 mm thick and provides a barrier between the radiation source and the provider. This form of shielding should be updated occasionally and is ideally fitted to the individual. Shielding can be compromised if the apron is ill-fitted or outdated, as the lead shielding elements could be fractured. Most current two-piece aprons are considerably lighter than older models, offering more comfortable shielding with less associated musculoskeletal aches and pains. An extension of the lead apron is the thyroid shield, which should also be at least 0.5 mm thick and worn consistently during fluoroscopic procedures. Lead garments should ideally be imaged annually to look for cracks or defects in the shielding. Any defective shields should be updated. Leaded eyeglasses should complete the shielding assembly. Although their effectiveness in preventing radiation-induced cataracts may be debated, some form of protective eyewear is required for compliance with universal precautions and leaded glasses should be the component of choice.

SELECTED READING

Delichas M, Psarrakos K, Molyvda-Athanassopoulou E, Giannoglou G, Sioundas A, Hatziioannou K, et al. Radiation exposure to cardiologists performing interventional cardiology procedures. *Eur J Radiol*. 2003;48:268-273.

Lipsitz EC, Veith FJ, Ohki T, Heller S, Wain RA, Suggs WD, Lee JC, Kwei S, Goldstein K, Rabin J, Chang D, Mehta M. Does the endovascular repair of aortoiliac aneurysms pose a radiation safety hazard to vascular surgeons? *J Vasc Surg*. 2000;32:704-710.

Pei H, Cheng SWK, Wu PM, Ting ACW, Poon JTC, Cheng CKM, Mok JHM, Tsang MS. Ionizing radiation absorption of vascular surgeons during endovascular procedures. *J Vasc Surg*. 2007;46: 455-459.

Disease-Specific Logical Care Outlines

CHAPTER 13

Great Vessel and Carotid Occlusive Disease

Today, the incorporation of medical management and that of open and endovascular therapies for cerebrovascular disease makes the vascular specialist an integral member of the health care team treating these patients. The necessity of this involvement has been proven by the success of carotid, aortic arch branch, and vertebral artery revascularizations for the relief of symptomatic, stenotic, or ulcerated arterial lesions, aneurysms, and vascular tumors located in these vessels. The vascular and endovascular surgeon may also be consulted to evaluate patients with asymptomatic cerebrovascular disease, to provide a risk assessment as well as to help determine the appropriateness of intervention for stroke-risk reduction. Currently, evaluation and analysis of the selection and performance of carotid angioplasty and stenting (CAS) versus carotid endarterectomy (CEA) and medical management continues to alter the landscape in which extracranial cerebrovascular disease is treated.

In this chapter, common clinical presentations that suggest extracranial brachiocephalic, carotid, or vertebral artery disease are discussed. Certain principles of current care that facilitate an appropriate, smooth, and safe procedure for the patient are highlighted. Finally, the management of the most common early and late complications of carotid interventions is summarized.

I. **Common clinical scenarios.**
  A. **Symptomatic carotid disease.** Symptomatic carotid occlusive disease consists of **transient ischemic attacks (TIA)** and **stroke, or cerebrovascular accident (CVA)**. The socio-economic, health care administrative, and individual health care importance of stroke is clear. In the United States, over 700,000 cerebrovascular accidents occur annually and result in 160,000 deaths. In the United States there are roughly 4 million stroke survivors with varying degrees of disability and the yearly economic burden of stroke is around 45 million dollars. Worldwide stroke is the second leading cause of death, estimated to occur in just over 5 million people per year. Approximately two-thirds of cerebrovascular accidents are due to thromboembolic events, and extracranial atherosclerosis is

the major contributor. The anatomic distribution of cerebrovascular atherosclerosis has been studied, and the breakdown by location in those with disease is as follows: carotid bifurcation 38%, intracranial 33%, arch-branch based 9%, and proximal vertebral 20%.

1. **Symptom classification.** Classically, a **TIA** is defined as acute neurologic symptoms lasting less than 24 hours that completely resolve. However, the duration usually is measured in minutes, not hours. The term reversible ischemic neurologic deficit **(RIND)** has been used to describe neurologic symptoms that last longer than 24 hours but then rapidly resolve. **CVA** is defined as neurologic symptoms lasting longer than 24 hours with evident structural infarction. The term **crescendo TIA**, or stuttering TIA, is used when TIAs occur more frequently (progressive over 24–48 hours), yet there remains complete reversal of neurologic symptoms in between. **Stroke-in-evolution** is when there is no resolution of symptoms, but rather they wax and wane indicating ongoing neuron ischemia and neural tissue at risk of infarction. These are highly unstable situations. Symptoms reflective of thromboembolic events due to disease in the carotid artery or anterior circulation include hemiparesis, hemiparesthesias, transient monocular blindness **(amaurosis fugax),** or difficulties with speech **(aphasia).**

2. **Outcomes of TIA.** Approximately 75–80% of patients who suffer a stroke have had no type of preceding transient neurologic symptoms. However, the corollary is that if a patient experiences a TIA, the risk of stroke is significant. Studies have delineated a 30–50% 5-year risk of stroke once TIA occurs. In fact, recent evidence suggests that a significant proportion of this risk occurs within the first several weeks after TIA with, perhaps, a **10–25% risk of CVA within 1 month of the event**. Some have even suggested that 5–10% of this risk is within hours of the event. It is, thus, critical to identify and evaluate these patients. Unfortunately, TIAs are not specific for the presence of significant carotid artery stenosis or ulcerated plaques. Only about 50% of patients with TIAs will have a tight, or hemodynamically significant, carotid stenosis (<2 mm; ≥50%), occlusion, or ulcerated plaques. The remaining 50% of patients have thromboembolism from other sources such as the heart, aortic arch, intracranial vascular disease, or no clearly evident etiology. TIAs from alternate site thromboembolism or hypercoagulability also commonly lead to stroke. However, patients with no evident etiology for their TIAs and relatively normal carotid arteries on evaluation usually follow a more benign course; they seldom suffer a stroke.

TIAs may be either hemispheric or retinal in nature. In approximately 25% of patients presenting with symptomatic carotid bifurcation atheroma, visual disturbances are the presenting symptom. **Amaurosis fugax (AF)** is the most common of these ocular manifestations. Transient hemianopsias and other subtle visual field defects occur less frequently. Classic amaurosis is described as a "shade coming down over the eye" for a few seconds to minutes at a time and is due to embolism to the ophthalmic artery. While the natural history of AF is somewhat more benign than hemispheric TIAs it is still significant. The stroke risk once AF arises is roughly 6–8% per year, or roughly half that in those with cerebral TIAs. And, in those experiencing visual symptoms due to cerebrovascular disease, a significant group (25%) will ultimately suffer permanent visual loss.

3. Stroke recurrence. The importance of identifying those with CVA and cerebrovascular atherosclerosis, particularly within the extracranial arteries, is due to the significance of stroke recurrence. Without treatment, those with CVA will have another stroke at a rate of between 10–20% per year, thus the 5-year gross risk is somewhere between 50% and 100%. The mortality associated with this second CVA is a staggering 35%, and events beyond the second are more than 60%. Hence, the institution of therapy is imperative.

4. Unusual presentations and symptoms of cerebrovascular disease. Rarely, deterioration in visual acuity may be due to chronic ocular ischemia (COI). Severe bilateral occlusive disease leads to a supply/demand mismatch in the retina with an increase in metabolic demand. COI is the name of the constellation of signs and symptoms related to this. Findings may include eye pain, venous stasis retinopathy, central or branch retinal artery occlusions from stagnant flow, ischemic optic neuropathy, narrowed retinal arteries, retinal microaneurysms, retinal hemorrhages, iris neovasularization (**rubeosis iridis**) with neovascular acute angle glaucoma, iris atrophy, corneal edema, and cataracts. This syndrome only occurs in 3–4% of those with cerebrovascular disease. Without treatment permanent blindness occurs uniformly. Another rare ocular symptom that may occur is "**bright light amaurosis fugax**." This occurs because of the poor retinal blood flow causing complete white out blindness when the retina is stressed, such as going outside into the sunlight. Frequently, the vascular specialist may be asked to comment on the presence of **Hollenhorst plaques** and retinal artery occlusions seen on fundus examination without evidence of COI. Less than 10% of these patients will have significant carotid stenosis ipsilateral to these findings.

There are a few other uncommon symptoms of cerebrovascular disease that may be attributed to significant carotid occlusive disease. One is jaw claudication with eating due to poor ECA flow to the masseter muscle. Focal seizure activity has been noted due to atheroembolism from carotid artery disease. Pre-syncope or syncope, sometimes called drop-attacks and cognitive impairments, may rarely occur secondary to poor perfusion from significant bilateral cerebrovascular disease.

B. Asymptomatic carotid disease. Extracranial cerebrovascular disease may also be identified in those who have no symptoms directly attributable to their arterial stenoses. Overall, only 1% of the population over the age of 65 harbors carotid occlusive disease. Yet, when focusing upon those with cardiovascular risk factors such as hypertension, hyperlipidemia, and cardiac disease this figure rises substantially to nearly 20%. This is the reasoning behind cerebrovascular screening programs, which allow recognition of those at highest risk of stroke, followed by the initiation of therapy for stroke-risk reduction. The most common initiating event for those undergoing evaluation for asymptomatic carotid stenosis is bruit on physical examination. **Carotid bruits** are present in approximately 5% of the general population over 50 years of age. However, only 23% of bruits are found to be associated with a hemodynamically significant stenosis (≥50%), and less than half of significant stenoses occur in the presence of a bruit. There is no correlation between the loudness of a bruit and the degree of narrowing. Thus, a bruit is neither sensitive, nor specific for significant carotid stenosis; still, with the ease of noninvasive imaging, the status of the carotid artery when a bruit is detected is relatively simple. A neck bruit may originate from the carotid arteries or be transmitted from the aortic arch or heart, such as with transmitted murmurs (Fig. 13.1).

Also, not infrequently, vascular specialists are asked to consult on patients with atypical symptoms, and noninvasive imaging is performed to establish the status of the carotid arteries. Usually, the symptoms are found to be unrelated to the carotid arteries, yet a stenosis is identified. When asymptomatic carotid stenoses are identified, some 10–15% will progress to a severe category. Therefore, the management of those

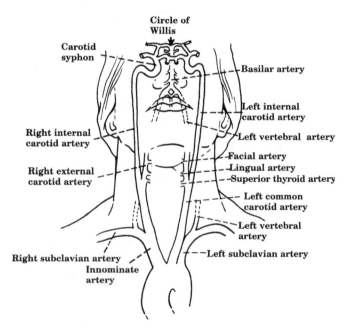

Figure 13.1.   Anatomy of the aortic arch and extracranial cervical arteries. The internal carotid artery has no branches in the neck.

with asymptomatic carotid artery stenosis has become a very germane issue.

II. **Imaging of cerebrovascular disease.**

A. **Duplex ultrasound.** With the advent of noninvasive vascular laboratories and the establishment of duplex ultrasonography, this is the initial imaging modality of choice for most patients in which a diagnosis of carotid artery disease is entertained (see Chapter 6). Duplex ultrasound combines brightness-mode (B-mode) ultrasound with pulsed-wave Doppler to produce a real time gray-scale image of the arteries, as well as spectral analysis of flow (Figure 13.2). Many criteria have been espoused that attempt to identify and quantify the degree of carotid stenosis using duplex ultrasound. This is an ongoing process and requires regular correlation with other imaging modalities in order to solidify each noninvasive laboratory's exactness. When performed by skilled vascular technologists, this imaging approach is quick, sensitive, specific, and highly accurate, and also carries no risk. Indirect evidence of arch-based and intracranial stenosis may be present but no direct imaging in these areas is possible. Transcranial Doppler may be performed in conjunction to further ascertain intracranial disease, but it cannot delineate lesion anatomy or true disease burden. The authors use the modified University of Washington criteria (Table 13.1). A greater understanding and study of duplex ultrasound in carotid occlusive disease, as well as its ease, has led to sensible surveillance regimens in those with cerebrovascular disease. This is now standard practice both in those found with moderate carotid stenosis and after carotid surgery (Table 13.2).

B. **Computed tomography (CT/CTA) and magnetic resonance arteriography (MRI/MRA).** Anatomic definition and direct imaging of the brain, intracranial vasculature, arch-branches, and aortic arch are valuable benefits of CTA and MRA (Fig. 13.2). Up to 10% of the time, arch-branch based disease is found to be present. In 2–5% of carotid bifurcation stenoses, either a tandem intracranial stenosis or intracranial aneurysm exists distal to the carotid lesion. Further, the status of the brain and recent or past CVA can be identified, which is particularly important in symptomatic cerebrovascular disease. With CTA, infarction cannot always be identified immediately as it often takes 24 to 48 hours for evidence of stroke to be present using this imaging modality. A benefit of CTA is the imaging of intracranial bleeding. Atherosclerotic calcification can limit CTA's ability to characterize stenoses. MRA, on the other hand, using diffusion weighted technology, can illustrate and describe infarction immediately. A drawback to MRA is its notorious overrepresentation of stenoses. This is due to the fact MR technology depends on electron polar changes with magnetic field pulses. In standard magnetic resonance, blood flow is thus represented as signal dropout or a black appearance, since electrons do not stay in one place in the blood. If not timed appropriately, flow attributes may not be portrayed correctly, so this technology is highly institution and personnel dependent.

C. **Arteriography.** The stroke risk associated with cerebrovascular arteriography is 1–2%. Access site and other com-

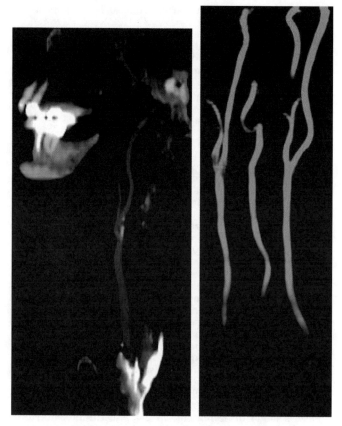

Figure 13.2.   CTA/MRA: Reconstructed CTA of the left carotid system *(left)*. **MRA of bilateral carotid bifurcations** *(right)*. **CTA, computed tomography; MRA, magnetic resonance arteriography.**

plications can occur in up to 3%, which led to the development of other less invasive methods of imaging. Yet, there remain several situations where arteriography is helpful and finalizes cerebrovascular imaging. These include discordant or unreliable noninvasive studies, a high carotid bifurcation, no clear lesion endpoint seen, concern for either intracranial or arch-based/great vessel disease, the possibility of nonatherosclerotic etiologies of disease, suspected posterior circulation disease as the symptom cause, recurrent stenosis, and the potential indication for endovascular treatment such as CAS or vertebral origin stenting.

III. Treatment of carotid occlusive disease.

A. Medical therapy. Risk factor modification is clearly indicated in patients with cerebrovascular disease (see Chapter 7). Many already have risk reduction therapies in place for hyper-

Table 13.1. Modified Washington duplex criteria

Stenosis	PSV	EDV	Spectrum
Normal	<125 cm/s		Normal with no plaque
1–15% (B)	<125 cm/s		Normal with plaque
16–49% (C)	<125 cm/s		Broadening
50–79% (D)	>125 cm/s	<140 cm/s	Broadening
80–99% (D+)	>125 cm/s	>140 cm/s	Broadening
Occluded (E)	No flow	No flow	No flow

PSV, peak systolic velocity; EDV, end diastolic velocity; cm/s, centimeters per second; CCA, common carotid artery; ICA, internal carotid artery; ECA, external carotid artery.
EDV: 80cm/s ~ 60%; 100 cm/s ~ 70%
ICA:CCA PSV ratio: 3.2 ~ 60%; 4.0 ~ 70%

tension, hyperlipidemia, and coronary artery disease at the time of diagnosis of carotid, great vessel, and vertebral artery disease due to the association with other cardiovascular processes. Statin therapy has been shown to be beneficial in carotid occlusive disease both in primary and post-procedural roles. Antiplatelet drugs such as aspirin and clopidogrel retard platelet aggregation and may prevent microemboli that cause TIAs and strokes. This has made these agents critical components of maintenance therapy after neurologic events and diagnosis of asymptomatic stenosis. Aspirin reduces the risk of continuing TIAs, stroke, and death by approximately 20%, compared to controls. In a randomized, blinded trial of clopidogrel (Plavix, Sanofi Pharmaceuticals, Inc., New York, NY, U.S.A.) versus aspirin in patients at risk of ischemic events (CAPRIE), clopidogrel (75 mg daily) reduced the relative risk for ischemic stroke, myocardial infarction and vascular death by 24%. After carotid endarterectomy, antiplatelet therapy reduces risk of stroke and to a lesser degree restenosis. It appears likely that antiplatelet therapies modestly reduce the risk of stroke in both symptomatic and asymptomatic individuals with cere-

Table 13.2. Standard carotid surveillance protocol

Clinical Group	Frequency of Surveillance Duplex
B lesion and C lesion	Every 1–2 years
D lesion without CEA	Every 6 months
Post CEA	Every 6 months for 2 years, then yearly or based on contralateral stenosis
Contralateral carotid occlusion	Every 6 months
Post CAS	Every 6 months

CEA, carotid endarterectomy; CAS, carotid angioplasty and stenting.

brovascular disease, and are indicated with minimal bleeding risk.

Heparin or warfarin sodium (Coumadin, DuPont Pharmaceuticals Company, Wilmington, DE, U.S.A.) can also control TIAs in at least 90% of patients with recent onset. Warfarin also has proved effective in reducing serious cerebral infarct from 45% in untreated patients to 24% in treated individuals over 5 years. Of course, the main disadvantage of long-term Coumadin therapy is compliance and bleeding complications in about 15% of patients. Indeed, the current recommendations from the multispecialty guidelines council has recommended heparin not be used in acute stroke due to the hemorrhagic risk.

B. Surgical therapy. Perhaps nothing in vascular disease has been scrutinized more closely than CEA. During CEA the carotid artery is clamped and opened, and the atherosclerotic plaque is removed. Large, multicenter prospective, randomized trials comparing this operation plus antiplatelet therapy to antiplatelet therapy alone have provided many insights into this surgical option. In patients with a hemodynamically significant carotid stenosis, who have had a TIA or a stabilized, nondisabling stroke and are candidates for operation, CEA reduces the risk of recurrent stroke. This was clarified in both the **North American Symptomatic Carotid Endarterectomy Trial (NASCET)** and the **European Carotid Surgery trial (ECST)**. The **Veterans Affairs Trial 309 (VA 309)** also found a trend favoring surgery, but was halted when the initial results of NASCET and ECST were reported. NASCET's evaluation of those with high-grade (≥70%) stenosis was stopped early as the risk of stroke at 2 years was 26% versus 9% (p<0.001), and mortality 12% versus 5% (p<0.01), in the medical and surgical arms, respectively. Stroke-risk reduction increased as the degree of stenosis became greater. Thus, those with the most significant degree of stenosis gleaned the highest degree of absolute benefit. For those with carotid stenosis of 50–69%, NASCET revealed a significant reduction in ipsilateral stroke (15.7% vs. 22.2%; $p = 0.045$) and any stroke or death (33.3% vs. 43.3%; $p = 0.005$) at CEA 5 years. Although still statistically noteworthy, the absolute risk reduction was less than in those with higher-grade stenoses and was not as evident until the later points of follow-up.

In ECST and the VA 309 similar outcomes were found. Data generated from the pooling of these three trials has confirmed the stepwise augmentation in stroke-risk reduction with CEA by increasing stenosis degree. Carotid stenosis of 50% was confirmed to be the point at which CEA yields significant absolute 5-year stroke-risk reduction compared with medical therapy. Above 60–70% was the degree to which significant 3-year absolute stroke-risk reduction occurred. Benefits of CEA in the symptomatic prospective, randomized trials appear to be greatest in men, those with recent stroke, and hemispheric symptoms.

When symptomatic patients are encountered, several questions can lead to sensible management.

1. Is there a significant carotid stenosis? The imaging modalities discussed earlier are used. Duplex ultrasound is the first-line modality, which helps to delineate degrees of carotid stenosis and important plaque characteristics such as ulceration, as well as indirectly attempting to find evidence of proximal arch-based disease and poor vertebrobasilar flow. Additionally, the anatomic location of the carotid bifurcation and the presence of an identifiable lesion endpoint with normal appearing distal internal carotid artery (ICA) are important features. The spectral analysis of flow may reveal a resistive pattern suggesting distal intracranial disease. In many patients, particularly those with TIA, carotid duplex scanning may provide enough anatomic and functional information to proceed with CEA without alternative imaging.

If any feature of the cerebrovascular circulation is not well appreciated, or there is concern for recent stroke, alternative noninvasive imaging is indicated. This may consist of an MRA or a CTA. Findings that may necessitate carotid arteriography after duplex and/or CTA/MRA are as follows: discordant or unreliable noninvasive studies (i.e., the studies conflict one another), a high carotid bifurcation precluding complete duplex imaging, absence of a visible lesion distal endpoint on duplex or CTA/MRA, concern for tandem disease in the intracranial or intrathoracic carotid segments, suspicion of posterior circulation disease and/or the presence of recurrent stenosis months or years following CEA. In one or more of these instances, arteriography will finalize imaging and evaluation of the degree of stenosis and lesion morphology. Today, some of these features may lead to endovascular therapies such as CAS at the time of diagnostic arteriography.

2. Are the symptoms actually consistent with TIA or CVA, or some other neurologic or psychosomatic complaint? Are they attributable to events ipsilateral to the carotid stenosis? These questions are not always easy to answer. As noted, carotid distribution symptoms classically include unilateral hemiparsis, hemiparesthesias, speech disturbance, or amaurosis fugax. The symptoms that present confusion in determining whether a true TIA, or potential CVA, is being experienced are atypical complaints, especially dizziness, lightheadedness, presyncope, and unsteady gait. These posterior circulation type symptoms are rather common in elderly patients who may experience postural hypotension when arising quickly from a lying, sitting, or stooping position and other etiologies that produce these sensations. If a psychosomatic problem is suspected, a careful inquiry about family or work situations may disclose emotional stress that initiates the symptoms. If the patient is unsure of the symptoms, a family member who may have observed an attack can be very helpful.

3. Are the neurologic symptoms chronic and stable or repetitive and progressive, and has the patient had a stroke? If they represent TIA and are not suggestive of CVA and are not progressive, a more elective/urgent outpatient evaluation is appropriate. Remember, however, the newer, more worrying up-front risks of TIA. If the symptoms are concerning for a new or recent stroke or are progressive and repetitive, suggesting either crescendo TIA or stroke-in-evolution, immediate or urgent assessment is indicated. Thorough evaluation for TIAs may also require electrocardiographic monitoring (Holter monitor) to detect arrhythmias or echocardiography to rule out diseased heart valves or mural thrombus. Transesophageal echocardiography may also reveal ulcerative atherosclerosis of the aortic arch as a source of thromboemboli in some patients. Moreover, electroencephalography (EEG) is appropriate if a seizure disorder is suspected. Consultation with a neurologist or ophthalmologist may be helpful in evaluating patients if atypical neurologic or retinal symptoms are present. In those with atypical symptoms, or concern for stroke, computed tomography (CT/CTA) or MRI/MRA of the brain is useful to not only better clarify the extent of cerebrovascular disease, but to identify stroke and check for hemorrhage. MRI with diffusion weighting is particularly useful for this. It can identify stroke immediately while CT takes several days for the stroke to be evident.

If the patient has had a stroke, particular aspects are relevant to possible intervention and surgical therapy. First, it is important to understand how significant and debilitating the CVA has been and if there is still brain tissue at risk for infarction. In those with dense, complete deficits such as hemiplegia and/or loss of speech, it makes little sense to put the patient at risk for an operation if there is little hemispheric function left to lose. Indeed, the prospective, randomized trials studying CEA for symptomatic patients only included those with TIAs and "nondisabling" stroke. Poor outcomes due to hemorrhagic conversion in those with stroke and immediate surgical intervention were encountered before CT and MR technology were developed. Since that time, there has been much controversy with regard to radiographic features of CVA and the timing of CEA. No clear consensus has been reached with regard to the timing of CEA following hemispheric stroke. What is clear is that the larger the CVA the more likely the patient is to have a permanent deficit. If there is any evidence of parenchymal hemorrhage associated with the stroke, or it is larger than 2–3 centimeters in size, it is probably wise to wait 4 weeks before CEA. If the stroke is small without hemorrhage, an earlier operation (within 14 days) can be performed.

Fortunately, scenarios where more emergent intervention is necessary are rare. Those with **crescendo TIA** should be immediately hospitalized for anticoagulation with heparin (loading dose of 5,000 to 10,000 units, with a continuous hourly infusion of 750 to 1,000 units) to achieve an aPTT of 60–90 seconds or an antifactor Xa level of 0.4-0.7 IU/ml. If the patient's condition is stable, an urgent MRA or CTA in conjunction with a duplex ultrasound usually is performed within 24 hours after admission. Arteriography is indicated if previously discussed features are present. Operative candidates with severe (>70%) carotid stenosis or shaggy, mobile, irregular ulcerative plaques undergo carotid endarterectomy when the surgical and anesthesia teams are optimized.

Management is more difficult if the neurologic symptoms are progressing, or waxing and waning, without complete resolution. These patients should be considered to have a **stroke-in-evolution**. Anticoagulation and emergent duplex ultrasound followed by immediate carotid surgery for severe carotid lesions and those with ominous plaque features may reduce the stroke severity and mortality in this group. However, the differentiation between a **stroke-in-evolution** and **completed stroke** is not always clear. This aggressive surgical strategy for crescendo TIA and stroke-in-evolution is related to a poor stroke and mortality rate with medical therapy alone in these patients. The reported mortality with these events is 50–80%, with up to 75% of survivors having a moderate to severe permanent neurologic deficit. Less than 5–10% will completely recover. With the institution of the treatment paradigm described, perioperative stroke and death rates of approximately 10–20% can be anticipated. While this is a considerable event rate after CEA it may be the patient's best alternative. Also, **treatment of acute ischemic stroke with intravenous thrombolytic therapy (tissue-type plasminogen activator) is approved for selected patients with no evidence of intracranial hemorrhage or other contraindications when started within 3 hours of onset of symptoms.**
4. What is the patient's operative risk? Combined 30-day mortality and stroke in NASCET and ECST was 5.6% and 7.0%, respectively. In general, stroke/death rates for CEA in symptomatic patients should be 5–6% or less in order for the operation to make stroke-risk reduction sense. If the patient is a poor surgical risk from a comorbidity standpoint, carotid angioplasty and stenting can be entertained. Antiplatelet and/or Coumadin therapy are medical alternatives that may be considered in this difficult scenario. Surgery or intervention should be reconsidered if antithrombotic/anticoagulant therapy fails to control the TIAs.

Based upon obtained imaging and surgical candidates with classic anterior circulation, carotid territory TIAs, or nondisabling stroke, we recommend CEA along with antiplatelet therapy for surgical correction of a stenotic plaque with ≥70% diameter reduction that correlates with the exhibited symptoms. In those with 50–69% diameter reduction, a more circumspect approach is used owing to the more modest risk reduction at later time points. If the patient clearly is healthy and has significant longevity, whereby they will glean the benefits that an operation can provide, CEA is undertaken. Other considerations causing us to lean toward surgical therapy include plaque morphology, such as ulceration or shaggy thrombus, contralateral ICA occlusion, and male gender, all of which may portend an increase in stroke risk for symptomatic patients. In those with less than 50% stenosis in the carotid artery, operation is not indicated except in very rare instances of ominous plaque morphology.

C. Surgical therapy in asymptomatic patients. The rationale for prophylactic carotid endarterectomy for high-grade asymptomatic carotid stenosis began with the classic observations of Dr. Jesse Thompson of Dallas, Texas. In his nonoperated group, 26.8% eventually had TIAs, 15.2% experienced a nonfatal stroke, and 2.2% had a fatal stroke. On the other hand, 90% of operated patients remained asymptomatic. Only 4.5% of the operated patients developed TIAs and 2.3% experienced a nonfatal stroke.

Subsequently, Strandness and colleagues at the University of Washington used duplex prospectively to study the natural history of carotid arterial disease in asymptomatic patients with carotid bruits. The presence of or progression to a greater than 80% internal carotid stenosis was highly correlated with development of TIA, stroke, and asymptomatic internal carotid occlusion in 46% of patients compared to those lesions of 0% to 79% stenosis (1.5%). The majority of adverse events occurred within 6 months of the findings of an 80% to 99% stenosis.

Trials comparing surgical and medical therapy for carotid stenoses in those without symptoms have also been accomplished. The risk of stroke with both medical therapy and operation is less in patients who are asymptomatic. Overall, the **Asymptomatic Carotid Atherosclerosis Study (ACAS), The Veteran's Affairs Asymptomatic Carotid Stenosis study, and the Asymptomatic Carotid Surgery Trial (ACST)**, have indicated that in those with ≥60% asymptomatic stenosis, the risk of CVA at 5 years with antiplatelet therapy alone is 9–12%, or roughly 1.5–2% per year. With CEA added to antiplatelet therapy, this risk is reduced by half to 1% per year or 4–6% at 5 years. In ACAS, all in the surgical arm were required to undergo arteriography, yet some did not. In those who did, the risk of stroke with cerebral arteriography was 1.2%. The 30-day risk of stroke and death in the CEA group was 2.3% and this was estimated to be 2.7% if all had an arteriogram. Thus, arteriography accounted for about half of asymptomatic perioperative events. In the ACST, enrollment was based upon duplex ultrasound. Arteriography was not required but some did undergo arteriography prior to CEA. The 30-day stroke and death rate was 2.8% in the surgical arm and 3.1% in all CEA procedures. As with the symptomatic trials, benefit with operation was not suggested in women.

Several points should be highlighted. First, duplex ultrasonography is an important diagnostic tool in asymptomatic patients, particularly when able to be used as a single modality prior to carotid surgery or to select those in whom the risk of arteriography is acceptable. It is worth noting that duplex criteria suggesting a stensois of ≥80% correlated with an arteriographic lesion of 60% in ACAS. Second, the yearly risk of stroke in those with no symptoms is small. While the relative-risk reduction obtained with CEA is on the order of 50%, absolute stroke-risk reduction is only 1–2% per year. Therefore, to gain advantage from operation patients must be selected well. They must be otherwise healthy and have a life expectancy of at least 5 years. Lastly, women must be looked at with some skepticism when evaluating them for prophylactic CEA and compelling reasons must be present. We believe that CEA in asymptomatic individuals with a carotid stenosis of over 60% is an essential component of therapy, particularly in men and those without considerable cardiac, pulmonary, renal, or other comorbidity, and the duplex ultrasound suggests the lesion to be 80%. This remains true only when the perioperative stroke and death rate can be 3% or less. Some physicians may be hesitant to recommend CEA for asymptomatic patients, but the natural history of this group does not appear to support this approach in otherwise healthy adults with good life expectancy.

D. Controversies in carotid occlusive disease.
   1. Asymptomatic ulcerated plaque. The natural history of asymptomatic ulcerated carotid lesions is not easy to define. Carotid ulceration is difficult to detect with duplex ultrasound and is usually large when seen with this modality. This imaging technique can define plaque morphology (homogeneous versus heterogeneous), but these characteristics do not always correlate with surface ulceration. Despite these limitations, some reports suggest that echolucent plaque, detectable by duplex ultrasound, increases the likelihood of future symptoms. Recent technological advances have improved duplex resolution, but it remains overall a somewhat insensitive method to characterize ulceration. Arteriography also is not particularly accurate in defining ulceration, which may vary from a slight nonstenotic irregularity to a complicated ulcerated stenosis.
   While carotid atherosclerotic ulceration has been shown to correlate independently with neurologic symptoms, the risk associated with lesions found in those who are asymptomatic remains somewhat controversial. Dr. Wesley Moore and colleagues classified asymptomatic ulcers without associated hemodynamically significant stenoses by their two-dimensional area on lateral arteriography: A, less than 10 mm^2 ; B, 10–40 mm^2 ; C, more than 40 mm^2 . They found the yearly risk of stroke was less than 0.5% for A ulcers, 4.5% for B ulcers, and 7.5% for C ulcers. CEA was recommended for C lesions, and for B lesions if the patient was a reasonable operative candidate with good life expectancy. In general, ulceration may predict increased risk of neurologic events and should be considered in the treatment plan for those with carotid occlusive disease.
   2. Is a patient with cerebrovascular disease scheduled for other major surgery? Controversy continues over whether patients with asymptomatic carotid stenoses are at increased risk for perioperative stroke at the time of other major surgery, especially any operation in which prolonged hypotension may occur. The major surgery of most concern has been cardiac and aortic operations. Many perioperative strokes occur in patients who were not suspected of having carotid disease prior to surgery. These strokes also are more commonly diffuse than focal. Less than 2% of patients with no prior stroke or TIA undergoing major general or cardiovascular surgery suffer a perioperative stroke.

With a history of prior neurologic event this rate may increase to 4–6%. In those with a known hemodynamically significant carotid stenosis, the stroke risk for major surgery is 3%. With bilateral ≥50% carotid stenosis, this risk may increase to 4–5%. This risk can be as high as 7–9% in those undergoing coronary artery bypass grafting (CABG) with either carotid occlusion or prior stroke.

How then to proceed in patients undergoing major surgery with carotid occlusive disease? First, noninvasive carotid testing is performed to determine the hemodynamic significance of the carotid stenosis if this is not known. It is well established that there is little stroke risk in those undergoing general surgery if the patient is asymptomatic, and they should proceed to the intended operation. A caveat may be poorly compensated lesions, such as asymptomatic, severe bilateral disease, particularly in those in which the general surgery caries no immediacy. These should be surgically corrected before elective vascular surgery is attempted. The authors' stance has been to entertain carotid revascularization on at least one side prior to major general surgery. It seems logical to carry out CEA prior to any other surgery in those who are CEA candidates and would otherwise undergo carotid endarterectomy as this may, perhaps, negate any possible risk. This approach is unproven.

The issues surrounding those with cerebrovascular disease requiring heart operations, such as coronary artery bypass or valve replacement, deserve special mention. Roughly half of strokes during CABG in those with a significant carotid stenosis are ipsilateral to narrowing and can be attributed to its presence. This special situation is confounded by the ability to perform these procedures in a combined fashion. In centers that carry out many combined CEAs with cardiac surgical procedures, the results are acceptable and can be quite good. However, this is not generalizable, and most evaluations suggest the stroke/MI and death rate with staged procedures are likely superior to combining them. The first principle dictates to treat the symptomatic vascular territory first. Combined procedures are reserved for patients symptomatic in both territories, or those with severe bilateral asymptomatic carotid disease or contralateral ICA occlusion. Most surgeons agree that patients with symptomatic carotid disease should have CEA before other elective surgery is performed.

3. Asymptomatic contralateral carotid artery stenosis. Another controversial area in carotid surgery is the management of patients with the asymptomatic contralateral carotid artery stenosis following a carotid endarterectomy. These patients may be at increased risk of TIAs and stroke. The outcome of such lesions again may depend on the hemodynamic significance of the asymptomatic lesion. Conservative management of nonoperated vessels opposite an endarterectomy appears appropriate until symptoms develop or a lesion greater than 80% is detected. We generally repair a hemodynamically significant contralateral carotid stenosis as a staged procedure. The endarterectomies are performed at least 5 to 7 days apart, although most patients require a longer recovery period between operations. If the contralateral stenosis is not hemodynamically significant, if the patient is not a good surgical risk, or if the first endarterectomy was complicated by cranial nerve injury, we follow the patient until symptoms occur or noninvasive studies document progression of the stenosis.

Study of duplex after CEA has informed us of several things. Progression of carotid stenoses is not uncommon and mandates surveillance in order to identify those who do progress. Further, flow velocity characteristics of the carotid artery contralateral to a severe carotid stenosis or occlusion may be artificially elevated due to increased blood flow demand on the "more open" side. The degree of stenosis by flow criteria may actually be lessened after CEA of the severe, contralateral side.

4. Acute internal carotid artery occlusion. It is uncertain whether thromboendarterectomy of an occluded internal carotid artery is advisable. Certainly, surgical repair of a thrombosed internal carotid artery in the setting of a completed stroke may be associated with intracranial hemorrhage and a high mortality risk. The natural history of untreated carotid occlusion is still debated. Approximately 25% of patients have TIAs, and 10% to 20% have a stroke with occlusion. Many patients, however, remain asymptomatic. Anticoagulation for 3–6 months followed by antiplatelet therapy remains the mainstay of the treatment paradigm.

A few reports indicate that thromboendarterectomy of a totally occluded internal carotid artery can be achieved with a reasonable morbidity and mortality rate and a 65% to 70% overall patency in severely symptomatic patients. Some have suggested that although the morbidity and mortality of operation in this setting is higher than without occlusion, these outcomes are better than without surgery. Not everyone agrees with this. Retrograde filling of the ipsilateral intracranial internal carotid artery to its petrous or cavernous segment appears to be a good sign of operability. Timing of such surgery seems critical. Operation within 4 hours of acute symptoms has been recommended if this course of action is entertained.

An uncommon approach to management of the persistently symptomatic patient with an occluded internal carotid artery is external carotid artery (ECA) endarterectomy. ECA revascularization may relieve symptoms by increasing both the total and regional cerebral blood flow. The best results of external carotid endarterectomy are achieved when it is performed in the setting of an ipsilateral internal carotid artery occlusion and external carotid artery stenosis with demonstrated "internalization" of the ECA on duplex spectral flow analysis and identification of intracranial collateralization of the ECA on arteriography. In this setting, this procedure is usually performed to relieve retinal symptoms such as retinal TIA, bright light amaurosis, rubeosis iritis, or neovascular glaucoma. The ECA-ICA collaterals develop in the periorbital area to the ophthalmic artery, temporal area via leptomenigeal branches, and the dural vessels.

Finally, symptomatic patients with total internal carotid occlusion also may be relieved by extracranial-to-intracranial (EC-IC) anastomosis of the temporal artery to the middle cerebral artery. EC-IC bypasses generally are performed by a neurosurgeon experienced in microsurgical technique. We continue to see gratifying results in rare, select patients. However, the international randomized EC-IC bypass study failed to confirm that EC-IC anastomosis is effective in preventing ischemic stroke in patients with atherosclerotic disease in the carotid and middle cerebral arteries. Consequently, EC-IC bypass is rarely performed anymore. However, resurgence of its theoretical benefits in certain situations has led to prospective, randomized trials currently ongoing in difficult cerebrovascular cases. It remains a mainstay in the rare, surgical treatment of progressively symptomatic ICA dissection when extracranial reconstruction becomes prohibitive.

E. CAS. Although the medical and surgical treatment of carotid occlusive disease has been well studied and effective treatment paradigms developed, the last decade has seen the emergence of endovascular therapies as an alternative for treatment of cerebrovascular diseases. **CAS** has been promoted as the preferred option in those who are "high-risk" for CEA. There has been much debate as to what constitutes high-risk individuals in this relatively low-risk operation, and ongoing deliberations focus on what clinical factors may produce a scenario when CAS may be favored over other modalities of treatment.

To this end many investigations have focused on noninferiority of CAS versus CEA in certain patient subgroups. Problems with these have been encountered, and center around differences in indications and devices used. Most have been industry sponsored and are specific to stent and embolic protection devices, in addition to combining endpoints and patient presentations. The most stirring study to date is the Stenting and Angioplasty with Protection in Patients at High Risk for Endarterectomy **(SAPPHIRE)** trial. This study was supported by Cordis Endovascular (a branch of Johnson & Johnson) and Cordis stents and embolic protection devices were used. It pitted CEA against CAS with embolic protection in those who were symptomatic with a $\geq 50\%$ stenosis or asymptomatic with a $\geq 80\%$, and had features that would place them at high risk for CEA. The main outcomes of stroke and death were not statistically different at 30 days and 1 year, thus CAS was not found to be inferior to CEA. However, when this endpoint was combined further to include MI, there was a trend favoring CAS in the perioperative 30-day period, and this added to the incidence of stroke or death in 1 year was reported to favor CAS (12% vs. 20%; $p = 0.05$). The occurrence of cranial nerve palsies was significantly less with CAS and the need for revascularization of the carotid artery within 1 year of the treatment was statistically higher in those receiving CEA (4.6% vs. 0.7%; $p = 0.04$).

This seems to indicate that CAS is competitive with CEA in the early and midterm treatment of carotid stenosis (Fig. 13.3). Against the background of conflict in the prior literature, the U. S. Food and Drug Administration used this report to usher in the era of approval of CAS devices. There are justified criticisms of SAPPHIRE concerning both the trial endpoints and the enrollment process, but this is the best information we have to date. The late stroke-risk reduction achieved and the later restenosis with stenting remain unknown. These are critical pieces of information that are needed as the physiologic outcome of CEA and CAS may ultimately be different. CEA removes the embolic source and relies on appropriate and "normal" healing of the endarterectomy and CAS pushes, opens, and constrains the embolic source against the diseased arterial wall.

Stroke after CAS seems to occur more often in the contralateral hemisphere compared to CEA, which is likely due to arch manipulation. Embolic protection devices do make a difference in the embolic rate during CAS. **Current indications for CAS** are being better defined (Table 13.3). Anatomic factors in the carotid artery, aortic arch, descending aorta, and iliofemoral systems are very germane and may alter, or support, one treatment plan over another. Other issues, such as prior neck pathology requiring radiation or tracheostomy, are more easily dealt with using CAS. Those with poor cardiopulmonary reserve may be better served with CAS. If the procedure seems anatomically feasible with minimal structural prohibitions, certain indications have become clearer. Restenosis, prior radical

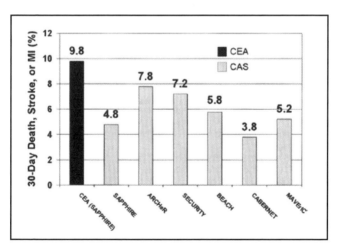

Figure 13.3.   Representative outcomes of industry-supported carotid angioplasty and stenting trials. (Needs Permission: From Narins CR, Illig KA. Patient selection for carotid stenting versus endarterectomy: A systematic review. *J Vasc Surg*. 2006;44:661-672.)

Table 13.3.   **Current recommendations and potential preferences for CAS vs. CEA**

CEA strongly recommended	CEA Preferred	CAS Preferred	CAS Strongly Recommended
Age >80 y	Inability to use EPD	High carotid bifurcation	Prior neck radiation
	Difficult aortic arch or carotid anatomy	Recurrent stenosis	Prior radical neck surgery
		Neck immobility	Tracheostomy stoma
	Difficult vascular access	Significant cardiac or pulmonary disease	
		Contralateral recurrent laryngeal nerve dysfunction	

CEA, carotid endarterectomy; CAS, carotid angioplasty and stenting; EPD, embolic protection device.

(From Narins CR, Illig KA. Patient selection for carotid stenting versus endarterectomy: A systematic review. *J Vasc Surg.* 2006;44:661-672.)

neck surgery, an adverse neck due to tracheostomy and/ or radiation, high carotid bifurcations at the C1-2 level making surgical exposure difficult, and significant cardiopulmonary comorbidities are reasons to proceed with CAS. It also appears that those patients who are 80 years of age or older do worse with CAS. This may be due to more atherosclerotic disease and arch angulation in older people.

IV. Vertebrobasilar insufficiency (VBI). Symptoms of **VBI** are characterized by ischemic events in the midbrain and cerebellum. These include ataxia, dysarthria, diplopia, dysphagia, vertigo, dizziness, drop attacks and gray outs with head rotation, instability of the patient in the upright position, visual changes, and bilateral paresthesias with occasional paresis. These may result from emboli (vertebrobasilar TIAs, or thromboembolic VBI) or hypoperfusion of the basilar artery and its branches (hemodynamic VBI). Overall, it appears that hemodynamic VBI is more common. Stroke in the posterior circulation accounts for 25% of CVAs and the risks of stroke and related mortality after verterbrobasilar TIA appear similar to that of the carotid territory. However, vertebrobasilar stenosis and its treatment are much less well studied in contrast to the anterior circulation and carotid occlusive disease.

Left subclavian stenosis proximal to the left vertebral artery or stenosis of the origin of either vertebral artery may decrease vertebrobasilar flow. Additionally, only half of individuals have a "normal" circle of Willis and collateral intracranial circulation between the anterior and posterior supplies may be compromised. Thus, hemodynamic VBI is especially likely to occur when carotid occlusive disease along with either vertebrobasilar or subclavian stenosis is present and collateral flow via the circle of Willis is inadequate.

In such cases, we generally repair the carotid lesions first, in the hope that increased collateral flow will alleviate the VBI. However, if both carotid and vertebral artery disease is present, consideration can be given to concomitant correction of both. Without significant carotid occlusive disease, or if the circle of Willis is not intact and appears to provide no considerable collateral flow, direct extracranial vertebral artery reconstruction should be considered. Proximal subclavian stenosis is usually corrected by carotid-subclavian bypass, subclavian-subclavian bypass, or subclavian-to-carotid trasposition. Stenosis at the origin of either vertebral artery may be managed by endarterectomy or reimplantation of the vertebral artery into the side of the common carotid artery. Anterior-to-posterior bypass grafts may be performed at either the low vertebral level, or at the skull base. Transposition of external carotid artery branches to the vertebral artery at the skull base have also been described. EC-IC anastomosis also may improve the posterior cerebral circulation. Finally, percutaneous balloon angioplasty and stenting of focal subclavian stenosis and vertebral artery lesions can be successful. Their utilization is well described but not well studied.

V. Great vessel disease and subclavian steal syndrome. Stenoses in the arch-based brachiocephalic vessels can lead to stroke, anterior or posterior circulation TIA, "watershed" ischemia of the brain noted during times of relative lowering of blood pressure, subclavian-steal, and thromboembolic events or claudication in the arms. Indications for treatment of these lesions are based primarily in the symptomatic in order to prevent recurrent TIA, stroke, and upper-extremity tissue loss. Similar to the treatment of lower-extremity claudication, arch-based disease therapy may improve quality of life.

Left subclavian stenosis or occlusion is a common atherosclerotic lesion. Generally, it is asymptomatic and is discovered because the left arm blood pressure is lower than the right. Left arm claudication seldom is a significant problem, since the collateral flow to the left arm usually is well developed. However, for a few patients proximal left subclavian occlusion may cause subclavian steal syndrome. Its clinical features are those of VBI such as dizziness, syncope, visual blurring, or ataxia, classically associated with vigorous left-arm exercise. The mechanism of the syndrome relates to retrograde flow from the left posterior cerebral circulation down the left vertebral artery to the distal subclavian artery and arm. This "stealing" of blood from the brain to the left arm causes intermittent posterior cerebral ischemia. Another common scenario today is due to the standard use of the left internal thoracic artery for coronary artery bypass grafting. When a significant left subclavian artery stenosis develops proximal to such a LIMA graft, vigorous left arm use may lead to angina pectoris or "subclavian-coronary" steal. Should the stenosis become severe enough, unstable or early angina may develop regardless of arm use. This is clearly a more pressing issue in order to prevent acute myocardial infarction.

In our experience, classic subclavian steal syndrome is uncommon. Although many patients with subclavian occlusive disease have retrograde left vertebral flow on duplex, few have cerebral symptoms with arm claudication owing to the vast collateral flow in both the brain and the arm. If they do have cerebral ischemic symptoms, we perform a standard duplex carotid examination and either an MRA or CTA in order to further interrogate the arch and brachiocephalic vessels in addition to both the carotid and vertebrobasilar systems. Arteriography is utilized for evaluation when either the disease anatomy remains unclear or an endovascular option is entertained. Subclavian-steal syndrome sometimes is relieved simply by correcting a severe left carotid stenosis, which improves collateral flow via the circle of Willis to the posterior brain. Significant arm claudication may be relieved by carotid-subclavian bypass, subclavian-subclavian bypass, subclavian-to-carotid transposition, transluminal angioplasty and stenting, or direct anatomic reconstruction.

Overall, the treatment of arch-based disease has evolved as endovascular therapy has progressed. Anatomic surgical revascularization for arch-based symptomatic atherosclerotic lesions requires a median sternotomy and bypass grafting from the ascending aorta to each of the vessels beyond the blockages. Thus, it is imperative to have a CT of the aorta to confirm the ability to use proper side-biting cross clamps for the proximal anatomosis. If lesions are focal in nature, classically the innominate artery, endarterectomy may be used. Arch-based grafting can be performed in conjunction with standard carotid bifurcation endarterectomy. Dacron and expanded polytetrafl:uroroethylene (ePTFE) prosthetic grafts are used.

Extra-anatomic open revascularizations such as the ones mentioned here for subclavian-steal may also be used and are lower-risk procedures. Additionally, carotid-carotid bypass can be done. Should autogenous conduit for any of these open revascularizations be required, superficial femoral vein or paneled greater saphenous vein is an option if available. Patients undergoing operative revascularizations, particularly those based on the ascending aorta, must be evaluated for significant cardiopulmonary disease and risk stratified accordingly (see Chapter 8).

Endovascular methods, particularly balloon angioplasty and stenting, have been shown to achieve excellent immediate and midterm results. Due to this, operative anatomic reconstruction has been reserved for significant multivessel brachiocephalic disease. Creative techniques such as CEA with retrograde common carotid artery angioplasty and stenting are performed more commonly. The success of the neck-based extra-anatomic reconstructions and endovascular methods are particularly useful to avoid an increased morbidity and mortality with redo median sternotomy.

VI. Other cerebrovascular pathologies.

A. Pulsatile masses. Pulsatile masses near the carotid artery usually represent one of the following: true arterial aneurysms, carotid body tumors, local lymphadenopathy, or a prominent, tortuous carotid artery. After CEA, this may represent a patch pseudoaneurysm. Sonography, CT scanning, or MRI can generally differentiate between these etiologies. Carotid aneurysms are rare but dangerous since they may lead to rupture, cerebral embolization, thrombosis, and local pressure symptoms. The best surgical approach is resection and arterial restoration by direct end-to-end anastomosis or an interposition graft with either autogenous vein or ePTFE.

B. Carotid body tumors (CBT) are uncommon neoplasms of the neuroectoderm paraganglion cells, which make up the carotid body and are also referred to as paragangliomas. These tumors arise from the afferent ganglion of the glossopharyngeal nerve and are slowly progressive. CBTs are rarely malignant neoplasms. This occurs some 5–10% of the time and in 8% of cases they are bilateral. They can be associated with multiple endocrine neoplasia syndromes I and II, and, thus, familial tumors. Familial tumors have a higher incidence of being bilateral. Periadventitial resection or carotid artery replacement is recommended for all CBTs. The blood supply to these vascular tumors is from the external carotid artery and preoperative embolization may be helpful when the tumor is over 5 cm in size. Radiation therapy appears to be of little value in their management and observation is appropriate only for asymptomatic elderly patients who are poor surgical risks. The risk of stroke with CBT is 5%, and the risk of cranial nerve injury is significant with some suggesting up to 40%.

C. Carotid fibromuscular dysplasia (FMD) is a relatively benign, often incidental finding that rarely causes symptoms. Although carotid FMD may be associated with TIAs, the incidence of subsequent stroke is less than that seen with atherosclerotic carotid occlusive disease. Patients with FMD are more prone to internal carotid artery dissection. When neurologic or visual symptoms can be attributed to carotid FMD, they generally resolve without operation and recurrence is uncommon. We place these patients on antiplatelet therapy even when asymptomatic FMD is found. High-grade symptomatic FMD stenoses can be treated by operative probe dilation or internal carotid balloon angioplasty.

D. Carotid dissection may occur spontaneously or as a result of trauma with neck hyperextension. When spontaneous, it may be associated with hypertensive scenarios, inciting causes such as wretching or coughing, and connective tissue diseases. Most often, however, the causative piece remains unclear. Symptoms suggestive of dissection include headache, neck pain, and Horner's syndrome. Cranial nerve palsies and tinnitus, usually pulsatile, can also occur. Neurologic events arise due to either thromboembolic events or hypoperfusion. Initial treatment is anticoagulation as these are challenging to repair surgically. Serial duplex surveillance is suggested. With continued symptoms, either open repair, EC-IC bypass, or carotid stenting is indicated.

E. Carotid kinks and coils. Coils in the carotid artery arise from improper sequencing of cardiac descent and carotid uncoiling during embryologic development. Kinks are normally secondary to atherosclerotic plaque and arterial wall weakening with the degenerative process. Indications for surgical correction are the development of symptoms, significant stenosis falling within indications for CEA, or thromus formation. Several repair techniques have been described, but all include the component of resection and reconstruction. Should endarterectomy be necessary, eversion endarterectomy with ICA resection and straightening is an excellent option.

VII. Technical aspects of carotid interventions.

A. CEA is the most common open operation for extracranial cerebrovascular disease, and so we focus on principles of operative care for carotid reconstructions. These same principles also apply to other types of vertebral and subclavian revascularization.

1. Preoperative preparation. For elective cases, anticoagulants are discontinued 4–5 days prior to operation. Depending on the indication for Coumadin, either a heparin or lovenox window can be used. Aspirin is continued throughout the course of operation. Clopidogrel (Plavix) is usually discontinued at least 5 days before surgery and aspirin instituted prior to discontinuation. The main exception is a patient with multiple recent TIAs or a severe carotid stenosis (<2 mm), who usually remains on heparin or clopidogrel accepting a slightly higher hematoma rate for a presumed decrease in neurologic events. There is mounting evidence that, if the patient is not already on statin medications and beta-blockers, these should be instituted in the perioperative period to reduce cardiac events.

Although neck infection is rare, several preventive measures are taken. The chin, neck, and anterior chest are shaved on the side of endarterectomy. This area is washed with a surgical scrub solution within 6 to 12 hours of operation. Preoperative parenteral antibiotics are started when the patient goes to the operating room; the antibiotic of choice usually is a cephalosporin or semisynthetic penicillin to cover skin flora.

The patient is given non per os (nothing by mouth; NPO) status after midnight prior to operation. Stable or asymptomatic patients are admitted on the morning of operation. Some symptomatic patients will already be hospitalized for heparin anticoagulation. An intravenous infusion of balanced salt solution (e.g., 5% dextrose in Ringer's solution at 100 to 125 mL/h) is begun to maintain hydration. General narcotic premedications that may cause hypotension are avoided.

On the day of surgery, a responsible member of the operating team is present in the operating room from the time the patient enters the room until the patient is transported to the recovery area. When the operation is complete, the surgical scrub remains sterile and the team maintains room preparation. An arterial line is generally inserted in the operating room. Occasionally, selected patients with severe cardiac disease (see Chapters 7 and 8) may also receive a Swan-Ganz catheter. A Foley bladder catheter is optional but may assist with blood pressure control since bladder distention may exacerbate hypertension in a labile patient.

2. Operative principles.

a. General endotracheal anesthesia is our preference, since it both provides the best control of the airway and best facilitates management of cardiorespiratory function. Other experienced surgeons prefer regional

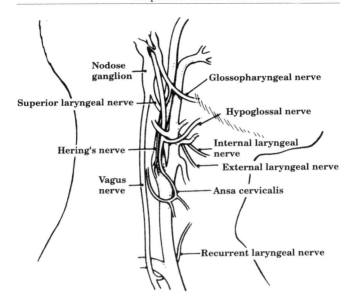

Figure 13.4.   Nerves that may be encountered or injured during carotid endarterectomy and their typical relationship to the carotid arterial system.

cervical block and local anesthesia. They believe this provides a better hemodynamic course and direct neurologic monitoring.

b. Carotid exposure must be gentle and meticulous to avoid venous or nerve injury and dislodgement of atheromatous material from a plaque. Figure 13.4 demonstrates the relative positions of the major nerves of the neck that surround the carotid artery.

(1)   Branches of the **ansa cervicalis** (ansa meaning loop) provides innervation to the strap muscles and may be divided for better exposure, without a resulting neurologic deficit.

(2)   The **hypoglossal nerve** usually crosses the carotid artery at or near the carotid bifurcation. Most hypoglossal injuries are caused by retraction of the nerve. Clamp injuries may occur if the hypoglossal nerve is not dissected free from the common facial vein before this venous structure is divided. Hypoglossal injury results in weakness of the tongue on the operated side, with tongue deviation toward the side of the injury. This deficit may cause biting of the tongue while chewing, and the patient may have some difficulty swallowing or speaking. Bilateral hypoglossal nerve injury may be life threatening, since the tongue may prolapse posteriorly and obstruct the airway when the patient is supine.

(3)   The **vagus nerve** usually runs in the posterior carotid sheath behind the carotid artery. In 3–5% of

cases it swings anteriorly along the anterolateral surface of the carotid artery (anterior vagus nerve). The nerve must be dissected frcc from the carotid artery, especially at the proximal and distal extent of carotid dissection, where clamps may accidentally injure it.

(4) Vagal injury is most commonly manifested by hoarseness, as the **recurrent laryngeal nerve** normally originates from the vagus in the chest and runs back to the vocal cord in the tracheoesophageal groove. This cranial nerve injury is touted as the most common during CEA. The recurrent laryngeal nerve loops around the subclavian artery on the right side and the ligamentum arteriosum on the left. In roughly 1% or fewer cases, the laryngeal nerve is nonrecurrent and originates from the vagus nerve in the neck and passes posterior to the carotid artery.

(5) The **external branch of the superior laryngeal nerve** travels behind the carotid bifurcation to the true vocal cord. This nerve innervates the cricothyroid muscle, which maintains the tone of the vocal cord. Injury may be avoided by careful dissection around the external carotid and superior thyroid arteries. Injury results in voice tone fatigue, especially after prolonged speaking or singing.

(6) The **greater auricular nerve** is a sensory nerve to the skin overlying the mastoid process, the concha of auricle, and the earlobe. It lies on the anterior surface of the sternocleidomastoid muscle and may be injured when the neck incision is carried toward the mastoid process. Injury results in skin numbness around the lower ear and earlobe. This is the most common nerve injury during CEA.

(7) The **mandibular branch** of the facial nerve runs forward from the angle of the mandible and parallel to the mandible. Injury results in weakness of the perioral musculature on the injured side. The patient may have a facial droop and drool from the corner of the mouth.

(8) With very high internal carotid exposures, the **glossopharyngeal nerve** is at risk for injury. Injury to this nerve is rare but devastating and results in difficulty swallowing, which may preclude oral feeding and necessitate placement of a gastrostomy feeding tube. The glossopharyngeal nerve also provides a branch to the carotid sinus called **Hering's nerve,** which usually traverses posterior or deep to the internal carotid artery (Fig. 13.4). Use of local anesthetic to temporarily denervate the carotid bodies can help with blood pressure and heart-rate control during CEA if dissection around the bulb causes bradycardia and hypotension.

c. Prevention of thromboemboli obviously is essential if neurologic deficits are to be avoided. Thromboembolism is the most common etiology of postoperative stroke with CEA. The following measures should be taken to avoid thrombus accumulation and embolism.

(1) During gentle carotid dissection, **suction** is used rather than blotting with sponges to keep the operative field dry. Vigorous manipulation of the carotid bifurcation may dislodge loose atheromatous material from an ulcerated plaque. We therefore prefer sharp dissection during carotid exposures and minimize any spreading maneuvers.

(2) Before carotid clamping, **heparin** is administered intravenously and allowed to circulate for at least 3 minutes. Our usual dose is a 5,000-unit bolus. Others use 100 units per kilogram for dosing.

(3) The inside of the carotid artery is **irrigated** with heparinized saline to wash out any loose atheroma or clot both before a shunt is inserted and before the internal carotid artery is reopened.

(4) Bleeding of the internal and external carotid arteries (back-bleeding) and forward bleeding of the common carotid artery flush out any thrombus or atheroma that may accumulate behind vascular clamps. Carotid blood flow also is reinstated up the external carotid artery for a few cardiac cycles before opening the internal carotid artery. This sequence of reopening the carotid branches should allow any thromboemboli to go out through the external carotid artery and not directly to the brain.

d. Cerebral protection from clamp ischemia probably is best achieved by two methods: careful blood pressure control and cerebral monitoring of some type in conjunction with either selective or compulsory shunting. Clamp ischemia is based upon the limits of cerebral perfusion and is a lesser cause of stroke with CEA. Infarction of brain tissue occurs when the flow rate is reduced to 10cc/100g tissue/min for several minutes. Electrical quiescence takes place at 15cc/100g tissue/min.

(1) Cerebral perfusion is directly related to **mean arterial blood pressure**, which was discussed in Chapter 8. Therefore, prior to carotid clamping, we remind the anesthesiologist to maintain the blood pressure in a normotensive to mildly hypertensive range (140–150 mm Hg systolic; mean arterial pressure of at least 80 mm Hg). If continuous EEG monitoring is used, a diffuse slowing pattern often can be eliminated by simply raising the patient's mean arterial pressure.

(2) **Shunting** during carotid endarterectomy remains controversial. Experienced surgeons have demonstrated that with or without shunting, carotid endarterectomy can be performed with a low incidence of permanent postoperative neurologic deficit (1% to 3%). The key question is how to identify the few patients who will not tolerate carotid clamping long enough for the surgeon to complete endarterectomy without a shunt and, thus, allow for selective shunting. There are risks associated with shunting,

which include thrombus formation with potential embolism and dissection. Under general anesthesia, the two most common methods to assess adequate cerebral perfusion during carotid clamping are carotid stump pressures and EEG monitoring. Our experience suggests that carotid stump pressures may not correlate with adequate cerebral perfusion as indicated by EEG monitoring. Consequently, we insert a shunt after carotid clamping if focal EEG changes occur and are not corrected by manipulation of anesthetic agents or blood pressure. If EEG monitoring is not available, a mean carotid stump pressure below 50 mm Hg may indicate inadequate cerebral collateral flow during carotid clamping.

Even without EEG changes, we often insert a shunt to allow for an unhurried endarterectomy and to provide an intraluminal stent which, in our experience, facilitates a better closure of the internal carotid artery. For these reasons, in a teaching situation, we are more likely to use shunting. We also believe that routine shunting is advisable when the contralateral internal carotid artery is occluded and when the patient has had a recent stroke. Finally, in patients in whom the internal carotid plaque extends high into the carotid artery, an intraluminal shunt may make endarterectomy excessively difficult. In such cases, the endarterectomy of the distal plaque probably should be performed without a shunt in place. A shunt may subsequently be inserted to complete the operation.

Other techniques described for cerebral monitoring during CEA include the use of spectral analysis monitors, evoked potential monitoring, and cervical block, awake anesthesia. Spectral analysis quantifies bilateral hemispheric EEG tracings. Ischemia is manifest as lower number on the affected hemisphere. Evoked potentials may be motor (cortical) or sensory (peripheral) and search for latency and reduced strength or amplitude in peripheral nerve conduction. Monitoring and stump pressures all lead to a shunting rate above what is necessary clinically. One very successful strategy to maintain adequate cerebral perfusion during CEA that minimizes excess shunt use while avoiding hypoperfusion is use of regional cervical anesthesia in an awake patient. Problems are patient tolerance and the amount of dissection required to achieve a safe and complete operation.

e. The **endarterectomy technique** should achieve the two main goals of carotid artery reconstruction (Fig. 13.5). The first goal is adequate removal of the stenotic or ulcerated plaques. The carotid arteries are clamped sequentially and a longitudinal arteriotomy is made from the distal common carotid past the stenosis to normal ICA. Since atherosclerotic lesions involve the intima and media, we generally remove the plaques down to the external elastic lamina. In our experience, such a deep

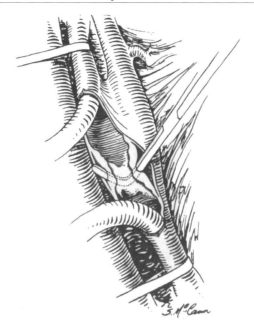

Figure 13.5.   Standard longitudinal CEA with shunt. CEA, carotid endarterectomy.

endarterectomy plane has resulted in the removal of retained media fibers, which may cause recurrent myo-intimal restenosis, but it has not been associated with late aneurysm formation. In those with rough residual carotid artery walls **dextran-40** is instituted for antiplatelet purposes during the procedure at a rate of 25–50 ml/hour. This is continued as the patient's only IV fluid for 24 hours postoperatively. Its use must be selective for several reasons. It is highly hypersomolar and fluid overload and cardiac failure have been described. Prior to administration a test dose must be given as anaphylaxis is also a known entity secondary to dextran.

The second goal is closure of the arteriotomy so that stenosis or thrombosis does not occur. A primary closure of the arteriotomy is usually adequate for very large (>6 mm) internal carotid arteries. Patches are used when primary closure would cause stenosis or in cases of redo endarterectomy. Patch angioplasty may protect against early thrombosis, and there has been a substantial trend toward more patching by all surgeons in the recent years. Recent clinical trials indicate that patching is extremely beneficial in the following situations:

1. Small internal carotid artery (<3.5 mm)
2. Long internal carotid arteriotomy (>3 cm)
3. Women who tend to have small arteries
4. Reoperative endarterectomies.

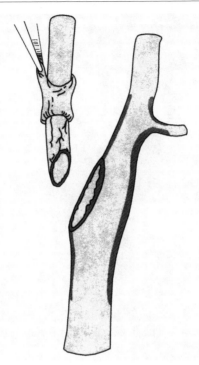

Figure 13.6. Eversion CEA. CEA, carotid endarterectomy.

Further trials have now clearly noted that recurrent stenosis is reduced with the use of patch angioplasty.

An alternative technique is **eversion CEA** (Fig. 13.6). In this procedure, the origin of the internal carotid artery as obliquely amputated at the carotid bulb. A circumferential endarterectomy is started in a similar plane and extended beyond the stenosis with the elevator. The ICA is then everted upon itself beyond the stenosis where an endpoint is identified and the plaque gently amputated or removed. Potential advantages of this technique include no need for prosthetic and the ability to resect redundant, kinked, or coiled portions of the ICA and essentially straighten it. Proponents believe it to have less restenosis than traditional, longitudinal CEA, and perhaps less stroke risk. Disadvantages include a more challenging shunting technique and complete bulb dissection with more lability in blood pressure and heart rate afterward.

In our opinion, low-power magnifying glasses (magnification of 2 to 4) help us perform a more meticulous endarterectomy and arterial closure. Flow through the internal and external carotid arteries is assessed by a sterile continuous-wave Doppler probe. Absence of flow or an obstructed, monophasic signal indicates thrombosis or stenosis, which requires immediate thrombectomy and a patch. Other methods of intraoperative assessment include arteriography or duplex ultrasound. Completion duplex ultrasound has become standard in many institutions and is an excellent, noninvasive way to further investigate the CEA site.

f. Recognition of postoperative neurologic deficit ideally is made in the operating room if the anesthesiologist can awaken and extubate the patient early. This is the reason that the surgical technician and the back table as well as those in the operating room should maintain strict sterile methods until the patient appears neurologically intact. Otherwise, the patient is moved to the recovery area and a neurologic examination of general motor function is made as soon as the patient is responsive. In our experience, the earliest signs of a neurologic deficit may be severe hypertension, difficulty in being awakened from anesthesia, or clumsiness of fine hand movement. This can be a tricky evaluation in those with recent stroke as it is not uncommon for them to awake with an exacerbation of their stroke symptoms. This is due to the ischemic penumbra of neurons surrounding the area of infarction whose metabolic function is affected by the decreased blood flow experienced, yet they are viable. This typically resolves in the first several hours to days after the operation.

The proper management of an **immediate postoperative neurologic deficit** must be individualized, however, the general tenet when this occurs is return directly to the operating room.

(1) First, the patient's general **cardiorespiratory status** must be stabilized expeditiously. This includes stabilization of heart rate, blood pressure, pulmonary ventilation, and blood oxygenation.

(2) Treatment then depends on the **location** of the neurologic deficit.

(a) If the deficit is a **contralateral hemiparesis,** a technical problem at the endarterectomy site may exist. We generally have returned these patients immediately to the operating room to examine the endarterectomy site. Two tests may help determine whether the arteriotomy should be reopened. First, duplex ultrasound is a sensitive method to ascertain carotid thrombosis or a major filling defect due to thrombus or a technical problem (e.g., residual plaque). Second, an intraoperative carotid arteriogram may also be done if ultrasound is not available or equivocal. If these tests are not satisfactory, reexploration of the artery remains the only way to rule out technical error.

(b) If the neurologic deficit is diffuse, the patient may have suffered an **internal capsule stroke,** usually caused by a hypotensive episode. Patency of the carotid arteries should then be assessed with duplex ultrasound. If the operated side is occluded, then reoperation is appropriate. If both carotid arteries appear widely patent, the patient should receive supportive care. CT/CTA of the brain should be performed once the patient is initially stabilized to search for hemorrhage and distal intracranial arterial patency, and again in approximately 12 to 24 hours to localize the cerebral infarct area and assess the amount of cerebral edema or hemorrhage.

Delayed deficits after CEA are typically defined as occurring 12–24 hours postoperatively. Duplex should be performed. If this appears to be fine, then CTA should be accomplished to evaluate the CEA site and the brain for hemorrhage and CVA. Any question of the CEA site should instigate arteriography. If this evaluation path reveals nothing, or CVA is seen on CT without concern for the CEA site, transthoracic and transesophageal echocardiography are done to assess for a cardiac source. Should no sources be identified, augmentation in antiplatelet therapy or anticoagulation can be instituted. Faults in the CEA site should lead to surgical correction and intracardiac thrombus treated with anticoagulation.

3. Postoperative care.

a. Day of surgery. All patients spend the first 12 to 24 hours after cerebrovascular surgery in an intensive recovery area, where vital signs and neurologic status can be continuously monitored. The head of the bed is elevated 30–45° to diminish edema and facilitate deep breathing. Antiplatelet therapy is continued without interruption and we generally try to keep the patient's systolic blood pressure below 150 mm Hg and above 100 mm Hg. This may require vasoactive intravenous medications the first 24 hours after CEA. The patient is kept NPO until the first postoperative morning since reexploration is occasionally necessary. While the patient is NPO, a maintenance intravenous infusion of 5% dextrose in water and one-half normal saline is run at 1 mL/kg/h. Antibiotics are continued for 24 hours postoperatively. Patients who have undergone staged bilateral carotid endarterectomies may be insensitive to hypoxia as a result of carotid baroreceptor trauma. Therefore, they must be observed for bradycardia, hypotension, and respiratory distress.

b. Postoperative Day 1. If a wound drain has been used, it is removed on the first postoperative day. Patients who are doing satisfactorily resume a normal diet and all preoperative medications. Clopidogrel can be safely started 24 hours after CEA if there are no concerns for neck hematoma. If patients have resumed normal activities without complications or hemodynamic instability, they are discharged later the first postoperative day. Older patients with labile blood pressure or other medical comorbidities may stay an additional night.

c. **Discharge instructions.** Most patients are discharged within 24 to 48 hours after operation. Because the patient's full physical strength may not recover for 2 to 4 weeks, we generally advise patients to convalesce for that period of time before resuming normal working activities. This is particularly true for activities that require active neck motion, such as driving. All patients are rechecked as outpatients 3 to 6 weeks after surgery. They return to their local referring physician for long-term management of any medical problems.

4. **Complications.**

a. **Early postoperative problems** are usually apparent on the day of surgery and require prompt recognition and treatment.

(1) **Immediate and delayed postoperative neurologic deficits** are discussed in the section on operative management (p. 187).

(2) **Hypertension** is a common postoperative problem that occurs in approximately 20% of patients who have carotid endarterectomy. Patients who were hypertensive before operation, especially if poorly controlled, are more likely to have severe postoperative hypertension. The incidence of neurologic deficit and death is significantly higher in these hypertensive patients. Therefore, we strive to maintain postoperative systolic blood pressure in a range mentioned earlier from the minimal normal preoperative recording to a maximum of 150 mm Hg. Chapter 9 discusses the use of nitroprusside and other antihypertensives in detail. Alterations in blood pressure due to carotid sinus dissection may require antihypertensive medication manipulation.

(3) **Neck hematomas** may compromise breathing and swallowing. Patients with large neck hematomas should be returned to the operating room for evacuation. If a patient's respiratory status and hematoma are stable, no attempt at intubation should be made until the surgical team is ready to operate. In cases where respiration is desperately compromised or bleeding is profuse, nasotracheal intubation and control of bleeding in the recovery room may be necessary to save the patient. Smaller neck hematomas may be left alone and usually resolve in 7 to 14 days. They seldom are complicated by infection. If a pulsatile mass persists after the major portion of the hematoma resolves, a pseudoaneurysm should be suspected and evaluated by ultrasonography.

(4) **Local nerve injuries** following carotid operations probably are more common than generally is recognized or reported. Some degree of cranial nerve dysfunction affects 5% to 20% of patients. The mechanism of injury usually is nerve retraction or clamping and not transection. Most cranial nerve injuries manifest as deficits in the recurrent laryngeal and the hypoglossal nerves. The injuries often are mild or asymptomatic and will not be detected unless one

specifically examines for them. For example, one-third of recurrent laryngeal nerve injuries will go unrecognized unless direct laryngoscopy is performed. **Therefore, all patients who undergo staged, bilateral carotid endarterectomy should be tested by direct laryngoscopy before the second operation.** Should dysfunction of the swallowing mechanism be suspected, formal swallowing study evaluation is indicated. Fortunately, most cranial nerve injuries resulting from retraction trauma will resolve in 2 to 6 months. Time and reassurance are all the treatment most patients require.

(5) Hyperfusion syndrome is a rare occurrence after CEA. It happens in 1–2% of cases and usually is seen 3–7 days after CEA. The complete syndrome occurs as a classic triad of headache, seizures, and intracranial hemorrhage. Hypertension usually accompanies the process. It is thought to be due to poor intracranial arterial autoregulation secondary to a significant period of time with reduced extracranial flow. Those at highest risk appear to be those with very high-grade carotid stenosis, severe bilateral carotid disease, and poorly controlled hypertension. Treatment is supportive and consists of blood pressure and seizure control, as well as evaluation for intracranial hemorrhage and significant cerebral edema by CT.

b. Late complications of carotid artery reconstructions are uncommon or at least seldom cause symptoms.

(1) Recurrent carotid stenosis that is symptomatic is rare, affecting only 1% to 3% of patients after carotid endarterectomy, and overall the need for either operative or interventional therapy after CEA is 4–5%. Asymptomatic restenosis is detectable in 10% to 20% of patients followed by noninvasive carotid testing, and is more common in women and active smokers. High-grade ($\geq$80%) restenosis is rare. The risk of a future stroke in this asymptomatic group appears to be low. Recurrent lesions have a striking predilection for the internal carotid artery near its origin and within the confines of the original endarterectomy site. Early recurrent lesions (<36 months) are predominantly a combination of intimal hyperplasia and surface thrombus. Features of recurrent atherosclerosis (abundant collagen, calcium deposits, and foam cells) are more pronounced in late recurrences.

An important feature that differentiates primary and recurrent atherosclerotic carotid lesions is the presence of surface and intraplaque thrombus in 90% of recurrent stenoses. Recurrent symptoms after carotid endarterectomy generally require repeat evaluation and arteriography. Recurrent stenosis is operatively repaired by repeat endarterectomy and patch angioplasty, or by patch angioplasty alone if an endarterectomy plane is not achievable. Segmental carotid resection and an interposition vein or ePTFE graft may also be performed. The rates of stroke and cranial nerve injury are slightly higher with reoperation. Alternatively, CAS can be utilized.

The need for long-term ultrasound surveillance of carotid endarterectomy sites is debatable. Since early restenosis is often a relatively benign process, asymptomatic restenosis does not mandate reoperation. However, contralateral atherosclerotic asymptomatic 50% to 79% stenoses have a significant risk of becoming symptomatic, especially if they progress. Consequently, we recheck carotid duplex scans on CEA patients every 6 months for 2 years and then yearly, and caution patients to report any ipsilateral, or contralateral neurologic or ocular symptoms. Since the late results of carotid stent angioplasty are unclear, these patients should be followed regularly (e.g., every 6 months).

(2) Carotid pseudoaneurysm may occur after primary arterial closure or patch angioplasty. In general, such pseudoaneurysms should be repaired since mural thrombus may accumulate and cause cerebral thromboembolism. Large pseudoaneurysms also may cause local pressure symptoms. These require interposition grafting.

c. Carotid angioplasty and stenting (CAS).

(1) It is imperative that the patient be fully awake with little sedation. Generally, only local groin anesthetic is used at the arterial access site. Yet, these procedures should be done with an anesthetist comfortable with cardiovascular anesthesia. A full array of antihypertensive medications, pressors, heparin, and atropine should be quickly available. Specifically, atropine is necessary to counteract the reflex bradycardia associated with carotid bulb angioplasty. In the past, transvenous pacemakers were placed prior to CAS, however, this in no longer advocated in the majority of cases.

(2) This procedure begins with safe and adequate aortic arch and selective carotid and intracranial arteriography. Several technically challenging aspects of CAS have been categorized (Table 13.4). Each of these plays a role in successful performance of CAS, and one or several may preclude CAS. The use of embolic-protection devices such as filters and occlusion-based technology is now considered standard and a stenosis that is not amenable to their use should be questioned (Fig. 13.7). Unprotected pre-dilation with a small balloon may facilitate proper positioning of the stent in certain cases of very severe stenosis. Arch anatomy may be especially challenging and has been graded based on degree of arch angle (Fig. 13.8). Specifically the distance between the uppermost aspect of the aortic arch and the origin of the innominate and left common carotid arteries is one reliable predictor of difficulty in positioning of the necessary sheath prox-

Table 13.4.   CAS Technical Challenges

Technical challenge	Category
High-grade stenosis precluding initial EPD	1
Complex arch anatomy	2
Compromised femoral access	3
Tandem stenoses	4
Circumferential calicification	5
Internal carotid tortuosity	6

CAS, carotid angioplasty and stenting; EPD, embolic protection device.
(Adapted from Choi HM, Hobson RW, Goldstein J, et al. Technical challenges
in a program of carotid artery stenting. *J Vasc Surg.* 2004;40:746-751.)

imal to the carotid stenosis. The greater this distance, the more acute the angle of the aortic arch and the more difficult the arch will be to maneuver. Type C arches represent the most difficult in this respect. Additionally, MRI/MRA data have shown that thromboembolic events leading to stroke during carotid stenting occur almost equally between hemispheres, which suggests that arch calcification and atheroma are important causes to consider. Although novel attempts at accomplishing carotid artery stenting with arm and neck access sites are described, this procedure is optimally performed from a standard groin access and approach. Anatomy contrary to this approach should lead to consideration for open operation. Long, tandem stenoses generally fare worse using CAS. ICA tortuosity may make the stent placement difficult if not impossible, to achieve appropriate wall apposition. Creation of an area of malapposition may become a nidus for thrombus development and thromboemolic complications. Circumferential calcium is an anatomic scenario that may limit stent expansion and is at higher risk of rupture with balloon angioplasty, and should give pause to the consideration of CAS.

Platforms for CAS are based upon 6 F. guiding sheaths and monorail systems (see Chapter 11). Bra-

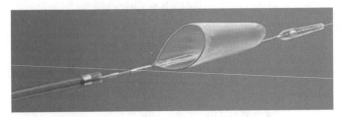

Figure 13.7.   Example of a filter anti-embolic device. (FilterWire EZ, Boston Scientific, Natick, MA, U.S.A.)

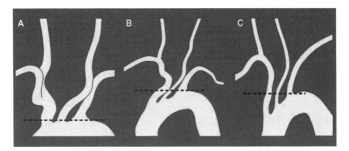

Figure 13.8.   Arch anatomic classification: (A) brachiocephalic vessels originate at level of superior arch; (B) more acute arch angulation and innominate and left carotid originate below superior arch level; (C) severe arch angulation with all brachiocephalic vessels originating below level of superior arch.

chiocephalic or common carotid artery access, trackability, and purchase may require 7–8 Fr sheaths. Systemic, intravenous heparin is given prior to selective catheterization of the brachiocephalic vessels. Activated clotting times can be monitored to keep this value above 250 seconds and further boluses may be necessary. Some use GIIb/IIIa inhibitors, yet these are associated with increased hemorrhagic complications. Clopidogrel is continued through the procedure. If the patient is not on this, they are loaded with 300 mg by mouth the day prior to CAS. Self-expanding stents are used during carotid artery stenting and may have either an open or closed cell configuration. Open cell configurations tend to be more flexible; however, closed cells provide somewhat more radial strength and are better at "jailing" atherosclerotic plaque against the vessel wall and potentially reducing emboli. Filter distal embolic protection devices allow antegrade flow during the procedure, whereas occlusion-based distal embolic protection devices act like a clamp and cease antegrade flow in the ICA during the procedure. Usually, stenoses require placing the stent across the origin of the external carotid artery. Tapered stents are now available designed for this purpose. We have avoided this if the ICA is straight enough and the lesion is higher in the ICA such as with restenosis.

(3) Unique complications associated with CAS compared to CEA include the potential for bilateral hemispheric events as mentioned previously due to aortic arch catheterization and manipulation and complications associated with the access site. These may comprise bleeding with hematoma, pseudoaneurysm, and arteriovenous fistula formation. These events occur in less than 4% of cases. If at all possible, one single stent should be used as multiple stents may increase the risk of thromboembolic complications.

However, arterial dissection and stent misplacement may require further stent placement. Soft balloon angioplasty is critical as profound bradycardia and hypotension can occur. A unique advantage of CAS is the ability to accomplish intracranial arteriography before and after the procedure. This is, in our opinion, mandatory to document the state of the cerebral vessels and aid in the provision of distal emoli. Should "neuro rescue" be needed with distal thromboembolization, useful tools may include catheter-directed thrombolytic therapy, remote catheter thrombectomy, and intracranial angioplasty and stenting. Proper antiplatelet therapy and anticoagulation cannot be stressed enough for CAS.

SELECTED READING

Adams HP Jr, del Zoppo G, Alberts MJ, et al. Guidelines for the early management of adults with ischemic stroke. *Stroke.* 2007;38: 1655-1711.

Blacker DJ, Flemming KD, Link MJ. The preoperative cerebrovascular consultation: Common cerebrovascular questions before general and cardiac surgery. *Mayo Clin Proc.* 2004;79:223-229.

Executive Committee for the Asymptomatic Carotid Atherosclerosis Study. Endarterectomy for asymptomatic carotid artery stenosis. *JAMA.* 1995;273:1421-1428.

Hans SS, Jareunpoon O. Prospective evaluation of electroencephalography, carotid artery stump pressure, and neurologic changes during 314 consecutive carotid endarterectomy performed in awake patients. *J Vasc Surg.* 2007;45:511-515.

Karkos CD, McMahon G, McCarthy MJ, et al. The value of urgent carotid endarterectomy for crescendo transient ischemic attacks. *J Vasc Surg.* 2007;45:1148-1154.

Luebke T, Aleksic M, Brunkwall J. Meta-analysis of randomized trials comparing carotid endarterectomy and endovascular treatment. *Eur J Vasc Endovasc Surg.* 2007;34:470-479.

MRC Asymptomatic Carotid Surgery Trial (ACST) Collaborative Group. Prevention of disabling and fatal strokes by successful carotid endarterectomy in patients without recent neurological symptoms: randomised controlled trial. *Lancet.* 2004;363: 1491-1502.

Narins CR, Illig KA. Patient selection for carotid stenting versus endarterectomy: A systematic review. *J Vasc Surg.* 2006;44:661-672.

North American Symptomatic Carotid Endarterectomy Trial Collaborators. Beneficial effect of carotid endarterectomy in symptomatic patients with high-grade carotid stenosis. *N Engl J Med.* 1991;325:445-453.

North American Symptomatic Carotid Endarterectomy Trial Collaborators. Benefit of carotid endarterectomy in patients with symptomatic moderate or severe stenosis. *N Engl J Med.* 1998;339: 1415-1425.

Rothwell PM, Eliasiw M, Gutnikov SA, et al. Analysis of pooled data from the randomized trials of endarterectomy for symptomatic carotid stenosis. *Lancet.* 2003;361:107-116.

Rothwell PM, Eliasiw M, Gutnikov SA, et al. Endarterectomy for symptomatic carotid stenosis in relation to clinical subgroups and the timing of surgery. *Lancet.* 2004;363:915-924.

Veterans Affairs Cooperative Studies Program 309 Trialist Group. Carotid endarterectomy and prevention of cerebral ischemia in symptomatic carotid stenosis. *JAMA*. 1991;266:3289-3294.

Yadav JS, Wholey MH, Kuntz RE, et al. Protected carotid-artery stenting versus endarterectomy in high-risk patients. *N Engl J Med*. 2004;351:1493-1501.

CHAPTER 14

Lower-Extremity Ischemia

Lower-extremity arterial disease involves a spectrum from intermittent claudication to limb-threatening ischemia. Up to 20% of those over the age of 55 have some degree of peripheral arterial occlusive disease (PAOD). **Intermittent claudication,** or functional ischemia, of the lower extremities is the most common manifestation of this PAOD. The term claudication comes from the latin *claudicatio,* "to limp." **Limb-threatening ischemia** occurs when there is tissue loss, such as ulceration or gangrene, or ischemic rest pain. Another term used to describe this is critical limb ischemia. Causes may include continual progression of chronic atherosclerosis or acute processes such as plaque rupture with thrombosis, or embolism. As the term limb-threatening ischemia indicates, if treatment is not pursued, there is a high likelihood of amputation.

Patients with claudication may limp or claudicate for several reasons. The patient's calf muscles may develop cramping pain with walking. The hip and thigh muscles may cramp or tire. Walking also may be limited because of a feeling of diffuse lower-extremity weakness, numbness, and heaviness. Although claudication usually is associated with vascular disease, degenerative hip disease or conditions of the spine such as spinal stenosis, or "pseudoclaudication," may cause similar symptoms. Therefore, in the evaluation of lower-extremity claudication, the physician must first question the underlying etiology. Is the claudication caused by arterial occlusive disease or some other problem? The history and physical exam often can answer this question (see Chapter 4). Noninvasive testing, including resting segmental pressures (e.g. ankle-brachial indices; ABI), exercise "stress" segmental pressures, accompanying pulse volume recordings (PVR), and duplex ultrasound of the aortoiliac, femoropopliteal, and tibial segments, provide objective data to support or refute the clinical impression (see Chapter 6).

If the initial evaluation suggests arterial occlusive disease as the cause of intermittent claudication, the next question concerns how management proceeds. Which levels of the arterial system are involved? Should therapy be medical, or should a procedure such as percutaneous balloon angioplasty, stenting, or atherectomy be entertained, or should an operation be recommended? And, if surgery is chosen, what operation should be performed? If acute or limb-threatening ischemia is present, what is the likely etiology? How quickly is assessment and treatment needed?

This chapter delineates answers to these issues and gives global evaluation, diagnostic, and therapeutic insight for assessment of those with lower-extremity vascular disease.

I. Patterns of disease. Vascular claudication of the lower limb generally is caused by an arterial stenosis or occlusion in two general regions (Fig. 14.1). A common location of stenosis or occlusion in the superficial femoral artery is at the adductor canal. In diabetics, infrainguinal disease classically involves the tibial arteries. The other large anatomic category of claudicants has occlusive disease localized primarily to the distal abdominal aorta and iliac arteries with open distal arteries, this is termed aortoiliac disease. Over time, collateral branches in the groin and around the knee become well developed when occlusive disease occurs (Fig. 14.1).

Patient history, physical examination, and noninvasive segmental leg pressures and pulse volume recordings usually can identify the primary location and objectify the severity of disease. Since therapeutic decisions are influenced by the location of occlusive lesions, we categorize patients into five patterns of peripheral arterial disease (Fig. 14.2).

A. Aortoiliac disease (type 1 and type 2). Type 1, the least common pattern (10% to 15%), is limited to the distal abdominal aorta and common iliac arteries. Patients with focal aor-

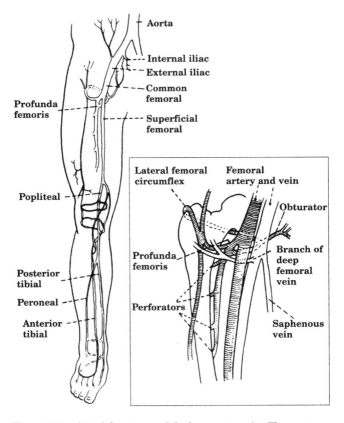

Figure 14.1.   Arterial anatomy of the lower extremity. The most common locations of atherosclerotic occlusive disease causing claudication are the aortoiliac region and the superficial femoral artery. Enlarged drawing of the femoral region demonstrates the major collateral channels of the profunda femoris artery. Enlarged drawing of the popliteal region shows the genicular collateral network around the knee connecting the distal SFA to the infragenicular arteries.

toiliac disease are characteristically between the ages of 35 and 55, with a low incidence of hypertension and diabetes but a high frequency of heavy cigarette smoking and hyperlipidemia. There has been an alarming increase in premature atherosclerotic aortoiliac disease in younger women (age 35 to 50) who have smoked since adolescence. These patients generally complain of proximal lower-extremity claudication involving the hip and thigh muscles with progression to the calf muscles. In about 15% of such patients, however, the claudication affects only the calves. Diminished femoral pulses and femoral bruits are characteristic physical findings. Weak pedal pulses often are palpable, since the femoropopliteal system is open. Some men have the tetrad of bilateral hip and buttock claudication, impotence, leg muscle atrophy and absent femoral pulses, which is called **Leriche's syndrome.** Patients with **type 2** disease (20%) have aortoiliac atherosclerotic lesions that also involve the external iliac arteries extending to the groin. Final definition of whether the patient has type 1 or 2 aortoiliac disease must be made by imaging. Classic findings of peripheral arterial disease may be present in either of these two categories of proximal aortoiliac occlusive disease as well as any of the remaining three categories to be discussed. Such findings include atrophic skin, dray and flaky skin include atrophic skin, dry and flaky skin (due to poorly functioning skin appendages), and hypertrophic toenails due to an ischemic cuticle. Dependent rubor is a late finding but is classic.

B. Combined aortoiliac and femoropopliteal disease (type 3). The majority of patients with lower-extremity claudication (66%) have combined aortoiliac and femoropopliteal disease (type 2), which usually occurs in patients with multiple cardiovascular risk factors: smoking, hypertension, hyperlipidemia, and sometimes adult-onset diabetes mellitus. These patients usually have more incapacitating, higher grade claudication than is seen in aortoiliac or femoropopliteal disease alone and often progress to more severe ischemia problems, such as rest pain, foot ulcers, or gangrene (i.e., critical ischemia).

C. Isolated femoropopliteal disease (type 4). Patients with isolated femoropopliteal disease generally present with calf claudication that starts after the patient walks for some time and is relieved by stopping for a few minutes. These patients are older (age 50 to 70) and have a higher prevalence of hypertension, adult-onset diabetes mellitus, and associated vascular disease of the coronary and carotid vessels than those with aortoiliac disease. Like patients with aortoiliac disease, they frequently are cigarette smokers. They generally have good femoral pulses but no palpable popliteal or pedal pulses. Their claudication usually is improved by a supervised walking program and remains stable for long periods of time if significant proximal aortoiliac disease is not present. In fact, the following observations support initial nonoperative management: Patients over 60 years of age with superficial femoral artery occlusive disease (a) have a low likelihood of limb loss (2% to 12% in a 10-year follow-up) if followed closely on conservative treatment, (b) can expect improvement in

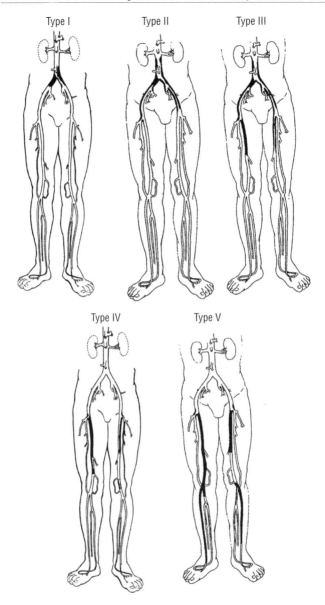

Figure 14.2.   Patterns of arterial occlusive disease of the lower extremitites. Type 1 is limited to the distal abdominal aorta and common iliac arteries. Type 2 is aortoiliac, involving the aorta, common iliacs and also the external iliacs. Type 3 involves these areas and the femoropopliteal region. Type 4 is isolated femoropopliteal disease with preserved aortoiliac inflow and poplitealtibial outflow. Type V is combined disease of the femoropopliteal and more distal tibial arteries.

symptoms (80%) if the initial ABI is greater than 0.6, and (c) should undergo evaluation for percutaneous treatment or reconstructive surgery if the ABI falls below 0.5. Five-year survival is 70% to 80%, and only 10% will require surgical revascularization.

D. Femoropopliteal-tibial disease (type 5). These patients are at highest risk of limb loss over time. This is due to the poor long-term outcomes with revascularization treatments for disease in the tibial vessels. Furthermore, within this particular pattern of disease patients are usually older (over 65) and have a significant prevalence of diabetes mellitus, smoking, and lipid abnormalities, all of which are significant factors in disease progression. Diabetes in particular has been implicated in disease progression and is causative in infrapopliteal disease. Some within this group have classically spared aortoiliac and femoropopliteal segments with diffuse, significant tibial disease. These are usually poorly controlled diabetics and noted to be of Hispanic and Native American ethnicities.

II. Common clinical scenarios. Understanding the spectrum of lower-extremity ischemia and how it is classified is vital. This practical classification helps to break down and define how the limb ischemia is approached therapeutically. Chronic limb ischemia (Table 14.1) and acute limb ischemia (Table 14.2) classifications are available and reveal the spectrum of chronic disease and help define the imminent viability of the limb, respectively. Lower limb ischemia in the great majority of cases is due to atherosclerotic disease, but a large spectrum of vascular diseases may cause the symptoms (Table 14.3).

A. Claudication (grade I; categories 1-3; Table 14.1) is a reproducible, consistent pain, ache, fatigue, heaviness, numbness and/or weakness of muscle groups due to exercise-induced ischemia. Symptoms are absent at rest and abate when exercise is stopped. In general, the symptoms occur in the muscle groups one level beyond the significant disease. Thus, calf claudication alone usually indicates superficial femoral artery disease. The addition of the thigh and buttock muscles points to aortoiliac disease. The disappearance of the symptoms is not positional as opposed to neurogenic claudication. The natural history of intermittent claudication due to arterial insufficiency is a benign one in general. Only 4-5% of those with true vascular claudication progress to a limb-threatening stage. Most actually die of associated cardiovascular morbidity, rather than from factors related to their leg ischemia. Similarly, many patients with asymptomatic but identified atherosclerosis of their lower-extremity arteries do not progress to develop symptoms if their condition is managed carefully. This being said, there are certain factors associated with advancement of PAOD to the critical point (Fig. 14.3).

B. Critical ischemia. Ischemic rest pain in the lower extremity may be the first symptom of severe ischemia (grade II, category 4; Table 14.1). There are many causes of leg and foot pain in which arterial perfusion to the foot may be normal. These include diabetic neuropathy, arthritis, venous insufficiency, and causalgia-type complex regional pain syndromes. Specific features suggest pain to be of ischemic origin. Ischemic rest pain is sharp and localized primarily to the fore-

Table 14.1.   Categories of chronic limb ischemia

Grade	Category	Clinical description	Objective criteria
0	0	Asymptomatic—no significant occlusive disease	Normal treadmill/ stress test[a]
	1	Mild claudication	Complete treadmill test[a]; AP after test >50 mm Hg
I	2	Moderate claudication	Between categories 1 and 3
	3	Severe claudication	Cannot complete tread-mill test[a]; AP after test <50 mm Hg
		Subcritical limb ischemia	
		No resting symptoms or tissue loss	Resting AP <50 mm Hg, ankle or metatarsal PVR flat or barely pulsatile; TP <40 mm Hg
		Critical limb ischemia	
II	4	Ischemic rest pain	Resting AP <40 mm Hg, ankle or metatarsal PVR flat or barely pulsatile; TP <30 mm Hg
	5	Minor tissue loss— nonhealing ulcer, focal gangrene and pedal ischemia	Resting AP <60 mm Hg, ankle or metatarsal PVR flat or barely pulsatile; TP <40 mm Hg
III	6	Major tissue loss— extending above TM level, functional foot no longer salvagable	Same as category 5

AP, ankle pressure; PVR, pulse volume recording; TP, toe pressure; TM, transmetatarsal.
[a]5 minutes at 2 miles per hour on a 12% incline
(Adapted from: Inter-society Consensus for the Management of Peripheral Arterial Disease (TASC II). *J Vasc Surg.* 2007;45(suppl S):S29A.)

foot below the ankle and the foot usually has dependent rubor and elevation pallor. Not uncommonly, patients are awoken by the pain at night and dangle their foot for relief. Palpable pulses are absent.

The reason ischemic rest pain is classified as limb threatening is clear. Once perfusion is so poor that rest pain develops, 95% of people will loose the limb within a year unless revascularization is instituted. An interesting group of patients has recently been identified as having "subcritical" ischemia. These patients have severe disease with no apparent symptoms,

Table 14.2. Categories of acute limb ischemia

Category	Description	Capillary refill	Muscle weakness	Sensory loss	Arterial Doppler	Venous Doppler
I. Viable	Not immediately threatened	Intact	None	None	Audible	Audible
II. Threatened						
a. Marginally	Salvageable if promptly treated	Intact, slow	None	Minimal (toes) or none	Often audible	Audible
b. Immediately	Salvageable with immediate revascularization	Very slow or absent	Mild, moderate	More than toes, associated with rest pain	Usually inaudible	Audible
III. Irreversible	Major tissue loss, amputation regardless of treatment	Absent (marbling)	Profound, paralysis (rigor)	Profound. anesthetic	Inaudible	Inaudible

(Adapted from Inter-society Consensus for the Management of Peripheral Arterial Disease (TASC II). *J Vasc Surg.* 2007;45(Suppl S):S41A.)

Table 14.3. Arterial diseases causing claudication

Atherosclerosis (PAD)

Arteritis

Congenital and acquired coarctation of aorta

Endofibrosis of the external iliac artery (iliac artery syndrome in cyclists)

Fibromuscular dysplasia

Peripheral emboli

Popliteal aneurysm (with secondary thromboembolism)

Adventitial cyst of the popliteal artery

Popliteal entrapment

Primary vascular tumors

Pseudoxanthoma elasticum

Remote trauma or irradiation injury

Takayasu's disease

Thromboangiitis obliterans (Buerger's disease)

Thrombosis of a persistent sciatic artery

usually due to inactivity, and a resting ankle pressure <50 mm Hg with a toe pressure <40 mm Hg. Some have nonspecific symptoms in their leg with exertion, which may be attributed to the degree of their ischemia but this is usually not clear. They are at increased risk for progression to limb loss as well, but almost one-third will still have their limb at one year with-

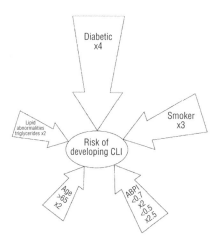

Figure 14.3.   Influence of risk factors on the development of critical limb ischemia (CLI) in those with peripheral arterial occlusive disease (PAOD). ABPI, ankle-brachial pressure index. (From Intersociety Consensus for the Management of Peripheral Arterial Disease [TASC II]. *J Vasc Surg.* 2007;45(suppl S):S10A with permission.)

out revascularization, and with comorbidities medical management may be appropriate.

Ischemic rest pain usually does not occur unless the patient has at least two hemodynamically significant arterial occlusive lesions (e.g., at least two levels of disease). Most individuals with rest pain will have one of two distinct anatomic patterns of occlusive disease that must be defined before an appropriate therapy can be selected:

1. Combined aortoiliac and superficial femoral arterial occlusive disease (type 3; Fig. 14.2)
2. Femoropopliteal arterial occlusion with distal tibial occlusive disease (type 5; Fig. 14.2)

C. Critical ischemia. Nonhealing ulcers of the distal foot may also be the result of arterial ischemia (grade III, categories 5 and 6; Table 14.1). Even with arterial perfusion, healing may be prevented by infection of bone or soft tissue, pressure from improper footwear, foot malformation, or improper medical treatment. In this situation the metabolic demand of the local process outstrips the arterial supply. A good history and physical should provide information for sorting out the reasons for poor healing. The sensory neuropathy associated with long-term diabetes makes diabetic patients susceptible to **neuropathic foot ulcers.** Such patients may not feel the initial sore and therefore not present until the ulcer is deep and infected.

D. Critical ischemia. Gangrene is a classic sign of ischemia in the skin and subcutaneous tissue (grade III, categories 5 and 6; Table 14.1). Dry gangrene is characterized by a noninfected black eschar, whereas wet gangrene has tissue maceration and purulence.

E. Microemboli cause bluish, mottled spots scattered over the toes **(blue toe syndrome)**, which may be painful. They also may be mistaken for local traumatic bruises, and their true significance overlooked. Microemboli may originate from any point in the proximal arterial system, most commonly from the heart, aneurysms, or ulcerated plaques.

F. Acute arterial ischemia (Table 14.2) is characterized by the sudden onset of extremity pain, pallor, paresthesia, pulselessness, poikilothermia, and sometimes paralysis. If the patient has a history of claudication or previous lower-extremity arterial graft, the symptoms may be caused by thrombosis of a stenotic artery, usually from acute atherosclerotic plaque rupture, or the arterial graft. **If the patient previously had no symptoms of peripheral vascular disease, the acute ischemia is more likely embolic.** The embolic source is usually the heart, followed distantly by more proximal atherosclerotic disease.

III. Management.

A. Claudication/functional ischemia. The following principles are crucial in determining the best treatment for a patient with intermittent vascular claudication. For most patients, initial treatment is nonoperative. As mentioned, only 5% to 10% of patients with claudication will require amputation of an extremity due to progression of the disease in 5 years, most of whom continue to smoke or who have diabetes mellitus. **Lower-extremity imaging can be accomplished by CTA,**

MRA, or duplex ultrasound. Arteriography should be viewed as an invasive intent to treat and is not usually necessary in the majority of patients with recent onset vascular claudication.

1. **Determination** of initial treatment is based on the duration, disability, and progression of the claudication. Initial management also is influenced by the patient's medical condition.

   a. **Duration.** If the leg claudication is of recent onset and is not incapacitating, a trial period of nonoperative therapy is indicated without the need for an imaging. This approach is recommended particularly for patients who are suspected of having a recent superficial femoral artery occlusion. Although they may experience sudden severe calf claudication when the artery occludes, their claudication usually improves in 6 to 8 weeks if profunda femoris arterial collaterals are well developed. In general, we prefer to follow patients with recent onset of claudication for at least 3 to 6 months to determine whether the claudication will stabilize, improve, or worsen.

   b. **Disability.** We generally ask two important questions of the patient about the disability imposed by the leg claudication: Does the leg claudication prevent normal activity, especially the performance of essential daily activities or a job? Does the claudication limit leisure activities that the patient enjoys? In our experience, the answers to these two questions are more helpful in determining patient management than is the distance the patient can walk before he or she is stopped by claudication, but this test may provide helpful insight to the severity of disease.

   c. **Progression.** It is extremely important to determine whether the claudication is stable or progressing. Patients who have noted rapid progression of claudication over 6 months to 1 year are more likely to need arterial reconstruction than are stable claudicants. Patients with progressive claudication also are more likely to appreciate any relief that revascularization may provide.

   d. **Assessment of the patient's general medical condition** is essential for determining the proper initial management of claudication. Elective operations for intermittent claudication should be reserved for patients who appear to have a low risk of mortality (2% to 3%) and morbidity. This assessment is discussed in detail in Chapter 8. Patients with multiple medical problems and stable leg claudication should be followed until symptoms become incapacitating or the limb is threatened by progression to rest pain, nonhealing ulcers, or gangrene (i.e., critical limb ischemia).

2. **Nonoperative management** includes a supervised, structured walking program and control or elimination of cardiovascular risk factors. Nonoperative management includes regularly scheduled follow-up assessments with noninvasive surveillance. This usually includes either ABIs or segmental pressures and PVRs. This also allows for

ongoing assessment of the patient's peripheral vascular system as many people with PAOD have concomitant cerebrovascular, coronary, and aneurysmal disease.

a. Regular lower-extremity exercise increases metabolic adaptation to ischemia due to walking and may enhance collateral blood flow. The result is stabilization or improvement of claudication. A variety of exercise programs can alleviate claudication. A relatively simple program that has helped 80% of our patients emphasizes the following concepts:

(1) Patients are asked to set aside a definite period and frequency for exercise in **addition** to normal daily activities (e.g., 30 minutes, 3 to 5 days per week). Exercise every day may be too much activity for many older patients; consequently, an every-other-day exercise program is ideal.

(2) Patients are instructed to walk at a comfortable (not too fast) pace and stop for a brief rest whenever claudication becomes severe.

(3) This walk–rest routine should be continued for 30 minutes. As the leg muscles adapt to anaerobic metabolism, the frequency and length of rest stops will decrease. After 6 to 8 weeks, most claudicants can double or triple their comfortable walking distance. In bad weather, the patient may use an indoor treadmill, walk inside a shopping mall, or use a stationary exercise bicycle.

b. Risk factor control. Chapter 7 describes the important and critical cardiovascular risk factors associated with PAOD. Smoking cessation, control of hyperlipidemias, diabetes mellitus, hypertension, and weight reduction are imperative if nonoperative management is to have a maximal effect. Failure of nonoperative management in the claudicant is usually due to the inability to quit smoking and control these other factors.

c. Pentoxifylline (Trental, Hoechst Marion Roussel, Kansas City, MO, U.S.A.) was the first drug approved by the U.S. Food and Drug Administration for the treatment of intermittent claudication. This rheologic agent is a methylxanthine that reduces blood viscosity by improving red blood cell membrane flexibility and inhibits platelet aggregation. Although the benefits of pentoxifylline are still debated, a recent meta-analysis concluded that the drug resulted in an average 29 m increase in initial claudication distance and a 48 m increase in absolute claudication distance compared to placebo.

d. Cilostazol (Pletal, Otsuka Pharmaceuticals, Rockville, MD, U.S.A.) is a more recent medication for intermittent claudication. It is a phosphodiesterase III inhibitor with vasodilator and antiplatelet activity. Three randomized trials have shown improvements in initial claudication distance and absolute claudication distance in the treated groups compared with placebo.

In our practice, pentoxifylline, 400 mg two or three times daily with meals, or cilostazol, 100 mg twice daily, have been combined with a walking program and smoking reduction for selected patients with mild to moderate claudication. If walking is improved after 6 to 8 weeks, the drug is often stopped to ascertain whether exercise and abstinence from tobacco will maintain improvement. If claudication worsens, the drug may be restarted. Common side effects of pentoxifylline are gastrointestinal upset and dizziness. Some patients can tolerate only 400 mg twice daily. For cilostazol, the most common side effects are headache and diarrhea. Cilostazol is contraindicated in patients with class III or IV congestive heart failure and a significant arrhythmia history. If used, the dose should be reduced to 50 mg twice a day for those on calcium channel blockers, ketoconazole, or erythromycin derivatives as these inhibit cilostazol's hepatic metabolism by the P-450 system. Increased drug concentrations potentiate its risk of atrial arrhythmias.

We emphasize that drug therapy with pentoxifylline or cilostazol cannot prevent the need for revascularization in patients with severe progressive claudication or critical ischemia.

3. Indications for invasive therapy in a claudicant. Patients must be selected carefully for percutaneous therapies or surgery for lower-extremity claudication. Impairment of occupational performance and significant lifestyle limitation on a low-risk patient are reasonable indications. In this situation, it is important that a favorable anatomic situation for percutaneous or surgical reconstruction be present. The best results are obtained when the occlusive disease is localized to the aorta and iliac arteries with open distal vessels. Isolated superficial femoral artery disease with good (two or more tibial vessels continuous to the foot) runoff is also a favorable anatomic lesion for treatment.

We generally discourage elective arterial reconstruction for stable claudication if the primary disease is (a) combined severe, diffuse aortoiliac and severe femoropopliteal arterial disease or (b) severe below-the-knee popliteal and tibial artery disease. Aortoiliac angioplasty/stenting or an aortofemoral bypass in the setting of a patent, large, well-collateralizing profunda femoris artery may significantly improve many patients. However, without this type of runoff the immediate or staged addition of a femoropopliteal bypass may be necessary to significantly relieve claudication when multilevel occlusive disease (type 3) exists. Thus, aortofemoral reconstruction for claudication in patients with combined aortoiliac and femoropopliteal disease should be recommended only when claudication is rapidly progressing and the aortoiliac disease has advanced to critical stenoses or occlusions and it is clear that normalizing inflow with reasonable outflow is likely to provide improvement in activity level. **Likewise, due to reduced durability compared to above-knee reconstructions, below-the-knee femoropopliteal or femorotibial bypasses should be limb salvage procedures, and rarely should they be used to treat claudication alone.**

Currently, the rapid advancement and use of endovascular therapies has led to readdressing the indications for intervention for claudication. In general, proponents of endovascular therapies for claudication believe that such interventions have lower associated risk to the patient and ultimately improve activity levels. In addition these proponents point out that in the majority of cases endovascular therapies do not "burn bridges" for future endovascular or open surgical reconstruction. At this time, as bodies of evidence are accumulating, we believe there is no definitive evidence that indications for intervention in claudication should be changed based solely on the availability of endovascular therapies (e.g., just because it can be done doesn't mean it should be done).

4. Preoperative evaluation.

a. The principles of assessing **operative risk** and stabilizing chronic medical problems are discussed in Chapter 8. Mortality for percutaneous, endovascular therapy should be negligible. Operative mortality for elective aortoiliac reconstruction or femoropopliteal bypass for claudication should not exceed 2-3%. The primary risk to life during vascular reconstructions is coronary artery disease. Significant coronary artery disease exists in at least 40% of patients with peripheral vascular disease. In general, we recommend that the necessary surgical procedures for significant coronary artery disease be performed before elective vascular intervention is attempted.

b. Before elective surgery, patients should be asked to make a commitment to **stop smoking** and to not resume tobacco use after recovery. They should be informed that the chance of graft failure approaches 30% in patients who continue to smoke regularly. Elective reconstruction for claudication in active smokers should be eschewed, but can be entertained once a significant and progressive reduction in smoking has occurred to the point of just a few cigarettes a day. Most of these individuals will quit completely after hospitalization.

c. Lower-extremity arteriography is performed only after the decision has been made to intervene with arterial reconstruction or percutaneous therapy. In our practice, we liberally use duplex ultrasound to delineate arterial disease prior to arteriogram to aid in determining the possibility of an endovascular revascularization option prior to arteriography. This is purely lab dependent. Intravenous contrast may, therefore, be minimized if inflow and outflow segments do not need dedicated arteriographic interrogation prior to intervention. Others use CTA and MRA in a similar manner, while some proceed directly to arteriography and make an on-table determination of therapeutic options. Ideally, at least a one-day delay should be allowed before open surgical revascularization to ensure that renal function does not deteriorate after the contrast load from the angiogram. Endovascular therapy can be instituted at the same sitting as diagnostic arteriography, or delayed in a staged fashion several days to weeks later.

Table 14.4. Aortofemoral graft for multilevel occlusive disease: Predictors of success and need for distal bypass

Emphasis of Evaluation	Predictors of Good AF-Only Result	Predictors of Need for Distal Bypass
Proximal disease	Absent or severely reduced femoral pulse	"Normal" femoral pulse
	Severe stenosis/occlusion (arteriogram) (positive femoral artery pressure study)[a]	Mild-moderate inflow disease (arteriogram) (Negative femoral artery pressure study)
Distal disease	Good outflow tract (arteriogram)	Poor outflow tract (arteriogram)
	Index runoff resistance <0.2	Index runoff resistance ≥0.2[b]
Intra-operative	Improved pulse volume recorder amplitude	Unimproved/worse pulse volume recorder amplitude profunda femoris diseased (origin ≤4mm and #3 Fogarty® embolectomy catheter (Edwards Lifesciences Corp., Irvine, CA) inserted <20 cm)
Clinical	Nonadvanced ischemic symptoms (i.e., claudication, rest pain)	Advanced ischemia (necrosis/sepsis)

AF, aortofemoral.
[a]Femoral artery pressure study. An iliac stenosis is significant when the resting pressure gradient across iliac segment is greater than 5 mm Hg or falls more than 15% after reactive hyperemia or directed injection with papaverine or nitroglycerin.
[b]Index runoff resistance = thigh-ankle pressure difference/brachial pressure
(Adapted from: Brewster DC, Perler BA, Robinson JG, Darling RO. Aortofemoral graft for multilevel occlusive disease: predictors of success and need for distal bypass. *Arch Surg* 1982;117:1593-1600.)

5. Selection of proper procedure in aortoiliac disease. The choice of operation or endovascular intervention for claudication depends on the general condition of the patient, the extent of the atherosclerotic process, and the experience of the surgeon/interventionalist. The preoperative arteriogram in conjunction with both resting and "stress" femoral artery pressure measurements, using techniques for distal vasodilation to unmask a stenosis, are the best determinants of which procedure to undertake in a given patient (Table 14.4). A well-trained vascular surgeon should understand the indications and limitations for the following procedures: aortoiliac endarterectomy, aortoiliac or aortofemoral bypass graft, femoropopliteal bypass, lumbar sympathectomy, transluminal angioplasty, angioplasty and stenting, and extraanatomic reconstruction such as axillofemoral and femorofemoral bypasses.

a. Aortoiliac endarterectomy. In patients with occlusive disease limited to the distal aorta and common iliac arteries, **aortoiliac endarterectomy** gives excellent long-term results, provided the patient eliminates or controls his or her vascular risk factors. Endarterectomy is contraindicated in the presence of (a) aortic or iliac aneurysmal disease, (b) aortic occlusion to the level of the renal vessels, or (c) any occlusive disease in the external iliac or femoral arteries. The 5- and 10-year patency rates are 95% and 85%, respectively. However, such focal aortoiliac disease is currently treated in most patients by percutaneous balloon angioplasty and stenting with excellent results at decreased procedural risk. This has relegated endarterectomy to almost a historical setting.

b. Percutaneous transluminal angioplasty/stenting is currently the initial treatment of choice for focal arterial lesions that cause claudication (see Chapter 11). While beyond the full scope of this discussion, the Trans-Atlantic Inter-Society Consensus documents on the management of PAOD (TASC I [2000] and TASC II [2007]) have provided anatomic recommendations on the use of endovascular revascularization (Fig. 14.4). These communications place the growing literature and changing technology into perspective. Suffice it to say that as atherosclerotic lesions become longer, more tortuous, and completely occluded, the more difficult are the endovascular solutions. Thus, a focal common iliac stenosis of less than 3 cm in length has been a lesion well suited to endovascular treatment (TASC A). Endovascular recanalization of long iliac occlusions and infrarenal aortic disease, and longer severely diseased iliac lengths (TASC C and D) are also commonplace as first-line therapy, yet surgery remains superior. Endovascular therapies, however, will only become more widespread as re-entry technology and stent engineering improves. Owing to their inferior durability, these reconstructions require close serial duplex surveillance and repeat intervention as necessary.

Angioplasty results in the iliac system are enhanced by the addition of stents. Balloon expandable stents are generally used in the common iliac where the plaque burden is usually bulky and significantly involved with calcification. The radial force of these stents is helpful in this case (Chapter 11). In the external iliac artery, self-expanding stents are generally used as they are more flexible in this variably tortuous area. This therapy has provided a primary patency rate of 70-80% at 4 years. Consequently, t**he primary limitation of aortoiliac endovascular therapy is restenosis,** which affects 20% to 30% of patients within 3 to 5 years. These current results indicate that repeated endovascular intervention may be required to achieve satisfactory, long-term relief of symptoms. The impact that newer technologies, such as cutting balloons, cryoplasty, re-entry devices, and both directional and laser-based atherectomy devices, may have on these results remains to be clarified.

TASC 2007 Classification of Aortoiliac Disease Lesions

Type A lesions

- Unilateral or bilateral stenoses of CIA
- Unilateral or bilateral single short (≤3 cm) stenosis of EIA

Type B lesions

- Short (≤3 cm) stenosis of infrarenal aorta
- Unilateral CIA occlusion
- Single or multiple stenosis totaling 3–10 cm involving the EIA not extending into the CFA
- Unilateral EIA occlusion not involving the origins of internal iliac or CFA

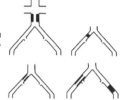

Type C lesions

- Bilateral CIA occlusions
- Bilateral EIA stenoses 3–10 cm long not extending into the CFA
- Unilateral EIA stenosis extending into the CFA
- Unilateral EIA occlusion that involves the origins of internal iliac and/or CFA
- Heavily calcified unilateral EIA occlusion with or without involvement of origins of internal iliac and/or CFA

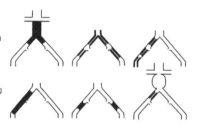

Type D lesions

- Infra-renal aortoiliac occlusion
- Diffuse disease involving the aorta and both iliac arteries requiring treatment
- Diffuse multiple stenoses involving the unilateral CIA, EIA, and CFA
- Unilateral occlusions of both CIA and EIA
- Bilateral occlusions of EIA
- Iliac stenoses in patients with AAA requiring treatment and not amenable to endograft placement or other lesions requiring open aortic or iliac surgery

Figure 14.4. TASC 2007 anatomic classification of aortoiliac disease lesions. Current recommendations for treatment include: endovascular results acceptable for type A, surgery superior for type D. For type B, endovascular treatment is preferred, while if a good surgical candidate, surgery is preferred for type C. The patient's comorbid condition, treatment preference after being informed, as well as the operator's experiences must be contemplated for a reasonable decision. (From Inter-society Consensus for the Management of Peripheral Arterial Disease [TASC II]. *J Vasc Surg.* 2007;45(suppl S):S49A with permission.)

c. **Aortofemoral bypass**. The majority of patients with incapacitating claudication due to diffuse, high-grade occlusive disease including the aortoiliac segments will ultimately require a **bypass graft of the aortoiliac segments** for durable relief (>5 years). Aortofemoral bypass grafts are preferred to aortoiliac bypass grafts, because, not uncommonly, the external iliac segment eventually becomes obliterated by progressive arteriosclerosis, albeit usually after the distal aorta and common iliac arteries. Subsequent downstream repair becomes necessary in approximately 25% to 30% of patients who are initially treated by aortoiliac bypass, compared to 10% to 15% of patients who undergo aortofemoral bypass initially. In selected patients with unilateral iliac occlusive disease, unilateral aortoiliac or aortofemoral bypass grafts or endarterectomy may be performed through a retroperitoneal approach. Five-year patency rates of 70% to 80% are encouraging and indicate that iliac-origin arterial grafts are useful in situations where one wants to avoid transabdominal, or retroperitoneal aortofemoral grafting or extraanatomic bypasses. The primary patency of aortobifemoral bypass grafts is 85-95% at 5 years. It remains one of the most durable reconstructions in vascular surgery.

d. Extra-anatomic axillofemoral or femorofemoral bypasses, in our practice, are useful only in a very limited group of patients with severe claudication. The most suitable candidates are those with the following:

1. Iliac occlusion on the symptomatic lower extremity and a normal contralateral iliac artery in the case of planned femorofemoral bypass or axillary artery in the case of planned axillofemoral bypass
2. Previous postirradiation intestinal obstructions or fistulas that discourage intra-abdominal aortofemoral reconstruction
3. Known extensive postsurgical abdominal adhesions
4. Significant cardiopulmonary comorbidities and category 3 claudication or subcritical ischemia

Direct aortoiliac reconstruction for claudication is preferable to extraanatomic bypass. As such, if the patient is a candidate for direct reconstruction but has the above drawbacks, retroperitoneal aortofemoral grafting, or thoracofemoral bypass are also excellent options. When done by experienced hands, aortoiliac reconstruction is safe and, as stated, provides a very durable result in 85% to 90% of patients at 5 years. In contrast, 5-year patency for femorofemoral bypass and axillofemoral bypass for claudication ranges from 50% to 75%.

e. Elective aortoiliac reconstruction for occlusive disease is generally **not combined** with other nonvascular, intra-abdominal operations. For example, we favor leaving asymptomatic gallstones alone despite the recommendations of others to do a cholecystectomy if there are no mitigating circumstances. Although the morbidity of adding cholecystectomy may be low, additional procedures do increase the risks of complications. Also, postoperative cholecystitis secondary to cholelithiasis is rare in our experience. Most postoperative cholecystitis is acalculous and occurs in patients who have been in shock and have the so-called splanchnic shock syndrome. Occasionally, however, we discover incidentally a gallbladder with cholelithiasis *and* chronic smouldering cholecystitis during operative exploration. If the aortic reconstruction goes well, we may perform cholecystectomy *after* the retroperitoneum and femoral wounds have been closed to cover the prosthetic graft.

f. Prior to hospital admission, complete history, physical examination, and routine diagnostic studies are performed. Baseline studies include a complete blood count, chest x-ray, 12-lead electrocardiogram (ECG), serum electrolytes, creatinine, blood sugar, liver function tests (bilirubin, serum glutamic-oxaloacetic transaminase, alkaline phosphatase, total protein, albumin), platelet count, prothrombin time (PT), partial thromboplastin time (PTT), fasting serum cholesterol and triglycerides, calcium, phosphorus, and pulmonary function tests in patients with chronic lung disease. Any preoperative consultations with other specialists are arranged before admission.

(1) The patient is typed and cross-matched for 2 to 4 units of packed red blood cells for aortic operations and typed, screened, and held for femoropopliteal and extra-anatomic reconstructions. If autotransfusion is planned, arrangements are made for its availability.

(2) Generally, we do not use bowel preparation for aortic surgery. Should supraceliac cross-clamping be anticipated, however, a prep is initiated as the liver ischemia in conjunction with gut ischemia and possible bacterial translocation has been implicated in operative coagulopathy. For bowel preparation, the patient receives clear liquids and a laxative (e.g., magnesium citrate, 120-250 mL p.o.) 24 hours before surgery in conjunction with a standard neomycin/erythromycin oral preparation.

(3) Since elective arterial patients may have chronic intravascular volume depletion from diuretics and acute dehydration from contrast loads and a bowel preparation, an intravenous infusion of Ringer's lactated solution at 100 to 125 mL/h is started before surgery. Depending on individual patient requirements, such hydration may take 6 to 12 hours prior to operation. Thus, selected patients will require hospital admission on the evening prior to aortic surgery.

(4) Skin preparation includes shaving hair in the operative field as close to the time of operation as possible to minimize bacterial colonization of the shaved areas. A shower with hexachlorophene, chlorhexidine gluconate, or povidone- iodine soap also is done as close to the time of operation as possible, usually just before the intravenous infusion is started.

(5) Patients are instructed in deep breathing and coughing, as well as in the use of an incentive spirometer. We also teach the patient leg exercises that are used as prophylaxis against deep venous thrombosis, for stimulation of lower-extremity blood flow, and for maintenance of leg muscle tone prior to ambulation.

(6) Preoperative prophylactic antibiotics are administered intravenously when the patient is called to the operating room. A semisynthetic penicillin or a cephalosporin is used. For patients with a history of penicillin allergy, the cephalosporins are avoided and the patient receives another antibiotic (e.g., vancomycin, 500 to 1,000 mg, or clindamycin 600 to 900 mg) with good coverage for hospital-acquired organisms.

g. Operative principles of aortofemoral bypass. The complete details of operative technique are beyond the scope of this handbook. Other operative atlases describe specific techniques for arterial reconstruction in a more detailed manner. Yet, certain principles of intraoperative care do warrant emphasis here.

(1) **Patient positioning.** The patient is kept in the supine position with the electrocautery ground beneath the buttocks. The arms generally are adducted to the sides. Ischemic heels are elevated or wrapped with a soft dressing to prevent pressure sores.

(2) **Skin preparation.** The operating room should be warmed (70°F to 75°F) during the skin preparation to reduce heat loss from the patient. The skin preparation extends from the nipples to the knees for aortofemoral reconstructions and to the toes for patients who may require an associated femoropopliteal bypass. Care must be taken to avoid pooling of the preparatory solution beneath the patient, especially in contact with the electrocautery ground. Full-thickness chemical skin burns can result from pooling and prolonged contact with the solution. After application of the antiseptic preparatory solution, the skin is covered with a plastic Steri-Drape (3M Health Care, St. Paul, MN, U.S.A.). Although Steri-Drapes may not reduce the incidence of wound infection, we recommend their use to prevent contact of graft materials with the skin, which may contaminate the graft.

(3) **Intraoperative monitoring.** All lower-extremity arterial reconstructions are monitored with a pulse volume recorder (PVR), or continuous wave Doppler for evidence of appropriate distal flow. As a general rule, PVR cuffs are placed one limb segment below the anticipated reconstruction site (i.e., at the calf for aortofemoral bypass and at the ankle for femoropopliteal bypass). A baseline recording is made. Additional recordings are made immediately following the arterial reconstruction and before the patient leaves the operating room. Sterile cuffs should be used in the operative field. Alternatively, objective changes in CWD signal characteristics are used.

(4) **Systemic anticoagulation.** Heparin is used for systemic anticoagulation while the aorta and distal arteries are clamped. Our experience has indicated that an adequate heparin dose is 3,000 to 5,000 units given intravenously 5 minutes before aortic clamping and an additional 1,000 U given every 45 minutes afterward unless clinical judgment speaks against this. Although monitoring of heparin effect may not

be necessary, we prefer to check an activated clotting time (ACT) before and after heparinization. An ACT of 200 to 300 seconds is adequate for most cases. Smaller additional doses of heparin (500 to 1,000 units) are given during regional irrigation of the iliac and major femoral artery branches. Reversal of heparin is optional at the termination of the procedure. In general, heparinization with the above doses does not require reversal, since the heparin effect diminishes in about 90 minutes. However, if one chooses to reverse heparinization, ACTs are the primary method used to monitor reversal with protamine sulfate (0.5 to 1.0 mg for every 100 U of heparin remaining).

(5) Intraoperative diuretics. Diuresis must be established prior to aortic clamping to keep urine output at 0.5 to 1.0 cc/kg/hour. Infrarenal aortic clamping diminishes renal cortical blood flow which can be prevented by intravascular volume expansion and administration of the osmotic diuretic mannitol. We give 12.5 to 25.0 grams of mannitol intravenously just before clamping the aorta. When needed, small (10 to 20 mg) doses of furosemide are added. In addition, dopamine (2 to 3 µg/min IV) may cause renal vasodilatation. In those with renal insufficiency, fenoldopam, a δ-1 selective receptor agonist, is advo-

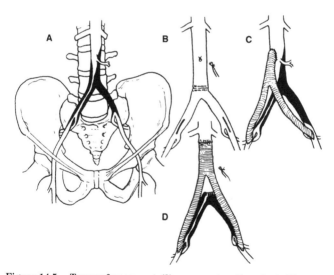

Figure 14.5. Types of open aortoiliac reconstruction. Aortoiliac endarterectomy (**B**) is an option for occlusive disease localized to the distal abdominal aorta and common iliac arteries. It has mostly been replaced by endovascular therapies for this focal pattern (**A**). For aortofemoral grafting, the proximal anastamosis may be performed end-to-side (**C**) or end-to-end (**D**). (Adapted from Darling RC, et al. Aorto-iliac reconstruction. *Surg Clin North Am.* 1979;59:565-579.)

cated to increase renal cortical blood flow and tubular filtration during aortic clamping and is used at 0.01-0.05 μcg/kg/min.

(6) Proximal aortic anastomosis. Controversy continues over whether the proximal aortic graft anastomosis should be end-to-end or end-to-side (Fig. 14.5). Our experience strongly favors end-to-end aortic anastomosis. Its primary advantages are as follows:

1. The origin of the graft is from a higher and less diseased part of the infrarenal abdominal aorta.
2. A better hemodynamic situation, as the aortic blood flow is direct through the graft without competitive flow from the distal aorta.
3. A more anatomic position and better retroperitoneal coverage as a segment of infrarenal aorta is resected prior to placement of the graft. The onlay or end-to-side aortic anastomosis leaves the graft protruding anteriorly. For this reason, the end-to-side graft seems more likely to adhere to adjacent bowel and cause aortoenteric fistula.
4. Exclusion of the diseased infrarenal and iliac segments is achieved and this may reduce the possibility of later atheroembolization.

Situations where an end-to-side is preferable relate to renal and gut perfusion and are as follows:

- When there are accessory renal arteries supplying significant parenchyma from the infrarenal aorta.
- A large inferior mesenteric artery is present and antegrade flow in the IMA is desired for adequate colon perfusion.
- When significant disease is mainly located in the external iliac arteries. In this situation, antegrade pelvic blood flow is preferred, as end-to-end will greatly reduce pelvic blood flow as retrograde flow will not exist.

(7) Distal anastomosis in aortofemoral bypass has a significant influence on graft patency. The leading cause of late aortofemoral graft failure is loss of outflow and this can be minimized if the correct distal configuration is chosen. There are five methods of distal anastomosis (Fig. 14.6).

Type 1, anastomosis to the common femoral artery, is preferred for patients with widely patent profunda femoris and superficial femoral arteries.

Type 2 anastomosis carries the graft onto the proximal superficial femoral artery and is recommended when the orifice of the superficial femoral artery is stenotic but the distal arteries and profunda femoris artery are otherwise normal.

Type 3 anastomosis (known as profundaplasty) carries the graft onto the profunda femoris artery and is recommended for patients with extensive superficial femoral artery disease or

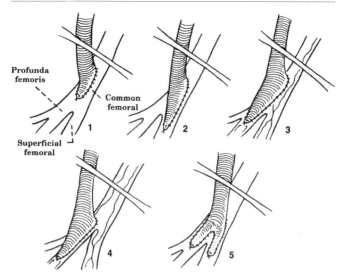

Figure 14.6. Types of femoral anastomosis for aortofemoral bypass grafts: **(1)** type 1 anastomosis to the common femoral artery; **(2)** type 2 anastomosis, in which the graft is carried onto the proximal superficial femoral artery; **(3)** type 3 anastomosis, in which the graft is carried onto the profunda femoris artery; **(4)** type 4 anastomosis, involving only the profunda femoris artery; **(5)** type 5 anastomosis, involving a patch angioplasty of both the superficial and deep femoral arterial orifices. (Adapted from Darling RC, et al. Aortoiliac reconstruction. *Surg Clin North Am.* 1979;59:565-579.)

occlusion. In most patients, the profunda femoris artery is of adequate diameter (3 to 4 mm) and length (15 to 20 cm) to maintain aortofemoral graft flow and perfuse the leg via collaterals.

Type 4 anastomosis is done only to the profunda femoris artery. It is necessary when the common femoral and superficial femoral arteries are extensively obliterated.

Type 5 anastomosis splits the hood of the graft to patch proximal stenoses of both the superficial femoral and the profunda femoris arteries.

The need for concomitant distal bypass in conjunction with aortofemoral bypass occurs in some 17-20% of cases, but these are in the scenario of limb-threatening ischemia and will be discussed subsequently.

(8) Revascularization of the inferior mesenteric artery (IMA), by either bypass or reimplantation, should be performed when the superior mesenteric artery is occluded and a large (>3.5 to 4.0 mm) inferior mesenteric artery is present. Also, if the IMA is patent but shows poor back bleeding at the time of aortic reconstruction, or an IMA pressure is transduced at ≤40 mm Hg, strong consideration to IMA reimplantation should be given.

6. Femoropopliteal bypass for stable claudication is being performed less frequently now than it was in the past. Long-term follow-up of patients with leg claudication from a solitary superficial femoral artery occlusion indicates that nonoperative treatment often stabilizes the problem. In addition, progression of proximal aortoiliac disease may lead to poor inflow to a femoropopliteal bypass and eventual hemodynamic graft failure, often within 5 years. Therefore, patients who undergo femoropopliteal bypass for claudication alone should have a good anatomic situation, which includes normal aortoiliac inflow, a patent popliteal artery above the knee with two- or three-vessel runoff, and a high likelihood of an available saphenous vein. All evidence continues to suggest autogenous saphenous vein remains superior to all other graft materials for durability of a femoropopliteal bypass. However, use of Dacron or ePTFE prosthetic for above-knee femoropopliteal bypass for claudication remains accepted. Today, endovascular therapies are also reducing the number of femoropopliteal bypasses performed. Hybrid procedures may be used to treat both the aortoiliac inflow with endovascular techniques such as iliac angioplasty and stenting with concomitant femoropopliteal bypass grafting. Alternatively, iliac disease may be bilaterally treated by endovascular means in one setting, with staged femoropopliteal endovascular intervention or surgical bypass.

7. Femoropopliteal percutaneous endovascular intervention for functional lower-limb ischemia is now commonplace. Purported benefits of endovascular SFA intervention include decreased morbidity and mortality, no incisions, no need for and preservation of autogenous conduit, decreased hospital stay and resource utilization, and, finally, less social and family stress. Further, early evidence suggests that there is a limited downside to endovascular therapy in that recurrent endovascular intervention is possible and surgical options and distal targets are not compromised.

Similar to aortoiliac disease, TASC 2000 and TASC 2006 have delineated the currently held treatment opinions on anatomic classification of femoropopliteal disease (Fig. 14.7). Endovascular therapy appears appropriate for more focal, simple (TASC A) lesions. The more lengthy, calcified, and recurrent a stenosis or occlusion (TASC D) is, the less amenable it is to endovascular therapy.

Some debate has centered on superiority of primary stenting in the SFA. With the advent of nitinol alloy stent engineering, it appears now that when using these self-expanding stents, restenosis, objective ankle pressure improvements, and clinical success are superior to angioplasty alone at 1 year. Moreover, the impact and indications for directional atherectomy, laser atherectomy, ePTFE covered stents, drug-eluting stents, cryoplasty, cutting-balloon angioplasty, new re-entry devices, and embolic protection devices in the SFA are currently being studied. Currently, even using nitinol stents, primary patency of SFA interventions is roughly 50% to 60% at 3 years. Assisted primary

TASC 2007 Classification of Femoropopliteal Disease Lesions

Type A lesions

- Single stenosis ≤10 cm in length
- Single occlusion ≤5 cm in length

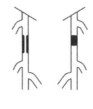

Type B lesions

- Multiple lesions (stenoses or occlusions), each ≤5 cm
- Single stenosis or occlusion ≤15 cm not involving the infrageniculate popliteal artery
- Single or multiple lesions in the absence of continuous tibial vessels to improve inflow for a distal bypass
- Heavily calcified occlusion ≤5 cm in length
- Single popliteal stenosis

Type C lesions

- Multiple stenoses or occlusions totaling >15 cm with or without heavy calcification
- Recurrent stenoses or occlusions that need treatment after two endovascular interventions

Type D lesions

- Chronic total occlusions of CFA or SFA (>20 cm, involving the popliteal artery)
- Chronic total occlusion of popliteal artery and proximal trifurcation vessels

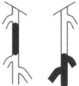

Figure 14.7.   TASC 2007 anatomic classification of femoropopliteal lesions. Current recommendations for treatment include: endovascular results acceptable for type A, surgery superior for type D. For type B endovascular treatment is preferred, while if a good surgical candidate, surgery is preferred for type C. The patient's comorbid condition, treatment preference after being informed, as well as the operator's experiences must be contemplated for a reasonable decision. (From Inter-society Consensus for the Management of Peripheral Arterial Disease [TASC II]. *J Vasc Surg.* 2007;45(suppl S):S51A with permission.)

patency has been shown to be improved compared to this, and the overwhelming majority of recurrent procedures necessary are also endovascular. Therefore, some feel that this type of therapy is comparable to prosthetic femoropopliteal bypass overall.

8. Lumbar sympathectomy alone is not considered adequate treatment of lower-extremity claudication. However, sympathectomy may be beneficial occasionally for ischemic rest pain, microembolic phenomenon, or foot sores when poor runoff and inadequate vein for a bypass are present and the ABI is greater than 0.35.

B. Critical/limb-threatening ischemia.

1. Prompt recognition of the signs of critical limb ischemia and timely initiation of therapy are necessary if the limb is to be saved (Table 14.2). The initial patient evaluation, therefore, must determine whether the patient needs emergent treatment or a less emergent diagnostic workup. This determination is based primarily on the patient history and physical examination supplemented by the results of noninvasive vascular tests and radiologic studies. In general, decompensation of longstanding ischemia due to atherosclerosis is less emergent than embolic acute ischemia due to significant collateral development in the former.

A number of diagnostic tests are available to quickly determine the best treatment plan for the threatened limb. Tests should be selected to provide the maximum amount of information with the minimum amount of discomfort and delay for the patient, who often is experiencing considerable pain.

a. Noninvasive vascular testing. Continuous wave Doppler and pulse volume recording (PVR) are simple yet accurate methods to determine criteria for ischemic rest pain and the likelihood of healing (see Chapter 6). Ischemic rest pain generally is associated with a Doppler ankle pressure below 35 mm Hg in nondiabetics (ABI of 0.3 to 0.4) and below 55 mm Hg in diabetics. Ischemic rest pain is unlikely when ankle pressures exceed 55 mm Hg in the nondiabetic and 80 mm Hg in the diabetic. Foot ulcers that are not infected and not associated with osteomyelitis have a favorable chance of healing if the ankle pressure is above 65 mm Hg in the nondiabetic and above 90 mm Hg in the diabetic. Ankle and forefoot PVRs that are less than 5 mm or flat, predict ischemic rest pain and poor tissue healing. Toe pressures of less than 20 to 30 mm Hg are also associated with advanced ischemia. A minimal TP suggesting adequacy for healing is 40 mm Hg. Resting supine transcutaneous oxygen (Tco_2) measurements of less than 20 to 30 torr are indicative of severe ischemia, especially if forefoot Tco_2 levels fall to less than 10 torr with leg elevation.

b. Plain radiograph of the bone underlying an ulcer may show signs of osteomyelitis, including bone rarefaction, periosteal elevation, and new bone formation. A bone scan or MRI is indicated when osteomyelitis seems likely but a plain radiograph is negative. Bone changes may not be apparent until osteomyelitis has been active for 2 to 3 weeks.

c. Cultures and **Gram's stains** should be made of all ulcers to identify any residing organisms and histologic stain also may reveal fungi.

d. An **ECG** is essential when arterial embolism is suspected, as atrial fibrillation is a common underlying condition. For cases in which intermittent arrhythmia is suspected, a 24-hour continuous ECG monitor (Holter) may be used.

e. An **echocardiogram** should be done as part of the diagnostic workup for arterial embolism that may originate from the heart. The echocardiogram may reveal a diseased valve or mural thrombus. Transesophogeal echocardiography (TEE) is indicated if cardioembolism is highly suspected.

f. Duplex ultrasound of the aortoiliac segment also should be performed in the evaluation of thromboemboli, since emboli may be shed from a thrombus in an abdominal aortic aneurysm, or significant occlusive disease. If a femoral or popliteal aneurysm is suspected as a result of physical examination, ultrasound is an accurate method to confirm peripheral aneurysms that also may act as the source of emboli or acute thrombosis. If Duplex is unremarkable a CT scan of the thoracic aorta may be necessary, as this segment can be diseased and lead to embolism.

g. Arteriography remains the definitive method to delineate the exact level of arterial occlusion and to define vascular anatomy before selecting a proper intervention (i.e., thrombolysis, other percutaneous therapies, or surgical revascularization). If the femoral pulses are weak or absent, an aortogram with runoff is needed. If femoral pulses are normal and the arterial occlusive disease appears localized to the leg alone, a transfemoral arteriogram of the affected leg may suffice. A femoral artery pressure study may be done to assess the adequacy of the proximal aortoiliac inflow (see Chapter 6). Contrast angiography with digital subtraction techniques can generally visualize distal tibial or plantar arch vessels. In the operating room, a sterile Doppler probe can be used to localize a tibial or pedal artery before surgical incision. Although the presence of a patent pedal arch on arteriography was once considered predictive of success for femorodistal bypass, more recent studies report reasonable patency rates and limb salvage in patients in whom the pedal arch appears absent or diseased.

h. Coagulation and **platelet function** should be analyzed in patients who present with atypical arterial thrombosis (See Chapter 3). This group includes young adults (age 20 to 40 years) with arterial occlusive disease and other individuals with recurrent arterial thromboembolism.

2. Management may begin after it has been determined whether the patient has acute or decompensated chronic limb ischemia. In our experience, the following principles provide the best chance of limb salvage. The general dictum of treatment is that ischemia of class IIb requires an immediate trip to the operating room for simultaneous evaluation and treatment. Class III ischemia should usually be treated with primary amputation. With lesser degrees of ischemia, individualization of diagnosis and treatment is recommended.

a. Acute limb ischemia is usually caused by a thromboembolus, popliteal aneurysm thrombosis, or a sudden arterial or graft occlusion. Thrombosis of a chronic arterial stenosis may cause temporary pain, pallor, and paresthesia, but usually it does not progress to paralysis. The acute symptoms often resolve because of previously developed collateral vessels.

(1) Immediate treatment should include systemic heparinization (5,000 to 10,000 units IV, then 1,000 units/h adjusted to maintain the APTT to twice baseline, usually 60 to 90 seconds) to prevent further propagation of thrombus. If leg pain is severe, a narcotic may be administered while further tests are arranged.

(2) Initial diagnostic tests should include routine blood counts, electrolytes, glucose, and baseline coagulation studies (prothrombin time, partial thromboplastin time, and platelet count). An ECG should be done to check for atrial fibrillation and any sign of acute myocardial infarction.

Continuous wave Doppler may be used to localize the level of obstruction and record ankle pressures. Absence of arterial signals at the ankle almost always means that urgent surgical intervention will be necessary (class IIb or III ischemia; Table 14.2). If the ankle has monophasic Doppler signals and the foot has sensation and movement (class I or IIa), 2 to 3 hours may be allowed for workup, initial therapy, and observation. If the leg does not improve during this time, urgent surgical intervention will generally be necessary.

(3) An emergency arteriogram usually is performed to determine the location of the arterial occlusion as well as the inflow and outflow on either side. This can be performed in a radiographic suite or the operating room. Today, newer endovascular operating rooms have been developed for just such clinical situations. However, arterial exploration in the operating room should be undertaken immediately if the acute occlusion is clearly an embolus. Intraoperative arteriograms can be performed if necessary. Time is important in acute arterial occlusion, as irreversible nerve and muscle damage may occur within 6 hours.

(4) The choice of procedure for an acute arterial occlusion will depend on the underlying etiology. **Thromboembolectomy** with Fogarty® embolectomy catheters (Edwards Lifesciences Corp., Irvine, CA) is the operation of choice for thromboemboli. Thrombectomy of the femoral or iliac arteries can be accomplished through a femoral arteriotomy. A popliteal embolus should generally be extracted through a popliteal arteriotomy, so that each tibial artery may be checked for clot. Passing a catheter from the groin will not clean out all of the tibial arteries. Extracted thromboemboli should be sent for pathologic examination, as occasionally arterial tumor embolism will be the first manifestation of an atrial myxoma or other vascular tumor. After embolectomy, the patient should be continued on heparin, followed by long-term warfarin sodium (Coumadin) therapy.

Bypass grafting of an arteriosclerotic occlusion of the iliac or superficial femoral artery may be necessary to salvage the acutely ischemic leg. In another example, a few seriously ill cardiac patients who are dependent on a transfemoral intra-aortic balloon assist device will develop limb-threatening ischemia. An emergency femorofemoral bypass may be necessary if the balloon must remain in place for cardiac support. Another difficult situation to deal with is acute popliteal aneurysm occlusion. Classically, operative bypass has led to 40-50% limb loss in these patients. The addition of preoperative thrombolytic therapy both to open the distal outflow and to allow a better distal target evaluation has reduced this to about 10% to 20% (Chapter 11).

If the acute arterial ischemia is caused by a graft occlusion, **regional thrombolytic therapy (urokinase or tPA),** either pulsed during operation (2-5mg tPA; 250,000 IU urokinase), or pulse spray with subsequent drip therapy (0.05-0.1mg/kg/hr tPA; 1,000-4,000 IU/hr urokinase) for 12 to 24 hours via a percutaneous thrombolytic catheter placed across the occlusion at the time of initial arteriogram may reopen the graft and reveal the cause of the occlusion (e.g., distal anastomotic stenosis, proximal inflow disease, or graft pathology or kinking). Some degree of systemic heparinization either intravenously or via the arterial sheath should accompany this process. Once the cause is identified, a more focused later staged operation or endovascular procedure (e.g., angioplasty $\pm$ stent, atherectomy, balloon angioplasty of graft stenosis, etc.) can be undertaken. Also, newer mechanical, rheolytic thrombectomy devices, which can suction and/or macerate/particularize thrombus, may be helpful in completely clearing thrombus from occluded grafts and arterial segments. Their practical application is currently being defined.

This same approach can also be used for treatment of acute native arterial occlusions, such as that mentioned above for popliteal aneurysm thrombosis. Data evaluating the use of thrombolysis in arterial occlusions are mixed and confusing, but with lower grade acute ischemia and significant thrombus burden, thrombolysis may be beneficial. Possible benefits include the opening and improvement of outflow, identification of a focal culprit lesion amenable to a less-invasive endovascular procedure, or influencing the level of distal anastomosis required with surgical bypass and thus affecting durability of the reconstruction. The trade is a higher likelihood of bleeding complications. Not uncommonly the limb appears to clinically deteriorate with drip thrombolytic therapy as thrombus becomes unstable, and particles embolize. This usually improves but close observation is required.

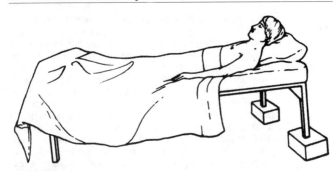

Figure 14.8. Bed position for patients with ischemic rest pain of the lower extremity. The head of the bed is elevated 6 inches to improve arterial perfusion of the pedal circulation by gravity. Sheets are draped over a footboard to alleviate pressure on the feet and either lambswool or gauze placed between the toes and egg-crate or Rooke boots used to protect the heels.

b. Chronic critical limb ischemia is usually associated with arteriosclerotic occlusive disease of the aortoiliac region, femoropopliteal segment, or distal tibial arteries.

(1) **Foot protection** from further injury is the first order of care. The heel should be protected from pressure sores by a soft gauze pad secured with a gauze roll, **not** tape. The heels themselves should either be elevated off of the bed surface or placed in egg crates or commercially made vascular "boots" (e.g., Rooke boot). Lambswool or gauze should be placed between the toes to prevent "kissing" ulcers caused by toes and toenails rubbing against one another. A lanolin-based lotion should be applied daily to the foot to keep the skin soft and prevent cracking, especially over the heel. If pressure bothers the foot, bed sheets may be draped over a footboard (Fig. 14.8). Elevating the head of the bed 6 inches may relieve ischemic pain by the effect of gravity on arterial perfusion. We do not recommend so-called metal bed cradles or tents, as a patient may inadvertently abrade the lower leg or foot against the metal frame, causing skin ulceration.

(2) **Local infection** should be controlled before insertion of synthetic bypass grafts. Local debridement and drainage of infected foot/toe tissue and parenteral antibiotics should precede graft procedures by several days. Otherwise, graft infection may occur in the groin, where lymphatics may be laden with bacteria. Deep-space infection is a particular problem in the diabetic population. If sepsis is present, guillotine amputation is indicated. If the patient is not toxic, drainage/debridement may be attempted. Large heel ulcers or significant areas of tissue loss may ultimately lead to amputation.

(3) Arteriography and other imaging were discussed earlier.

(4) The **choice of operation or percutaneous procedure** depends on the location of the occlusive disease and the condition of the patient.

i. Combined severe aortoiliac and femoropopliteal occlusive disease should be treated by inflow correction of the aortoiliac disease as described above. For those with rest pain, aortoiliac inflow correction may be all that is needed. Long-term limb salvage will be accomplished in most patients with multilevel occlusive disease by aortofemoral bypass or aortoiliac intervention alone (i.e., treatment of inflow disease).

When significant femoropopliteal disease is also present, determining which patients will need simultaneous femoropopliteal revascularization is not easy. Preoperative factors that suggest a combined procedure is indicated are extensive below-the-knee femoropopliteal-tibial occlusions combined with tissue loss and an ankle pressure below 30 mm Hg. Also, a poorly formed profunda femoris artery and modest inflow disease suggest that correction of inflow alone will not suffice for tissue healing. Should a procedure with an open groin be chosen, such as aortofemoral bypass, combined inflow and outflow endovascular therapy, or hybrid iliac stenting and surgical distal revascularization, the profunda should be intraoperatively interrogated to assure adequacy. If the orifice accepts a 4 mm probe and a #3 Fogarty® embolectomy catheter (Edwards Lifesciences Corp., Irvine, CA) can be advanced at least 20 cm the profunda is adequately developed. In high-risk patients, endovascular therapies and extraanatomic axillofemoral or femorofemoral bypass may be used to bypass severe proximal occlusive disease.

ii. Occlusive disease of the common femoral artery, profunda orifice, and superficial femoral artery may be managed by endarterectomy, profundaplasty, iliofemoral bypass bifurcation reconstruction. Profundaplasty is most likely to succeed when (a) aortoiliac inflow is normal, (b) the distal profunda femoris artery is normal and has developed collateral pathways to the popliteal artery, and (c) the popliteal artery is patent with at least two- or three-vessel runoff. The profunda-popliteal collateral index and the low thigh to ankle gradient pressure index have been described to assist with this decision, however, this anatomic situation is very rare, so we seldom use profundaplasty as the sole operation for limb salvage. Indeed, patients with this disease pattern usually require a bypass to a distal target potentially in conjunction with some type of common femoral or profuda femoris revascularization.

Currently, endovascular therapies in the common femoral and femoral bifurcation are not as effective or durable as in other anatomic sites.

iii. Femoropopliteal artery occlusion can be managed by bypass grafting, endarterectomy (open or remote), or percutaneous treatments. When performing femoropopliteal bypass for limb salvage we prefer greater saphenous vein for conduit, which is superior to endarterectomy and synthetic bypass. Greater saphenous vein above-knee femoropopliteal bypasses have an 80% primary patency. Below the knee, this is roughly 70%. Should adequate greater saphenous vein be unavailable, we use prosthetic conduit. Others espouse arm vein and spliced vein segments as femoropopliteal bypass constructs. Each of these has benefits and disadvantages.

Current synthetic choices for femoropopliteal bypass are Dacron, human umbilical vein (HUV), and polytetrafluoroethylene (PTFE). In the above-knee position ePTFE primary and secondary patency is 55-65% and 60-70% at 5 years, respectively. These grafts provide excellent long-term patency when the distal anastomosis is above the knee, but poorer patency is observed in below-the-knee bypasses. In a prospective randomized comparison of autologous saphenous vein to expanded PTFE grafts, primary patency of vein was clearly superior to PTFE for infrapopliteal bypass (49% versus 12% at 4 years). However, there was no significant difference in limb salvage (vein versus PTFE, 57% versus 61%). Although 2-year patency was similar for both grafts to the popliteal artery (64% to 70%), vein was superior at 5 years (vein, 68%; PTFE, 38%). HUV grafts have had a patency similar to PTFE, but manifest aneurysmal degeneration in long-term follow-up. Another option is cryopreserved allogenic vein graft, but results using cryopreserved vein have been disappointing and it is expensive. They are seldom used.

As described above, percutaneous SFA interventions such as transluminal angioplasty and stenting are now performed routinely with reasonable early and mid-term results. Small studies describe equivalence with surgical bypass at 1 to 2 years in critical ischemia. These therapies may be the procedure of choice in seriously ill patients who need limb salvage.

iv. The most challenging group of patients who require operation for limb salvage have **severe type V disease of the femoropopliteal and tibial levels.** Acceptable long-term patency (50% to 60% at 5 years) and excellent limb salvage rates (50% to 73% at 5 years) may be achieved by femorotibial, femoroperoneal, and pedal bypass grafts using greater saphenous vein (GSV). Multisegment femorodistal occlusive disease also has been successfully treated by sequential anastomoses of a vein graft to several patent segments. Adequate GSV is generally believed to be at least 3.5 mm in diameter when distended and without sclerotic segments or stenoses. **Patency of femoroinfrapopliteal vein bypasses is comparable for each tibial artery and is similar in diabetics and nondiabetics.** Whether in situ or reversed saphenous vein grafting is superior remains controversial.

Several factors have rejuvenated enthusiasm for in situ **saphenous vein bypass grafting** after its original description in 1962 (Fig. 14.9). Proponents claim a higher use of smaller veins, a

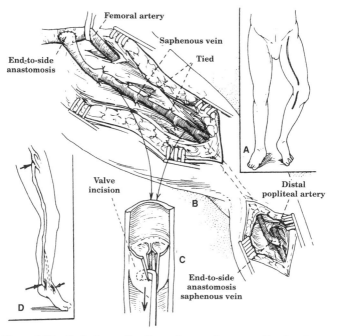

Figure 14.9. Technique of in situ saphenous femoropopliteal and tibial bypass grafting. **(A)** Greater saphenous vein may be exposed through one or two long incisions along the medial aspect of the thigh and calf. **(B)** Saphenous vein is left in its natural bed. Its valves are cut with special instruments "valvulotomes." **(C)** Its branches are tied to prevent arteriovenous fistulas. Proximal anastomosis is made to the common femoral or superficial femoral artery, and distal anastomosis is constructed to the distal popliteal artery or to the tibial or peroneal branches. **(D)** Long bypasses to the level of the ankle are possible by this technique. Incisions may also be limited to the groin and the level of distal anastomosis with side branches and vein defects identified with angioscopy, arteriography, duplex ultrasound and continuous wave Doppler. Side branches may then be ligated with small incisions or embolized via a distal side branch.

lesser degree of endothelial damage, better size match at the anastomoses, improved hemodynamics, and superior early and late patency. However, similar early and late patency rates for in situ versus reversed infrapopliteal bypasses (1-year, 87% to 90%; 3-year, 82% to 85%; and 5-year, 77% to 85%) have been shown in several studies. During in situ bypass, lysis of the valves with a valvulotome is blind. Identification of venous defects, as well as ligation of large side branches to prevent problematic arteriovenous fistulas is required. Several techniques to accomplish these are described.

Another good option for distal vein bypasses with targets at or below the trifurcation is nonreversed, translocated GSV. After harvest, the vein is distended and valvulotomes passed, similar to the technique for in situ bypass. However, with a nonreversed, translocated graft the vein is distended either by vein solution or after creation of the proximal anastomosis, but before placing the graft in the tunnel. We prefer the latter so as to have objective proof of good pulsatile flow with the graft completely exposed. Also, the pulsatile blood flow assists in finding problem areas on the vein that need either side branch ligation, repair, or resection and splicing. Usually two passes of the valvulotome are sufficient. The benefit of a nonreversed, translocated vein is for graft-artery size match at both the proximal and distal anastomoses, when a subcutaneous graft is not desired, or when anatomic or lateral subcutaneous tunneling are preferred. Regardless of the vein construct used, careful preparation of the vein and the meticulous technique of anastomosis are likely more important than position of the vein graft.

Because a vein remains the best conduit for early and late patency, extra effort to obtain a suitable vein seems justified. These options include the contralateral leg vein, arm veins, lesser saphenous veins, spliced vein-segment grafts, composite synthetic and vein, and shorter bypasses using less vein (e.g., SFA-tibial, popliteal-tibial, or tibiotibial bypasses).

Techniques of vein adjunct at the distal anastomosis when using prosthetic below the knee include **Taylor patch, Linton patch, Miller cuff, and St. Mary's Boot** (Fig. 14.10). These emphasize a long arteriotomy and placement of a cuff of vein using one of these techniques between the prosthetic and the target arteriotomy. These are known to greatly improve results of prosthetic-distal bypass. Although all of these conduit alternatives are generally not viewed as the first option, they represent reasonable choices when GSV is not available. But remember, tibial level revasculariza-

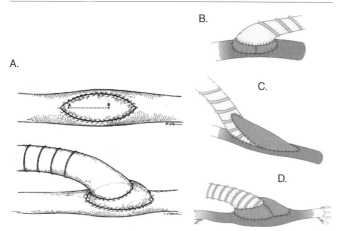

Figure 14.10. **Types of vein adjuncts at the distal anastomosis of infrageniculate prosthetic bypass grafts. (A) Linton Patch, (B) Miller Cuff, (C) Taylor patch, (D) St. Mary's boot. These adjuncts help to alter sheer stresses at the distal anastomosis and improve patency.**

tion using alternative autogenous reconstructions provide better long-term results than those based on prosthetic. Reports detail patencies of 50-60% at 4 years versus 30-40%, respectively.

Also, in our experience, vein grafts to isolated popliteal segments have been an acceptable alternative to femorodistal bypass in certain patients. These grafts have a 5-year patency similar to femorotibial bypasses (65% versus 66%, respectively). Provided that tissue necrosis is not extensive, such grafts are adequate to relieve severe ischemia, especially when a limited length of vein is available and the tibial arteries appear marginal for anastomosis.

Conduit selection is seldom this concrete though and the entire clinical picture, goal of revascularization, and status of the patient must be considered. Likewise, the proper selection of a distal target to maximize the patency, limb salvage and potential success of the bypass graft is important and depends upon many factors. The availability of conduit, outflow, degree of limb threat (rest pain vs. ulceration vs. gangrene), as well as collateralization, all play a role. In general, for critical ischemia, with all other things being equal, the best tibial (anterior or posterior) is chosen as they are in direct continuity with the foot's arterial arches. The peroneal artery is appropriate if (a) the tibial arteries are diffusely diseased (b) rest pain or minimal tissue loss is present (c) conduit will not allow a more distal bypass, and (d) there are well-developed collaterals from the distal peroneal branches to the pedal/ plantar arteries and arches.

Endovascular therapies in the infrageniculate popliteal and tibial level can be accomplished in concert with or without percutaneous intervention in the SFA. Similar to other lower extremity territories, a TASC classification has been developed to classify lesion anatomy in the tibial region. Single stenoses <1 cm are **TASC A**. Multiple focal lesions <1 cm are **TASC B. TASC C** refers to stenoses 1-4 cm in length or occlusions <2 cm while **TASC D** are diffuse, lengthy stenoses over 4 cm or occlusions over 2 cm.

Treatment of critical limb ischemia with endovascular methods in the popliteal-tibial region remains a considerable challenge. Results of angioplasty and stenting alone are mixed and generally over half fail in one year. Other techniques such as cutting balloon angioplasty, cryoplasty, and directional and laser atherectomy are reported to have better results, with over 90% limb salvage and 60 % to 75% patency at 6 months to 1 year. Some have reported excellent early results even with significant tissue loss using these technologies, but, to date, this is not a widespread experience. Currently, it is evident that while improvements in this therapeutic approach have occurred more study and refinements in technology are needed.

v. Patients presenting with **significant tissue loss or gangrene of the foot** deserve special mention. Attempts to salvage such a limb may require an extended hospitalization, significant effort at wound and foot care, and considerable expense. However, limb salvage is possible in 70% at 1 year and 60% at 3 years, but generally only about 30% at 5 years after surgery. Successful revascularization results in lower costs than primary amputation.

In patients over 80 years of age, limb salvage is comparable to younger groups, with a 3-year survival of about 50% and a limb preservation rate of 70%. Consequently, present data support an attempt at arterial reconstruction in most elderly patients with critical limb ischemia. Nonetheless, the individual patient as a whole should be considered. Those with significant comorbidities, dementia or neurologic degenerative disorders with minimal or no ambulation may be considered for primary amputation perhaps preceded by nonoperative management in those with dry gangrene.

Primary amputation is appropriate when gangrene extensively involves the forefoot and heel. Whether a failed below-knee femoropopliteal bypass changes the level of amputation depends on numerous factors, but generally an unsuccessful reconstruction does not alter final amputation level.

vi. Lumbar sympathectomy alone is not usually sufficient to salvage limbs that are at risk. However, relief of rest pain has been achieved when the preoperative ankle-brachial index is relatively high (i.e., >0.35). Results are less favorable when tissue necrosis is present. It is generally not considered today as a treatment option except in very rare cases.

vii. Creation of a **distal arteriovenous fistula** as an adjunct to maintaining arterial and synthetic bypass graft patency remains controversial. The physiologic advantage of this technique is questionable and we have not embraced it.

viii. Intraoperative angioscopy has been evaluated as an adjunct to *in situ* vein grafting, embolectomy, femoropopliteal bypass surgery, and laser recanalization. Clinical trials by Miller and colleagues at Harvard have supported its effectiveness, but this institutionally demanding technology has had a limited impact so far in most practices.

ix. Intraoperative duplex has also been advocated and used as immediate evaluation of the technical success of lower extremity revascularizations. It is easy to use in most vascular practices and may assist in the identification of technical errors, residual graft defects and clamp site injuries requiring attention.

6. Preoperative preparation. Lab tests for limb salvage cases are the same as those outlined for claudication previously. Skin preparation should include the abdomen and both legs, as an opposite leg vein is occasionally explored. A prophylactic antibiotic with good gram-positive skin coverage be given prior to the incision. In those with tissue loss, gangrene or diabetic foot infection, broad-spectrum antibiotics, such as vancomycin and an extended spectrum penicillin derivative should be used.

7. Patient positioning. Most lower-extremity arterial revascularizations are performed with the patient supine. The heels must be protected from pressure sores by elevating the calves on soft towels or placing soft pads on the heels. If PVR is being used for intraoperative monitoring of lower-extremity perfusion, the PVR cuffs should be placed at the ankles and baseline tracings should be recorded.

8. Surgical exposure. Certain features of surgical exposure facilitate performing the bypass graft anastomoses and prevent postoperative wound complications.

a. The incisions for exposure of the **GSV** must be made directly over the vein. There is a tendency to bevel the incision and bring it too far anterior to the course of the vein which results in skin flap necrosis. Leaving skin bridges along the saphenous vein harvest site may also alleviate skin flap necrosis. Some advocate subcutaneous, endoscopic vein harvest.

b. The **above-knee popliteal artery** can be exposed through a medial distal thigh incision going over the top edge of the sartorius muscle and beneath the adductor magnus tendon. **Three noteworthy anatomic features are present at the adductor magnus tendon: the superficial femoral artery becomes the popliteal artery, the supreme (descending) geniculate artery (an important collateral) originates from the proximal popliteal artery, and the saphenous nerve becomes superficial.** Injury to the nerve can result in bothersome chronic leg neuralgia.

c. The **below-knee popliteal artery** is exposed via a medial proximal leg incision. The medial head of the gastrocnemius muscle is retracted inferiorly. The popliteal vein and tibial nerve are medial and posterior to the artery. Extensive exposure of the popliteal artery may require detachment of the semimembranosus and semitendinosus muscle tendons. Insertions of the semitendinosis, gracilis and sartorius muscles form the **pes anserinus (foot of a goose)** on the medial surface of the tibia.

d. Occasionally, the entire popliteal artery requires exposure for repairs, such as for a popliteal aneurysm (Fig. 14.11). This exposure also allows for ligation of feeding collaterals into the aneurysm sac. Divided tendons can be anatomically reattached at the conclusion of the operation. Such an extensive exposure appears to increase postoperative leg edema but does not result in knee instability in most patients.

For focal mid-popliteal artery aneurysms or for popliteal artery entrapment, a posterior approach from a longitudinal knee incision provides excellent exposure without cutting normal tendons.

e. The **tibioperoneal trunk and proximal posterior tibial artery** can be exposed through the medial knee approach by detaching the soleus muscle at its arch on the posterior table of the tibia. Placing a right-angled instrument through the foramen for initial dissection is helpful. Exposure of the proximal **anterior tibial artery** generally requires a separate anterior lateral leg incision, which is made one finger-breadth lateral to the anterior edge of the tibia and carried 8 to 10 cm distally. The artery is located in the groove between the anterior tibialis and extensor digitorum longus muscles and can be approached the length of the leg in this groove. The **peroneal artery** can be approached from medial extending behind the tibia and over the posterior tibial vessels or laterally with a fibular resection.

f. Bypasses can also be taken to the **pedal arteries** (Fig. 14.12) in select patients. The most common pedal artery for distal anastomosis is the dorsalis pedis followed by the common and lateral plantar arteries. Incisions are directly over the pedal artery and, upon completion, the skin only is closed with interrupted permanent fine filament sutures. This decreases local tissue trauma in ischemic foot tissue.

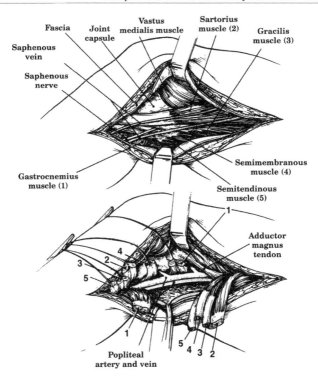

Fascia   Joint   Vastus   Sartorius
         capsule medialis muscle muscle (2)   Gracilis
                                                  muscle (3)
Saphenous
vein
Saphenous
nerve

Semimembranous
muscle (4)
Gastrocnemius
muscle (1)
Semitendinous
muscle (5)
1
Adductor
magnus
tendon
4
2
3
5
1
5 4 3 2
Popliteal
artery and vein

Figure 14.11.   Medial approach to the popliteal artery. The saphenous nerve should be gently retracted to minimize postoperative
saphenous neuralgia. Division of the medial knee tendons and
medial head of the gastrocnemius muscle provides clear popliteal
artery exposure with minimal morbidity. Most patients have a single
great saphenous vein, although an accessory saphenous vein may
be present as this illustration indicates. Tendons can be reapproxi-
mated with minimal morbidity and this exposure can be limited to
either the above-knee or below-knee aspects.

9. Preparation of the saphenous vein. Endothelial
damage during preparation of saphenous vein is an important factor in graft failure. Optimum preparation includes
gentle dissection of the vein, careful ligation of side
branches away from the vein wall, minimal warm ischemic
time if the vein is removed from the leg, and limited distention. Gentle dilation of the vein can be achieved with
vein solution. Immersion of the vein in solution should not
occur until ready for bypass and may minimize endothelial
damage. We use 500 cc Ringer's lactate with 10,000 U
heparin and 120 mg papaverine. If splicing of segments is
necessary after removing inadequate areas, the ends
should be beveled and fine suture (7-0) should be used create a widely open anastomosis.
10. Distal arterial control can be accomplished with
minimal damage to the arteries by using a **pneumatic**

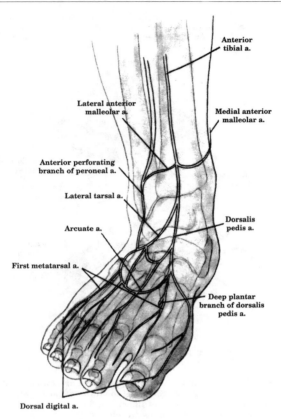

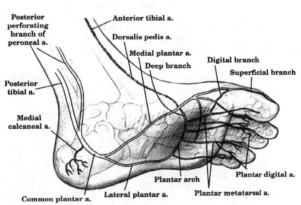

Figure 14.12.   Anatomy of the pedal arteries. **(A)** Dorsum of foot, **(B)** Plantar surface of foot. (Adapted from Gloviczki P, Bower TC, Toomey, et al. Microscope-aided pedal bypasses is an effective and low-risk operation to salvage the ischemic foot. *Am J Surg.* 1994; 168:76-84.)

thigh tourniquet after the proximal anastomosis is performed. The tourniquet is inflated to 300 mm Hg after the lower limb is wrapped tightly for exsanguination with an elastic Esmarch bandage while the leg is elevated. This is particularly useful when the arterial system is highly calcified and infrageniculate control with clamps unsavory.

11. Anastomotic technique should emphasize a long gentle anastomotic angle to minimize turbulence. Distal popliteal and tibial arterial anastomoses are constructed more accurately under low-power magnification. If prosthetic bypass is performed to tibial vessels, the use of a **vein adjunct** as mentioned previously may reduce intimal hyperplasia at the distal anastomosis and improve patency. Polypropylene permanent suture should be used. Size and strength of the suture should be chosen as appropriate for the size and amount of disease in the area. Generally, running anastomoses are used. Sometimes, when the target vessel is small or in an enclosed area where vision is difficult, we use several interrupted, horizontal mattress sutures at the toe of the anastomosis; securing them after placement and using a limb of the lateral-most suture to run the remaining portion. This improves accuracy and splays the distal hood of the graft and prevents a bunching of the graft toe which may become a nidus for intimal hyperplasia. Another helpful technique, particularly when the target vessel is fragile, is to place both the heel and a toe suture prior to beginning the anastomotic suture line. This assures proper length and distributes tension along the arteriotomy.

12. Wound closure is a critical component of lower extremity revascularization. We prefer interrupted polyglycolic-acid dissolving sutures in several layers. We have found running sutures to cause bunching and inaccurate closure. Virgin wounds are closed with a subcuticular closure and steri-strips. It is important to reapproximate the skin edges and not pull so much on this stitch to bunch skin with tension. This leads to skin edge ischemia and necrosis with skin breakdown. This may be a pathway for infection, or at least poor wound healing in these patients with poor skin to begin with. Interrupted nylon stitches are used for re-do skin closures, usually in a vertical mattress fashion with eversion and approximation of the skin edges. It is important to ligate lymphatic vessels to avoid a leak and appropriate. hemostasis with electrocautery and suture ligature to mitigate the potential for lymph leak, lymphocele and hematoma. Loose dressings of gauze wraps should be used and tape should be avoided.

13. Associated amputations. Some patients require an amputation after lower-extremity arterial bypass or endovascular revascularization to remove necrotic tissue present before surgery. This is usually foot-based when revascularization is attempted for limb salvage. Whether amputations should be done simultaneously with arterial reconstruction or staged afterward is debatable. Certainly, infected lesions or abscesses need debridement and drainage prior to grafting. Superficial dry gangrene may auto-amputate after foot circulation is improved. Thus, we normally wait several days after arterial reconstruction to perform necessary digital or foot amputations. This time allows better demarcation of the proper amputation level and perfusion to supply tissue with antibiotics and a granulation process to begin. Although this has been our general approach, we do combine revascularization with toe or forefoot amputations in select patients.

C. Postoperative care. Despite multiple medical problems and sometimes extensive operations, most patients who undergo aortic or lower-extremity based arterial reconstruction for occlusive disease can expect a reasonably uncomplicated recovery if certain principles of care are followed.

    1. Initial stabilization after aortic reconstructions should be done in an intensive care setting where vital signs, urine output, ECG rhythm, and respiratory status can be monitored continuously for 12 to 24 hours. On arrival to the intensive care unit the patient's blood pressure, heart rate and rhythm should be checked and arterial blood gases drawn for analysis. If the patient is intubated, ventilator settings should be adjusted after review of the initial blood gas. A plan for extubation should be established.

    After these vital functions have been stabilized, additional baseline tests may be obtained, including a portable chest x-ray to check endotracheal tube position and to ensure adequate lung expansion. In addition, formal 12-lead ECG should be compared with the preoperative ECG for any evidence of myocardial ischemia rhythm changes. Cardiac isoenzymes should be sent for study if intraoperative myocardial ischemia or arrhythmia was detected, however, in general, routine cardiac enzymes are unnecessary. Blood also should be sent for measurement of hematocrit, serum electrolytes, blood sugar, PT/PTT, and platelet count.

    After lower extremity revascularization, patients should remain under intensive observation for at least 6 to 12 hours. Similar laboratory evaluations should be accomplished. It is during this immediate postoperative period that most early graft occlusions occur. Hourly checks of pedal pulses, PVRs, or Doppler signals and ankle pressures should be made. To pharmacologically enhance early perioperative patency, one has several options. Antiplatelet therapy alone in femoropopliteal grafts with good outflow is appropriate. Another option is low molecular weight dextran 40 infused for the initial 24 postoperative hours. Our regimen has been 100 mL IV in the recovery room and 20 mL/h for one 500-mL bottle. Subsequently, patients receive aspirin, 80 to 325 mg daily, and low-dose heparin, 5,000 units subcutaneously, until discharge. For tibial reconstructions, or those requiring intraoperative revision, we use low-dose intravenous heparin (300 to 500 units per hour) in addition to aspirin. Long-term anticoagulation with warfarin and children's aspirin (80 mg) is often used for below-knee synthetic grafts or marginal quality vein grafts, revision grafts to the tibial arteries, or those with poor runoff (one or fewer vessels in continuity to the ankle). The clinical superiority of anticoagulation or antiplatelet therapy for graft maintenance postoperatively is debated and inconclusive.

2. Fluid management must be meticulous, as many vascular patients have significant heart disease and will not tolerate fluid overload. A few guidelines for fluid administration should make fluid management easy.

a. Patients leave the operating room after large amounts of fluid have been given. Most of this fluid is sequestered in interstitial spaces and will remain there until it is slowly mobilized and excreted in 48 to 72 hours In addition, inappropriate secretion of antidiuretic hormone results in sodium and water retention. Therefore, postoperative fluids should be limited to about 80 mL/h (1 mL/kg body weight per hour) of 5% dextrose in half normal saline with 20 to 30 mEq potassium per liter. When needed, the rate of intravenous fluid can be increased, or bolus fluid given.

b. Some patients are cold and vasoconstricted when they arrive in the recovery area. As they rewarm and vasodilate additional fluid may be necessary, indicated by decreased urine output, low filling pressures, and tachycardia. If the hemoglobin is less than 8 g/dL or hematocrit less than 25%, packed red blood cells should be transfused. Otherwise, volume replacement may be made with a bolus (5 to 10 mL/kg of a balanced salt solution, e.g., Ringer's lactated solution).

c. When patients begin to mobilize excess fluid on the **second or third postoperative day,** maintenance intravenous rates may need to be reduced or stopped. If the patient is edematous and urine output has not increased, a small dose (10 to 20 mg) of furosemide may initiate a good diuresis.

3. Postoperative pulmonary care is critical after extubation and is discussed in Chapter 9.

4. Pain management is a key component to early ambulation, pulmonary care, and gastrointestinal function. Epidural anesthesia with providing analgesia for 2-4 days after operation is an excellent method. Standard narcotic-based therapy is also used. See Chapter 9.

5. Antibiotics should be continued for 24 hours postoperatively unless otherwise indicated.

6. Gastrointestinal decompression with a nasogastric tube is often necessary for 24 to 72 hours after aortic-based revascularizations.

a. Gastrointestinal ileus may be prolonged after aortic reconstruction, especially if extensive lysis of adhesions or dissection of the duodenum is necessary. In our experience, most patients have sluggish intestinal peristalsis for 2 to 3 days after operation. Although nasogastric decompression was once used routinely for this entire period, the vast majority (90%) of patients can tolerate the removal of the nasogastric tube on the first postoperative morning. After removing the tube, we generally wait 24 to 48 hours to be certain that peristalsis is adequate before beginning a liquid diet, which is advanced to solids in the following 24 to 48 hours.

b. Appetite after aortic reconstruction usually is poor, and patients generally do not resume normal caloric intake for several weeks. A weight loss of 5 to 10 pounds is not uncommon in the first month following surgery. Patients who have marginal nutritional status prior to operation or a complicated postoperative course may not tolerate further weight loss, and their caloric intake may require enteral or parenteral supplementation.

7. Wound care requires special attention, since local infection may rapidly extend to a prosthetic graft or cause a bacteremia that could seed the graft surface. Initial dressings should be removed on the first postoperative day. If the wound is sealed, no further dressing is needed, but a simple gauze covering may be helpful to protect groin wounds and absorb sweat. If serosanguineous fluid is leaking from the wound, a sterile gauze dressing should be applied until the drainage stops. Lymph leaks from groin incisions may be treacherous, since infection of the deeper inguinal lymphatics may also infect an adjacent graft. Prolonged lymph leakage increases the risk of bacterial invasion of the perigraft lymphatics and may result in an early prosthetic graft infection. Most minor lymph leaks will resolve in 3 to 5 days. If a groin lymph leak is copious and not decreased or closed in 3 to 5 days, wound exploration, ligation of culprit nodes or lymph vessels, and reclosure done.

8. The proper time to **ambulate** a patient after aortic or other peripheral arterial reconstruction is another controversial area. Proper timing is individualized with consideration of the following.

a. Many patients after aortic reconstruction are not hemodynamically stable for 24 to 48 hours, and tachycardia with swings in blood pressure is not well tolerated. Incisional pain may also contribute to tachycardia and hypertension. Furthermore, within 48 to 72 hours, mobilization of fluid expands intravascular volume, placing additional stress on the heart. If hemodynamically labile patients attempt to ambulate before tachycardia is controlled and fluids are mobilized, they may experience myocardial ischemia. Myocardial infarction occurs most commonly on the third postoperative day. Patients with groin incisions are kept supine for at least 24 hours.

b. If the patient has an inguinal lymph leak, it is most likely to stop if lower-extremity activity is curtailed by bed rest. Since ambulation may be delayed for 24 to 72 hours, we insist that patients perform leg exercises (flexion and extension of calf and thigh muscles) for at least 5 minutes every hour. These exercises improve venous emptying from calf muscles and are prophylaxis for deep venous thrombosis. The leg exercise also increases blood flow to the legs and consequently through any graft. Finally, these exercises help maintain leg muscle tone prior to ambulation. In our experience, delayed ambulation in some patients has not increased either pulmonary complications or venous thromboembolism, provided coughing, deep breathing, appropriate mechanical and pharmacologic DVT prophylaxis and footboard exercises are performed routinely. No pneumatic compression devices should be placed on legs after an infrageniculate bypass, or endovascular procedure.

c. **Edema** can be a problem after revascularization and is multifactorial owing to lymphatic trauma, reperfusion, and dysfunctional vasoregulation. However, usually, after 2-4 days it is manageable. When not ambulatory, the patient should be supine with the leg elevated. If reconstruction is above the knee, compression hose may be helpful. Infrageniculate and pedal bypass may require longer periods of bed rest as tissue loss and incisions may be compromised by significant edema. Aggressive management is warranted in these individuals. Prolonged sitting is to be avoided. Not uncommonly, edema after lower extremity revascularization may last for several weeks to months, and fitted graded compression hose and elevation are useful.

9. After **endovascular procedures** involving an intervention for lower-extremity occlusive disease, standard care usually involves maximal antiplatelet therapy including aspirin and clopidogrel. Similar to open reconstruction, certain infrageniculate interventions may warrant anticoagulation but this is not well defined. Patients with manual pressure used for hemostasis after sheath removal, should remain supine for 6 hours. If a closure device is used, we have them remain supine for 4 hours barring problems. Monitoring of the revascularization is similar to those mentioned above for open operation. We obtain Duplex ultrasound and pressure studies on lower extremity endovascular interventions prior to discharge in order to assess immediate patency and physiologic improvement. Patients are usually able to be discharged in 12 to 24 hours.

IV. Postoperative complications. Early graft-related complications following operations for lower-extremity occlusive disease affect about 3-5% of patients. Late complications such as anastomotic aneurysm, graft thrombosis, or graft infection are more common, involving approximately 10% of patients. We focus here on the recognition of such complications and the principles of management.

A. Early graft-related complications.

1. Hemorrhage from an arterial graft anastomosis is manifested by a groin or leg hematoma in femoral or popliteal anastomoses and shock in aortic or iliac anastomoses. Treatment is early reoperation, evacuation of the hematoma, and suture control of the bleeding site. Failure to follow this approach may result in infection of the hematoma, pseudoaneurysm formation, or death.

Postoperative hemorrhage usually occurs in two patterns. In the first and most common form, bleeding frequently occurs within 24 hours from the vein graft or an anastomosis. Early repair and hematoma evacuation usually do not lead to graft failure or infection. The second pattern of postoperative hemorrhage is rare and occurs from 3 to 28 days after operation and in most cases is caused by early and aggressive graft infection. Hemorrhage usually occurs at the proximal or distal anastomosis in conjunction with signs of local infection and possibly systemic sepsis. These patients are at greater risk of eventual limb loss.

2. Early thrombosis may be the result of a technical error at the anastomosis, an embolus, or inadequate runoff to maintain graft flow. Also, inadequate inflow may be the result of clamp injury or unrecognized disease on preoperative imaging. Other causes of early thrombosis may include graft kinking, extrinsic muscle or tendon compression, or an intimal flap. Occasionally, early graft thrombosis is due to a previously undiagnosed hypercoagulable condition. Routine perioperative vascular monitoring of the reconstruction (see Chapter 9) should recognize thrombosis or compromised inflow or outflow before severe ischemia occurs. Proper management includes anticoagulation, operative reexploration, thromboembolectomy, or graft revision. It often also includes operative arteriography. In our experience, the long-term prognosis of early graft failure has been poor, even if the graft is successfully reopened.

3. Infections of bypass grafts were classified by **D. Emerick Szilagyi who described three grades of infection: grade I, superficial involving the skin and dermis, grade II, involving the subcutaneous and fatty tissue but not the graft, and grade III, involving the graft** (Table 14.5). This grading system has important implications for the management of early infections involving arterial reconstructions. Early infections are usually due to virulent organisms and are very morbid complications. Grade I infections can be managed with close observation, local wound care, and antibiotics, while grade II infections require opening and irrigation in the operating room. Grade III infections may lead to anastomotic hemorrhage or graft erosion and therefore graft removal with extraanatomic bypass is the preferred method of management.

Table 14.5.   Clinical classification of infection associated with arterial reconstruction

Grade	Clinical description of infection	Management
I	Involving only the skin and dermis	Local wound care and antibiotics
II	Extending into subcutaneous and fatty tissue but not the graft	Exploration and washout of the wound in the operating room
III	Graft involved in the infection	Exploration and washout of the wound with graft removal and establishment of alternative route perfusion

(From Szilagyi DE, Smith RF, Elliott JP, Vrandecic MP. Infection in arterial reconstruction with synthetic grafts. *Ann Surg.* 1972;176:321–333, with permission.)

4. Colon ischemia may affect 1% to 5% of patients who undergo aortic reconstruction for occlusive disease and is more common than that associated with aneurysm repair. It usually affects the left or sigmoid colon. Ischemia may result from inferior mesenteric artery ligation, low cardiac output states and/or inadequate collateral blood flow from the superior mesenteric or internal iliac arteries. Very rarely it has been reported after lower extremity bypass due to ligation of common femoral artery branches which can supply the pelvis in patients with diffuse occlusions of their mesenteric and internal iliac arteries. Superficial mucosal or muscularis ischemia usually causes transient diarrhea and resolves spontaneously without mortality. Late colon stricture may occur. Transmural colon ischemia will progress to bowel perforation, sepsis, and death in at least 70% of cases.

Clinical manifestations vary with the severity of ischemia. Bloody diarrhea, lower abdominal pain, and unexplained fluid requirements or sepsis suggest colon ischemia. Flexible lower endoscopy may reveal changes of patchy hemorrhage, edema, congestion, or pallor. More severe signs include ulceration and mucosal sloughing. Mild cases need bowel rest, antibiotics, and hydration until the diarrhea resolves. Any clinical decline, presentation with fluid requirements and sepsis, or if symptoms and signs persist, resection of necrotic colon with formation of a colostomy is necessary. Any bowel movement within 48 hours of aortic reconstruction should prompt flexible sigmoidoscopy. Routine use of IMA reimplantation during aortic reconstruction is debated. The potential mitigating effect of IMA revascularization on the incidence of colon ischemia is not clear. Many individuals with aortoiliac occlusive disease have an occluded IMA negating need for reconstruction. If the IMA is patent then the factors mentioned previously, such as an enlarged IMA or associated internal iliac and SMA disease, should be scrutinized and reimplantation considered.

5. Compartment syndrome is caused by prolonged ischemia (>6 hours) before revascularization. After restoration of perfusion, edema forms within the calf muscles. Since these muscles are enveloped in fixed fascial compartments, swelling leads to increased pressure within the compartments leading to myonecrosis and permanent nerve damage. The anterior compartment is most susceptible to this ischemic syndrome. The earliest clinical signs are leg pain with sensory deficits on the dorsum of the foot and weakness of toe dorsiflexion. Treatment is fasciotomy. Prophylactic fasciotomy should be considered for all cases of acute arterial ischemia in which revascularization is delayed beyond 4 to 6 hours.

6. Femoral nerve injury may occur after groin operations, especially in repeat procedures or extensive dissections of the profunda femoris artery. The injury may not be apparent until the patient tries to ambulate and discovers that they cannot extend at the knee because of quadriceps weakness. Treatment requires a flexible knee brace. Many femoral nerve apraxias will resolve in 3 to 6 months. Sensory deficits such as numbness and paresthesias are much more common than motor ones and may be related to inflammation, edema and hematoma surrounding the cutaneous femoral nerve branches.

7. Early complications after endovascular reconstruction involve access site problems, early thrombosis, and rarely perforation. Acute pseudoaneurysm, local groin hematoma, retroperitoneal bleeding, acute site thrombosis with limb ischemia or thromboembolism, arteriovenous fistula and closure device infection are all described access site complications. In general, the more complicated the procedure and the more anticoagulation required the higher the incidence of these site problems. Access technique is crucial and when performed poorly may lead to dissection, intimal flaps and lacerations. Overall they occur in 1-10%. Acute failure at the endovascular intervention site may occur due to arterial dissection, incomplete therapy with residual stenosis, treatment of more complex (higher TASC) lesions such as occlusions and longer length stenoses, as well as smaller inflow and outflow vessels. Oversizing or undersizing of stents and angioplasty balloons is a technical consideration contributing to these etiologies.

B. Late graft-related complications are not uncommon and occur in about 20% of patients who undergo aortic reconstructive procedures for occlusive disease, and roughly 30% of those with reconstructions below the inguinal ligament.

1. Gastrointestinal hemorrhage, especially hematemesis, in a patient who has received a prosthetic aortic graft must raise the suspicion of an aortoenteric fistula. Although the initial hemorrhage ("herald bleed") may stop and not recur for days, untreated aortoenteric fistulas eventually lead to hemorrhage and death. Therefore, such patients should be resuscitated and undergo emergency endoscopy and CT scan. Aortography in cases of aortoenteric fistula is often normal, but is not the most helpful diagnostic test. If the source of hemorrhage is located in the stomach or duodenal bulb, appropriate therapy is instituted. However, if no gastric or duodenal lesions are evident and major bleeding with hemodynamic compromise continues, the patient should undergo emergency abdominal exploration for diagnosis and repair of a suspected aortoduodenal fistula. If this is not found, continued operative investigation for sources of small bowel bleeding is undertaken. Classically, repair of aortoenteric fistulas requires closure of the intestine and removal of the adjacent graft with extraanatomic bypass. However, if graft-enteric erosion is not associated with local abscess and gross infection, in situ graft replacement, bowel repair, and omental coverage of the new graft will succeed in 85% of patients.

If gastrointestinal hemorrhage is minor, and the patient stabilizes a more elective evaluation may be accomplished. An indium white blood cell scan and CT scan are sensitive tests for localization of an abnormality at the fistula site. CT scan will usually show adherence of adjacent bowel to the graft with no intervening fat plane. Although arteriography seldom shows the fistula, the arteriogram may demonstrate a local pseudoaneurysm and provides useful anatomic information for the reconstruction. It also may delineate other causes of hemorrhage, such as angiodysplasias of the intestine.

2. Chronic aortic or lower-limb graft infection may present as an aortoenteric fistula, femoral pseudoaneurysm, groin abscess, frank sepsis, or a chronically draining sinus tract (Table 14.5). Most infections of aortic prostheses originate in the groin and are commonly caused by *Staphylococcus*. Although infection may originate at one anastomosis, it rarely remains localized, and spreads along the perigraft plane to eventually involve the entire graft. CT scan or high-resolution ultrasound may show poor incorporation of the graft or perigraft fluid collections.

Sometimes the diagnosis of infection is difficult. Infections may be indolent, with no visible fluid collections, negative blood cultures, no fever, and no leukocytosis. An arteriogram should be done to define the involved anatomy and an indium white blood cell scan may demonstrate the infected site. Although removal of a focally infected segment of graft may succeed in eliminating infection, resolution of many graft infections will require extraction of the entire prosthesis and an extraanatomic bypass. Putting off or limiting operations often allows a local infection to spread, and eventually life-threatening graft hemorrhage or sepsis may occur. Graft preservation may be considered if (a) the infection does not involve a body cavity (b) the graft is patent (c) the anastomoses are not involved by gross infection and (d) the patient is not physiologically septic. These situations still typically require operative washout(s), muscle flap coverage, and often use of a negative pressure wound therapy device such as the VAC® (KCI, San Antonio, TX).

Patients with infected abdominal aortic grafts have discouraging 30-day and 1-year survival rates of 70% to 80% and 40% to 50%, respectively. Staged revascularization (i.e., axillofemoral bypass) followed by infected graft removal in 24 to 48 hours is the classically described treatment of aortic graft infection. The term sequential treatment is used when extra-anatomic revascularization precedes graft removal and aortic stump oversewing at the same sitting. Mortality is lower when a more remote revascularization precedes removal of an infected abdominal aortic graft or treatment of an aortoenteric erosion or fistula. These approaches substantially reduce major amputation from 40% when graft removal precedes revascularization to 5% to 10% when the extraanatomic bypass is done first. When extraanatomic revascularization precedes removal of an infected graft, subsequent infection of the new bypass has been rare.

In recent years, in situ reconstruction of the aorta with superficial femoral vein grafts (neo-aorto-iliac systems), rifampin soaked or silver impregnated prosthetic grafts, or allogenic aortic homografts have added another therapeutic option. In general, in situ reconstruction is appropriate for more indolent infections where the patient is stable. More aggressive infections with virulent organisms and sepsis require extra-anatomic reconstruction and graft removal.

3. Graft thrombosis that occurs within a few weeks to months of operation often is the result of a technical problem in graft placement or anastomosis. Graft stenosis or occlusion after this time, but before 2 years is generally due to myointimal hyperplasia. After 18 to 24 months, graft failure is caused by atherosclerotic progression.

Failed aortofemoral grafts are usually due to loss of outflow and limb thrombosis. Treatment usually involves limb thromboembolectomy or thrombolysis with some sort of outflow procedure. Reoperations to maintain patency of failing or thrombosed aortofemoral grafts succeed in nearly 80% of patients and result in long-term limb preservation in 60% to 70%. Operative mortality for revision of femoral anastomotic problems is 1% to 2%.

Special discussion about lower extremity graft failure is warranted. Increasing evidence documents that alterations in the vein graft itself may also lead to graft thrombosis. Mills and colleagues have emphasized that 10% to 15% of reversed saphenous vein grafts develop significant inflow, intrinsic graft or outflow stenosis at a mean follow-up of 2 years. The peak incidence of early hemodynamic graft failure occurs within 12 months of graft implantation. Intrinsic graft stenoses cause the majority of failures (60%). These lesions are usually focal intimal hyperplasia distributed equally at the proximal and distal anastomoses. The remaining causes are inflow failure (13%), outflow failure (9%), muscle entrapment (4%), and hypercoagulable conditions (4%).

If these vein graft alterations are detected before graft thrombosis occurs, successful repair and long-term patency can be accomplished. Results are much poorer after thrombosis occurs. **Late cumulative vein graft patency is 75% to 80% for revised grafts, and 5% to 15% for thrombosed grafts at 5 years. Thus, current emphasis is on detecting failing grafts before they occlude.** Periodic reevaluation (every 3 to 6 months for 2 years; then annually if normal) should focus on any recurrent symptoms, such as return or progression of claudication, and objective signs of a failing graft. These signs include reduced segmental pressures and a 0.15 fall in the ankle-brachial pressure index. Important duplex ultrasound criteria predicting graft failure are now defined, and duplex should also be accomplished at these times (Chapter 6). Specifics include an increased peak systolic velocity across a stenotic area (two to three times the normal graft velocity), plus a decrease in peak systolic flow velocity to less than 45 cm/s in the graft beyond the area of stenosis. Collectively, these duplex findings and clinical warning signs may be an indication for arteriography to define correctable lesions before graft thrombosis occurs (Table 14.6).

Today, when lesions intrinsic to vein grafts are found on surveillance, treatment may include balloon angioplasty or open revision. While improved outcomes with surveillance of prosthetic grafts are not as conclusive, many still proceed with a surveillance program. One reason for this is that

Table 14.6   Graft surveillance criteria

Category	High-velocity criteria		Low-velocity criteria		ΔABI
I. Highest risk	PSV >300 cm/s or Vr >3.5 or EDV >100 cm/s	and	PSV <45 cm/s	or	>0.15
II. High risk	PSV >300 cm/s or Vr >3.5	and	PSV >45 cm/s	and	<0.15
III. Inter-mediate risk	300 cm/s >PSV >200 cm/s or Vr >2.0	and	PSV >45 cm/s	and	<0.15
IV. Low risk	PSV <200 cm/s or Vr <2.0	and	PSV >45 cm/s	and	<0.15

Duplex surveillance criteria for vein bypass grafts of the lower extremities. Category I should be admitted and heparinized for immediate revision. Category II should have elective arteriography±revision. Category III should have intensified surveillance (every 3 mo.) and Category IV is considered appropriate for continued standard surveillance.
PSV; Peak systolic velocity; EDV, end diastolic velocity; cm/s, centimeters per second; Vr, velocity ratio= PSV in stenosis/ PSV of normal proximal area.

when prosthetic grafts occlude they are associated with loss of outflow, whereas with vein grafts this is less frequent. Thus, if a culprit lesion is noted, treatment can be important.

When infrainguinal bypasses fail, reoperative surgery can achieve limb salvage in about 50% of patients. Once a vein graft is occluded for several weeks a new bypass graft is inserted as compared to thrombectomy and patch angioplasty of the original graft. Some patients may benefit from endovascular therapy. As mentioned previously, directed thrombolytic therapy of graft thrombosis can be helpful in certain acute circumstances. There is suggestion that thrombolytic therapy can improve limb outcomes and limit the magnitude of surgical revision if graft thrombosis is less than 14 days old. This comes at an apparent increased risk of stroke, embolism and bleeding. Once graft occlusion is over 14 days old, repeat surgical bypass appears superior.

4. Anastomotic pseudoaneurysm occurs most frequently at the common femoral artery. The causative factors are complex and include atherosclerotic deterioration of the artery and anastomotic disruption due to inadequate suturing, infection, graft dilation, and suture deterioration. Clinically, asymptomatic anastomotic aneurysms of less than 2.5 cm may be safely followed by observation. However, large false aneurysms or symptomatic aneurysms should be electively repaired before they are complicated by thrombosis, distal emboli, or rupture. Most late groin pseudoaneurysms are degenerative in nature. However, an infection must be clearly ruled out. One must be prepared to treat a graft infection when taking on reoperation for pseudoaneurysm.

5. Sexual dysfunction in men following aortoiliac operations may be manifested by impaired or absent penile erection and retrograde ejaculation after otherwise normal coitus. This may occur in up to some 25% of men. Previously normal sexual function may be altered by the interruption of preaortic sympathetic fibers, the parasympathetic pelvic splanchnic nerves, or the internal iliac artery flow. It is obvious that the surgeon must know whether any sexual dysfunction existed before surgery. If impotence is a significant problem to the patient postoperatively, he may be referred to an urologist for evaluation and treatment.

6. Spinal cord ischemia following operations on the abdominal aorta is rare, occurring in less than 0.5%. It is considered unpredictable. However, a recent review emphasized that the problem appears to occur in patients in whom internal iliac artery perfusion was impaired, when atheromatous embolism is evident, and when early postoperative hypotension or low cardiac output may further compromise marginal spinal cord perfusion.

7. Late complications of endovascular reconstructions of the lower extremities center around intervention site restenosis, thrombosis and failure, as well as progressive stenosis of the access site. The main drawback to iliac stenting is restenosis. There is some evidence that the main limitation of SFA intervention is restenosis allowing later percutaneous reintervention without negative consequences on the distal outflow and loss of surgical options. Some refuting data exists, however, and there is no clinical equipoise to date. Tibial intervention is hindered by restenosis and thrombosis. Some now advocate endovascular intervention of the extremity using embolic protection devices to decrease atheroembolic risk.

Surveillance has now also become part of the post-procedure protocol for lower-extremity endovascular interventions. As mentioned earlier, study of SFA angioplasty and stenting and iliac interventions has suggested assisted primary patency for these procedures is significantly enhanced with repeat intervention. This makes the argument to surveille compelling. While criteria indicating significant restenosis are less well understood compared to vein grafts, these are active areas of study and more will be known soon.

SELECTED READING

Bates MC, AbuRhama AF. An update on endovascular therapy of the lower extremities. *J Endovasc Ther.* 2004;11(supp II): II 107-II 127.

Black JH, La Muraglia GM, Kwolek CJ, et al. Contemporary results of angioplasty-based infrainguinal percutaneous interventions. *J Vasc Surg.* 2005;42:932-939.

Brewster DC. Current controversies in the management of aortoiliac occlusive disease. *J Vasc Surg.* 1997;25:365-379.

Ferris BL, Mills JL, Hughes JD, et al. Is early postoperative duplex scan surveillance of leg bypass grafts clinically important? *J Vasc Surg.* 2003;37:495-500.

Fujitani RM. Revision of the failing vein graft: outcome of secondary operations. *Semin Vasc Surg.* 1993;6:118-129.

Gardner AW, Poelhman ET. Exercise rehabilitation programs for the treatment of claudication pain: a meta-analysis. *JAMA.* 1995;274:975-980.

Green RM, Abbott WM, Matsumoto T, et al. Prosthetic above-knee femoropopliteal bypass grafting: five-year results of a randomized trial. *J Vasc Surg.* 2000;31:417-425.

Hagino RT, Sheehan MK, Jung I, et al. Target lesion charateristics in failing vein grafts predict the success of endovascular and open revision. *J Vasc Surg.* 2007;46:1167-1172.

Hirsch AT, Haskal ZJ, Hertzer NR, et al. ACC/AHA Guidelines for the management of patients with peripheral arterial disease (lower extremity, renal, mesenteric, and abdominal aortic): A collaborative report from the American societies on practice guidelines (writing committee to develop guidelines for the management of peripheral arterial disease). *J Am Coll Cardiol.* 2006;47:1-192.

How TV, Rowe CS, Gilling-Smith GL, et al. Interposition vein cuff anastamosis alters wall sheer stress distribution in the recipient artery. *J Vasc Surg.* 2000;31:1008-1017.

Ihnat DM, Mills JL, Dawson DL, et al. The correlation of early flow disturbances with the development of infrainguinal graft stenosis: a 10-year study of 341 autogenous vein grafts. *J Vasc Surg.* 1999;30:8-15.

Kreienberg PB, Darling RC III, Chang BB, et al. Adjunctive techniques to improve patency of distal prosthetic bypass grafts: polytetrafluoroethylene with remote artertiovenous fistulae versus vein cuffs. *J Vasc Surg.* 2000;31:696-701.

Mills JL, Fujitani RM, Taylor SM. The characteristics and anatomic distribution of lesions that cause reversed vein graft failure: A five-year prospective study. *J Vasc Surg.* 1993;17:195-206.

Ouriel K, Shortell CK, DeWeese JA, et al. A comparison of thrombolytic therapy with operative revascularization in the initial treatment of acute peripheral arterial ischemia. *J Vasc Surg.* 1994;19:1021-1030.

Perera GB, Lyden SP. Current Trends in Lower Extremity Revascularization. *Surg Clin N Am.* 2007;87:1135-47.

Pereira CB, Albers M, Romiti M, et al. Meta-analysis of femoropopliteal bypass grafts for lower extremity arterial insufficiency. *J Vasc Surg.* 2006;44:510-517.

Schillinger M, Sabeti S, Loewe C, et al. Balloon angioplasty versus implantation of nitinol stents in the superficial femoral artery. *NEJM.* 2006;354:1879-1888.

Singh N, Sidaway AN, DeZee KJ, et al. Factors associated with early failure of infrainguinal lower extremity arterial bypass. *J Vasc Surg.* 2008;447:556-61.

TransAtlantic Inter-Society Consensus Working Group. Management of Peripheral Arterial Disease: TransAtlantic Inter-society Consensus. *J Vasc Surg.* 2000;31(Part 2):S54-75.

TransAtlantic Inter-Society Consensus Working Group II. Inter-society Consensus for the Management of Peripheral Arterial Disease (TASC II). *J Vasc Surg.* 2007;45(Supplement S): S5-S67.

Valintine RJ, Hagino RT, Jackson MR, et al. Gastrointestinal complications after aortic surgery. *J Vasc Surg.* 1998;28:404-412.

Veterans Administration Cooperative Study Group. Johnson WC. Comparative evaluation of PTFE, HUV, and saphenous vein in fempop AK vascular reconstruction. *J Vasc Surg.* 2000;32:267-277.

White JV, Rutherford RB, Ryjewski C. Chronic Subcritical Ischemia: A poorly recognized stage of critical limb ischemia. *Sem Vasc Surg.* 2007;20:62-67.

CHAPTER 15

Aneurysms and Aortic Dissection

Management of arterial aneurysms and aortic dissection requires an understanding of natural history, diagnosis, and treatment options. In recent years, these options have changed dramatically with the development of endovascular techniques. **Despite these changes, the best results continue to follow carefully planned elective treatment before complications of rupture, thrombosis, or embolism occur.** The contrast in mortality between elective (2–5%) and ruptured abdominal aortic aneurysm (AAA) repair (50–70%) remains one of the most striking examples of the importance of early recognition and proper treatment of these diseases.

Aortic dissections are a commonly encountered degenerative disease of the aorta, which are distinctly different from aortic aneurysms. This chapter focuses on the natural history, diagnosis, and management of aneurysms and aortic dissections. The hemodynamics of aneurysms are discussed in Chapter 1. Chapter 4 outlines the initial physical evaluation, and Chapter 6 outlines several useful diagnostic tests that may be used to diagnose and follow these conditions.

ABDOMINAL AORTIC ANEURYSM

I. Epidemiology. During the past 30 to 40 years, the incidence of AAAs has increased significantly. This is attributed to increased detection with the use of ultrasound and computed tomography (CT) and an aging population. The rising incidence has been tenfold for small AAAs (<5 cm), while the incidence for larger aneurysms has increased by a factor of 2. Small aneurysms account for 50% of all recognized AAAs, an important consideration given that much of the uncertainty surrounding appropriate management concerns aneurysms <5.5 cm.

II. Natural history and the evolution of evidence-based approach. Aortic aneurysms are a disease of the elderly diagnosed in the sixth and seventh decades of life. As many as 20% of patients with an AAA have a family history of aortic aneurysm. The expansion rate of AAAs is 2 to 3 mm per year and increases as the aneurysm enlarges. Twenty percent of aneurysms expand at a rate of more than 4 mm per year, while 80% grow at a slower pace. **Importantly, active cigarette smoking has been shown to be associated with an increased expansion rate and has been identified as an independent risk factor for aneurysm rupture.**

The natural history of AAA is expansion and rupture, an outcome that is related directly to aneurysm diameter. Less commonly, enlarging aneurysms may erode into the vena cava resulting in an **aortocaval fistula,** or into the intestine presenting as gastrointestinal bleeding (i.e., **aortoenteric fistula**). These concepts are controversial, not because of the risk associated with open surgery, but because experts have debated the size at which repair should occur. Initially, aneurysms <6 cm were considered appropriate for elective repair. Autopsy studies in the 1970s and 1980s suggested that even small aneurysms (4 to 5 cm) could rupture, which resulted in a more aggressive approach to repair. **Population-based studies in the 1990s showed that rupture risk did not increase until aneurysm diameter reached 5 cm** (Figs. 15.1 and 15.2). Rupture risk for small (<5 cm) AAAs was shown to be approximately 1% per year, 5% to 10% per year for medium-sized (5 to 7 cm) AAAs, and at least 10% to 25% per year for large (7 cm) AAAs. **The more recent U.K. Small Aneurysm** and **Aneurysm Detection and Management (ADAM) trials** were prospective randomized studies looking for survival benefit in early open repair of aneurysms between 4 and 5.4 cm. Findings from these trials confirmed the population-based studies of the 1990s, while showing no benefit to early open repair of aneurysms between 4 and 5.4 cm. Several caveats from these studies are worth noting. First, safe observation of aneurysms between 4 and 5.4 cm includes ultrasound every 3 to 6 months, which many feel is unrealistic for some patients. Second, in both studies two-thirds of patients in the "observation" group crossed over to eventual open repair once their aneurysms reached 5.5 cm during the study period. **Finally, in this era of endovascular aneurysm repair (EVAR) it is important to remember that both the U.K. Small Aneurysm and the ADAM trial compared observation to early open aneurysm repair and not to EVAR.** What makes this relevant is that the mortality associated with open repair in these two trials was 5.8% and 2.7% respectively, which is higher than recently reported for EVAR.

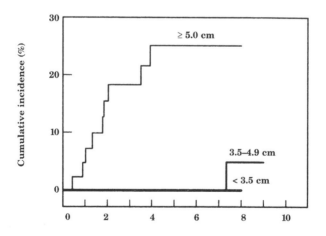

Years after initial ultrasound examination

Figure 15.1.   Cumulative incidence of rupture of abdominal aortic aneurysms according to the diameter of the aneurysm at the initial ultrasound examination. (From Nevitt MP, Ballard DJ, Hallett JW, Jr. Prognosis of abdominal aortic aneurysms: a population-based study. *NEJM*. 1989;321:1009-1014, with permission.)

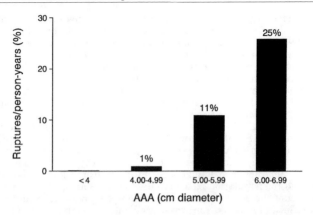

Figure 15.2.   Rupture risk of abdominal aortic aneurysm (AAA) per year for size diameter. (From Reed WW, Hallett JW Jr, Damiano MA, et al. Learning from the last ultrasound: a population-based study of patients with abdominal aortic aneurysm. *Arch Int Med.* 1997;157: 2064-2068, with permission.)

In 1997 the U.S. FDA approved the first device for EVAR. More than a decade later, the expanded use of this procedure seems to have had a positive impact on the mortality associated with AAA repair. Information from the Medicare database recently revealed that in the first 3 years of this decade the number of AAA repairs in the United States had not changed (approximately 60,000 per year). However the percentage of AAAs treated with EVAR did increase and, with an operative mortality of less than 2%, this less invasive approach appears to have reduced the overall mortality associated with AAA repair; something that had not been possible in this country for decades. How this shift in the treatment of AAAs impacts recommendations for repair in relation to AAA size remains to be seen and is the topic of significant clinical and epidemiologic research.

From these decades of clinical study, one can be assured that nearly all AAAs that rupture have enlarged to over 5 cm in diameter. Unfortunately, the prevalence of rupture remains unchanged, and even today 70% of patients with ruptured AAA are unaware of the diagnosis until the day of rupture. This statistic has been used as an important rallying cry for those advocating for the wider use of ultrasound screening to detect AAAs in targeted populations.

III. **Indications for operation.**
    A. **A practical approach using aneurysm diameter.** Currently in our practice, patients with asymptomatic AAAs <5 cm are followed with ultrasound. For these patients, CT scans are typically not obtained and aneurysm repair not recommended unless part of a clinical trial or if the most recent measurement confirms rapid expansion (i.e., more than 6 mm in 6 months or more than 1 cm in one year). Aneurysms <5 cm may occasionally be repaired as part of treatment for symptomatic aortoiliac occlusive disease with open (e.g., aortobifemoral bypass) or endovascular techniques.

Good-risk patients with aneurysms between 5 and 5.4 cm receive a contrast-enhanced aortic CT to define the size, shape, and extent of the aneurysm. Such patients are provided a summation of our clinical understanding of aneurysm observation versus repair, open and EVAR. Patients are made aware that although it is safe to observe aneurysms <5.5 cm, close surveillance will be required and it is likely that within 1-3 years the aneurysm will expand and repair will be required. Repair of asymptomatic aneurysms between 5 and 5.4 cm is not rushed and is strongly influenced by individual patient factors, such as medical comorbidity (e.g., risk of anesthesia), ability to commit to close surveillance, candidacy for EVAR, and level of patient anxiety regarding the aneurysm. **If these individual factors weigh in favor of repair, good-risk patients with AAAs between 5 and 5.4 cm are offered an operation either open or EVAR.** Finally all good risk patients who present with an aneurysm of 5.5 cm or larger receive a contrast-enhanced aortic CT and are offered repair, open or EVAR, in an expeditious manner.

For high-risk patients or those with more limited life expectancy and aneurysms greater than 5 cm we defer to less invasive EVAR if aneurysm morphology permits. If such high-risk patients are not endovascular candidates, we most often delay any open operation until the aneurysm expands to 6 cm or becomes symptomatic.

B. A less common but more urgent indication for AAA repair is evidence of **peripheral emboli** in the lower extremities of patients with aneurysms.

C. Urgent aneurysm repair is also indicated for patients with a known aneurysm that has become tender or is associated with abdominal or back pain. These patients should be hospitalized and considered to have a symptomatic aneurysm, even though their vital signs may be normal and their abdominal symptoms nonspecific.

D. Patients with ruptured aneurysms and shock should be taken directly to the operating room for resuscitation and operation. An increasing number of series now report the treatment of ruptured AAAs by endovascular means (i.e., EVAR), an option that has become more viable with increased experience, improved devices, and more complete "on-the-shelf" endovascular inventories.

IV. Preoperative evaluation. The preoperative evaluation for an elective AAA should define the size and extent of the aneurysm, associated medical risks, and associated vascular disease.

A. Size and extent of AAA. The reliability of the abdominal exam to detect and measure an AAA is poor. Information from the ADAM trial showed that the accuracy of the physical exam to detect an aneurysm in an individual with an abdominal girth of 38 inches or more was around 50%. The simplest and least expensive test to diagnose and measure an AAA is ultrasound. Measurement of the anterior–posterior diameter is more accurate than the transverse diameter; reliably measuring to within 2-3 mm. Ultrasound is also the favored method to follow changes in aneurysm diameter over time (i.e., aneurysm surveillance).

Although some prefer routine CT scan for patients with suspected or known small AAAs, this imaging modality costs more than ultrasound and carries morbidity associated with contrast administration. In our practices, contrast-enhanced aortic CT is reserved for aneurysms that are >5 cm or in which repair is actively being planned. In addition to assessing the size of an AAA, a common reason to obtain a CT is anatomic evaluation for EVAR (Figure 15.3). **In this regard, CT assesses the following characteristics of the proximal aortic and distal iliac artery seal or landing zones where the endograft is fixed, thereby excluding the aneurysm from flow and pressure:**

1. **The diameter and length in relation to branch arteries (e.g., renal and internal iliac arteries)**
2. **The degree of circumferential calcification and/ or thrombus**
3. **The degree of tortuosity or angle**
4. **The length of aneurysm in relation to the aortic bifurcation and branch arteries**

In addition, an aortic CT is indicated when a suprarenal or thoracoabdominal aneurysm is suspected. One must remember that CT scan may occasionally overestimate the diameter of an aneurysm because the measurements are made perpendicular to the body axis, which introduces some error if the aorta is tortuous. **This error can now be corrected for by use of modern CT software, which allows for calculations referred to as center line measurements of aneurysm length and diameter**.

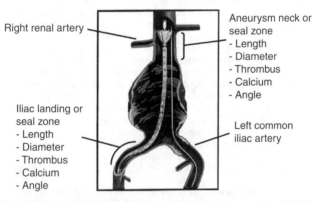

Figure 15.3.   Evaluation for endovascular aneurysm repair (EVAR) includes evaluation of the landing or seal zones of the endograft, which include the aortic neck below the renal arteries as well as the iliac arteries. These zones of endograft fixation are evaluated for their length, diameter, degree of thrombus, degree of calcification, and degree of angle or tortuosity. If any one of these four variables or a combination of one or more is unfavorable, the likelihood of an effective seal is reduced and the aneurysm should not be considered a candidate for EVAR. Depending on the experience of the institution, somewhere between 50 and 75% of AAAs are anatomic candidates for EVAR.

B. Aortography is not reliable for determining aneurysm diameter, as luminal thrombus obscures the outer limit of the aneurysm wall. Aortography prior to aneurysm repair, open or endovascular, should be used selectively for the following criteria:

1. Decreased peripheral pulses or symptoms of lower-extremity claudication
2. Poorly controlled hypertension or renal insufficiency indicating renal artery occlusive disease
3. Suprarenal or thoracoabdominal aortic aneurysms requiring delineation of visceral and intercostal arteries
4. Symptoms of intestinal ischemia suggesting visceral artery occlusive disease
5. Suspected horseshoe kidney with multiple renal arteries on ultrasound or CT

Although once commonplace, aortography prior to EVAR is now rarely indicated because of the high quality of dynamic, contrast-enhanced aortic CT. One or more of these criteria for preoperative aortography is present in fewer than 10% of patients with AAA, making this invasive preoperative test uncommon.

C. Medical risks. Most medical comorbidities can be detected by the performance of a thorough history and physical exam, both of which are outlined in more detail in Chapters 4 and 7. As many as 50% of patients with AAAs have some degree of coronary artery disease. Evidence-based guidelines offered by the American Heart Association (AHA) and the American College of Cardiology (ACC) in regard to evaluation prior to AAA repair are outlined in Chapter 8. These guidelines include recommendations for preoperative cardiac testing and selective preoperative cardiac revascularization. **In the context of these guidelines, traditional open aortic aneurysm repair is categorized as a high-risk procedure (see Table 8.5) because of the need for an abdominal or retroperitoneal incision and cross-clamping of the aorta**. Endovascular aneurysm repair should be considered an intermediate risk procedure (see Table 8.5) as it may be done under regional anesthesia, does not require aortic cross-clamp, and can even be performed percutaneously in many cases. In our experience, adherence to the AHA/ACC Clinical Guidelines contributes to a low elective operative mortality for open (3-4%) and endovascular (<2%) AAA repair.

A more aggressive approach to AAA repair in older or high-risk patients has been advocated by some. EVAR now clearly offers an option that is safer for many of these patients although they must still be carefully selected and treated by an experienced anesthesia and endovascular team. Under these conditions, EVAR in high-risk patients can now be accomplished with an operative mortality of <5%. If not repaired, many of these high-risk patients with larger AAAs will succumb to aneurysm rupture.

D. Associated vascular disease. Approximately 10% of patients with an AAA will have associated carotid occlusive disease in the form of an asymptomatic carotid bruit or symptoms such as TIA or stroke. In our practice, these patients undergo carotid duplex to determine the significance of the carotid disease (Chapter 6). Patients with symptomatic carotid stenoses undergo expeditious treatment of the carotid prior to AAA repair even if the aneurysm is large. In these cases, the timing of the AAA repair depends on the size of the aneurysm and, unless it is quite large (>7 cm) or symptomatic, the aneurysm repair is performed a week or two after treatment of the symptomatic carotid. Patients with asymptomatic carotid stenoses may undergo elective AAA repair prior to carotid endarterectomy. Exceptions to this are patients with asymptomatic unilateral preocclusive stenosis or bilateral high-grade stenoses, in which case it is reasonable to treat the carotid prior to AAA repair. However, patients with symptomatic or large aneurysms (>7 cm) should undergo AAA repair without delay for carotid surgery. Overall, the risk of perioperative stroke from carotid occlusive disease during AAA repair is low, and clinical evidence supporting preoperative carotid treatment is lacking.

V. Preoperative preparation for elective AAA repair is now occupied mostly by study of aortic CT reconstructions in consideration of EVAR. Suitability for EVAR, type of endograft, and specific endovascular approach all require significant consideration and planning. To this end it is our practice to have more than one set of eyes evaluate the aortic CT prior to final decisions regarding EVAR. This is productive when in the form of discussion within our vascular and endovascular surgery group, but may also be accomplished with experienced radiologists or even trusted clinical specialists employed by industry. Careful evaluation of the aortic CT in these forums helps the endovascular specialist anticipate and plan for "trouble spots" during EVAR before starting the case. This type of disciplined preoperative preparation before EVAR maximizes the likelihood of a successful treatment and minimizes the chances of a misguided endovascular attempt.

VI. Management of a ruptured aneurysm. Although EVAR has been utilized to treat ruptured AAAs, in some specialized institutions the most common form (>90%) of management remains emergent open repair. The key to successful management of a ruptured AAA with open or endovascular techniques is expeditious movement of the patient to the operating room. Delay in the emergency or radiology departments often results in deterioration and death from hemorrhage.

Operative mortality associated with ruptured AAA has remained unchanged for some time, although, just as in elective AAA repair, there is some early evidence that EVAR may improve mortality in certain groups of patients with ruptured aneurysm. Overall, only about half of patients with a ruptured AAA who arrive at the hospital will be discharged alive. Factors predicting poor outcome or death are profound shock, cardiac arrest (need for CPR), preexisting cardiac or renal disease, and technical complications during the operation. Several factors, however, can enhance the likelihood of survival for a patient with a ruptured AAA.

A. Rapid transport. Patients with suspected AAA rupture should be transported rapidly to a hospital, where a surgical team should be waiting for assessment and resuscitation. An operating room should be readied as the patient arrives.

B. Resuscitation should include two large-bore (14 or 16 gauge) intravenous lines, a nasogastric tube, and a Foley catheter. Blood should be typed and cross-matched for packed red blood cells. Crystalloid solutions are acceptable for initial volume administration, however emergency release type O negative or cross-matched blood and fresh frozen plasma should be given at a 1:1 ratio to patients with evidence of shock (i.e., component blood therapy). **In a strategy referred to as** *permissive hypotension* **, blood pressure should be maintained only to a level to support urine output and mental status.** Systolic pressures of 100 mm Hg are adequate if the patient is awake with some urine output. Inotropic agents, vasopressors, and overuse of crystalloid with the goal of achieving a normal blood pressure will worsen the situation by causing hemorrhage before bleeding can be controlled in the operating room.

If available, a rapid autotransfusion device (i.e., cell saver) should be set up in the operating room. Arterial and central venous lines can be placed and prophylactic antibiotics administered in the operating room.

C. Accurate diagnosis. If the patient has no previous diagnosis of AAA or the diagnosis is in question, ultrasound in the emergency department is the most expeditious method to determine the presence or absence of AAA. If the patient has shown no evidence of hemodynamic compromise, or if EVAR is an option at the institution, an abdominal CT scan should be considered. An ECG should also be performed to rule out acute myocardial infarction.

D. Immediate operation. A patient who has had hemodynamic compromise (e.g., syncope or shock) and has a pulsatile abdominal mass or a known AAA should be taken directly to the operating room. Performance of a contrast CT in this setting is risky and should only be performed if directed by an experienced endovascular surgeon who is present and who is considering emergent EVAR for ruptured AAA.

E. Temperature control. Patients with a ruptured AAA and shock become hypothermic quickly. Those with a body temperature below 33°C develop capillary leak syndrome necessitating more volume, manifest a diffuse coagulopathy, and slip suddenly into life-threatening cardiac arrhythmias. The three useful means of preventing hypothermia are **(1) warming the operating room to 70° to 80°F before the patient arrives, (2) using the Bair Hugger warming tent over the upper thorax and head, and (3) use of high volume, countercurrent warming infusing systems for all administered intravenous fluids.**

F. Aortic control can be obtained by open aortic clamping or with insertion of a large compliant aortic occlusion balloon from a femoral or brachial artery sheath. Since blood pressure can decrease precipitously with induction of anesthesia, the patient should be prepped, and the necessary arterial sheaths and occlusion balloons positioned prior to the patient being anesthetized. If open repair is pursued, a midline incision is the most direct approach. If the retroperitoneal hematoma is massive, initial aortic control should be gained by compression or clamping of the aorta at the diaphragm (Fig. 15.4). In many patients, however, the aorta can be clamped below the renal arteries. At this site, care must be taken to avoid injury to the duodenum and left renal vein. Rarely, a patient with multiple prior abdominal operations may need a left thoracotomy for initial aortic clamping. Prior to clamping, mannitol (25 g) may be given as a diuretic and free-radical scavenger.

G. Anticoagulation. Administration of heparin during ruptured AAA repair may be problematic. If the patient is hypothermic and in shock, a coagulopathy may already exist. On the other hand, lower-extremity thrombosis is not uncommon during ruptured AAA repair. Consequently, smaller systemic doses of heparin (2,500 to 3,000 units) or regional administration of heparin into the iliac arteries may decrease lower-extremity thrombosis.

H. Assessing limb and vital organ perfusion. Lower-extremity perfusion must be assessed before leaving the operating room. This can be achieved by palpating pulses, listening for Doppler signals, or by using calf plethysmographic pulse waveforms. If a significant thrombus or embolus is suspected to either lower extremity, thromboembolectomy should performed using a Fogarty® embolectomy catheter (Edwards Lifesciences Corp., Irvine, CA). In these instances, removal of the thrombus or embolus and restoration of flow to the extremity is best achieved by exposure and opening of the femoral artery of the affected leg as opposed to attempts from the abdomen.

Likewise, the colon should be inspected for viability. If questionable, intravenous fluoroscein can be given and the bowel inspected with a Wood's lamp. When the abdomen is massively distended, a tight primary closure may compromise renal or visceral perfusion. In such instances the abdominal fascia should not be closed and the abdominal contents covered with a temporary abdominal closure. Delayed closure of the fascia can be accomplished in 48-72 hours when patient physiology and abdominal edema has improved.

VII. Technical aspects of AAA repair. The following section briefly reviews some of the technical aspects involved with open and endovascular aneurysm repair (Fig. 15.3).

A. Open aneurysm exposure may be performed through a midline or left retroperitoneal approach (Fig. 15.5). Both exposures have certain advantages and use of one over the other tends to be specific to the institution or surgeon. Those who prefer a midline incision and the inframesocolic transperitoneal approach cite the excellent exposure of the entire aneurysm—both renal arteries and both iliac arteries. The disadvantage of the transperitoneal approach is the open exposure of the bowel contents and a larger, more painful incision. The retroperitoneal exposure is touted by some to be less painful and to produce less physiologic stress because it avoids exposure of the bowel contents, which remain in the peritoneal sack. The disadvantage of retroperitoneal exposure is that it provides limited exposure of the right renal and common iliac arteries, which may be particularly important in some cases. For aneurysms that extend to the renal arteries, transperi-

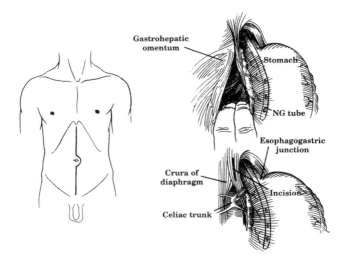

A

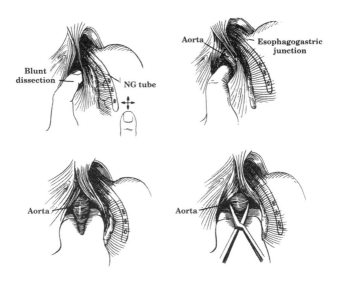

B

Figure 15.4.   Supraceliac aortic clamping is useful for large ruptured abdominal aortic aneurysms and huge retroperitoneal hematomas that obscure the proximal aneurysm neck at the renal level. NG, nasogastric. (The Mayo Foundation, with permission.)

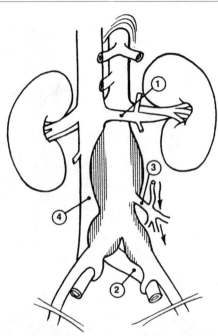

Figure 15.5.   Anatomic trouble spots in abdominal aortic aneurysm exposure. (1) The left renal vein or one of its branches (left renal lumbar, gonadal, or adrenal) may be injured during exposure of the aneurysm neck, especially with ruptured aneurysms. In 5% of cases, the left renal vein lies posterior to the aorta and may be injured in any attempt to encircle the proximal aorta for control. (2) The common iliac veins are usually adherent to the iliac arteries and may be injured during dissection. (3) The inferior mesenteric artery should be ligated on or within the aneurysm sac to avoid ligation of critical collateral vessels from the marginal artery of Drummond. (4) Dissection of the aneurysm sac from the vena cava is usually unnecessary.

toneal exposure of the renal arteries and suprarenal aorta may be facilitated by division of the left renal vein, leaving the adrenal and gonadal veins as outflow for the left kidney. Another alternative is extensive mobilization of the left renal vein by division of the adrenal, gonadal, and lumbar branches, allowing the vein to be retracted up or down to expose the suprarenal aortic segment. Those who advocate the retroperitoneal approach point out that this exposure facilitates visualization of the suprarenal aortic segment without manipulation of the left renal vein, as the left kidney including the left renal vein is reflected up with the peritoneal contents away from the aorta. After isolation of the proximal and distal clamp sites, intravenous heparin (100 u/kg) and occasionally mannitol (25 g) is administered and allowed to circulate for 5 minutes.

B. Flow through the aneurysm is arrested by proximal and distal clamping. This should be confirmed by palpating the aneurysm to assure the absence of pulsatility. Once this is confirmed, the aneurysm is opened, the layered mural thrombus removed, and the back-bleeding lumbar arteries suture ligated. Attention is also given to the inferior mesenteric artery, which most often has back bleeding into the open aneurysm sac. Depending upon the degree of bleeding from the inferior mesenteric artery (IMA) and surgeon preference, the IMA may either be ligated or temporarily occluded until the graft has been sutured in place and perfusion to the lower extremities reestablished. The prosthetic graft is sutured to the normal proximal aortic neck inside the aneurysm sac after the proximal aneurysm has been cut down to allow formation of a good sewing ring **(Creech technique)**. This sequence of steps from clamping, opening the aneurysm, occluding back-bleeding vessels, and suturing in a graft in the bed of the aneurysm to restore antegrade flow is referred to as **endoaneurysmorrhaphy.** In cases where the duodenum is adherent to the AAA **(e.g., inflammatory aneurysm)**, we do not dissect it from the aneurysm but attempt to work around it. If infection is suspected, the aneurysm should be cultured and completely excised. After the graft is in place, the clamps removed, and flow restored, perfusion to the colon is assessed and in most cases the inferior mesenteric artery may then be ligated. In instances where normal circulation to the bowel may not be present, such as a previous colon resection, the inferior mesenteric artery may be implanted onto the prosthetic graft.

C. Retroperitoneal coverage of the graft should be completed using the aneurysm sac to separate the graft from the intestine. If this is not done, the intestine, especially the duodenum, can adhere to the graft years later and result in an aortoenteric fistula.

D. EVAR was introduced by Parodi in the early 1990s and is now the operative approach for half of AAAs treated in the United States. EVAR involves the passage of self-expandable, covered stents (i.e., stent grafts) into the aorta through the femoral arteries. Precise positioning of the stent graft below the renal arteries and in the desired iliac "landing zones" is achieved using fluoroscopy and contrast arteriography. As the stent graft is fixed at normal arterial segments at the proximal infrarenal aorta (i.e., neck) and the iliac arteries, the AAA is excluded from flow and, therefore, arterial pressure. If appropriate fixation and seal is achieved, flow and pressure go through the graft, allowing the walls of the AAA to be depressurized and in many cases decrease in size or "heal" around the graft.

Incomplete positioning or sealing of the aneurysm sac following endograft placement results in endoleak. Endoleaks are categorized into four main groups according to their cause and may not be significant depending upon the category. **Type I endoleaks** result from failure of primary graft-artery seal points at the aortic neck or iliac arteries and are generally considered a technical failure of endograft placement. An example of a type I endoleak is failure to achieve a seal at the proximal aortic neck below the renal arteries resulting in antegrade flow around the deployed stent into the aneurysm sac. Type I endoleaks leave the aneurysm fully pressurized and should be corrected in the operating room. **Type II endoleaks** represent back bleeding into the aneurysm sac from patent lumbar arteries or the inferior mesenteric artery. Type II endoleaks are present at the conclusion of up to 25% of EVAR cases and are not immediately treated, as most do not pressurize the aneurysm sac and will resolve over time. Type II endoleaks are only relevant if they persist and if the aneurysm sac does not decrease in diameter over a period of 1 to 2 years. In these cases, type II endoleaks should be treated with the endovascular technique of coil embolization. **Type III endoleaks** represent flow into the aneurysm sac from junction points in the modular bifurcated endografts. Like type I leaks, type III leaks are viewed as a technical failure of the endograft and should be corrected when they are identified or soon thereafter, as the aneurysm sac remains pressurized. **Type IV endoleaks** represent flow into the aneurysm sac from flaws or porosity in the graft material itself. Type IV endoleaks are uncommon and are treated individually depending on their appearance on imaging studies (e.g., CTA or aortography) and whether or not the aneurysm sac is decreasing in diameter.

Although EVAR is successful, with a 98% technical success rate, and studies show lower morbidity and mortality with its use compared to open repair, it does have drawbacks. Specifically, following EVAR patients require more graft surveillance and even reintervention than patients who have undergone open repair. The follow-up of endografts is necessary to assess aneurysm size and the presence or absence of endoleaks. This follow-up regimen includes contrast-enhanced CT scans, which can lead to detrimental effects on renal function over years of surveillance. The use of contrast CT scans to follow endografts has been reduced in recent yeas with increased reliance on duplex ultrasound. Recent studies have shown that 25% of patients who have undergone EVAR will require some graft-related reintervention at 5 years, compared to 2% of patients who have undergone open repair. Nearly all of these interventions are performed with endovascular techniques and include treatment of endoleaks.

VIII. Concurrent intra-abdominal disease. As a rule we prefer not to combine elective AAA surgery with other intra-abdominal procedures that could be safely postponed. Therefore, if the coexisting pathology does not have an urgent need to be treated (e.g., asymptomatic gallstones) we proceed with the planned aneurysm repair, open or EVAR.

If the coexisting disease process has urgency, such as the case of gastrointestinal or genitourinary malignancy, we then consider the size of the AAA and whether or not it can be treated with EVAR. If the AAA is 5.5 cm or larger and EVAR is an option, we proceed with endovascular repair quickly, allowing full focus on treatment of the urgent malignancy or other disease process in the weeks that follow. If the aneurysm is 5-5.4 cm or is not an endovascular candidate and the coexisting process has urgency, we defer treatment of the AAA until after the other pathology has been addressed. This is especially the case in instances where the other disease process is symptomatic, such as cholelithiasis, cholecystitis, or an obstructing colon cancer. In these cases we follow the aneurysm closely in the perioperative period with ultrasound or even CT, as there have been anecdotal reports of aneurysm expansion following abdominal operations for other reasons.

On the rare occasion when intra-abdominal pathology is encountered during open AAA repair, the aneurysm repair should proceed as planned in almost all cases. This is particularly the case when the aneurysm is >5.5 cm. Even in cases where pathology is incidentally noted or palpated in the bowel or solid organs, the open aneurysm repair should be completed and note of the findings made in the operative dictation. Appropriate consultation, imaging, and endoscopy should be made in the early postoperative period in such cases. The only exception to this rule may be in a patient with an aneurysm <5.5 cm in whom an obstructing colon cancer is encountered at the time of open AAA repair. In such a case it would be reasonable to leave the aneurysm untreated and turn focus to the obstructing colon cancer recognizing that the aneurysm would require close observation in the perioperative period.

X. Postoperative complications. Early postoperative complications include cardiac or respiratory dysfunction, postoperative bleeding, and renal insufficiency (Chapters 8 and 9). Graft-limb thrombosis or lower-extremity embolization can lead to lower-extremity ischemia requiring urgent intervention. **Colon ischemia occurs in 1-2% of AAA repairs and usually manifests in the early postoperative period as a bloody bowel movement**. In these cases urgent lower endoscopy is indicated to make the diagnosis of colon ischemia and to allow appropriate treatment, such as broad spectrum antibiotics, aggressive resuscitation, or return to the operating room for removal of nonviable colon. Aortoenteric fistula, prosthetic graft infection, and sexual dysfunction are complications seen in the later postoperative period.

XI. Long-term follow-up. Long-term survival following elective AAA repair is 70-80% at five years and 50% at 10 years, which is less than that in age-matched controls without AAA. Studies have shown that long-term survival rates for patients undergoing EVAR are less than those having open repair, but this is a result of selection bias. Less fit patients were more likely to have had EVAR in these reports. The most important factor in long-term survival of patients following AAA repair is the presence or absence of coronary heart disease. Patients with clinically evident heart disease have a decreased survival of 50% at 5 years and only 30% at 10 years. Although less common than cardiac morbidity, stroke affects 5% of patients at 5 years and 10% at 10 years following aneurysm repair.

Late graft-related complications following AAA repair include graft limb occlusion, graft infection, and anastomotic aneurysm. These long-term complications are less frequent following open AAA repair (0.5-1% per year) than following EVAR (5% per year). Additionally, up to 25% of patients will develop aneurismal dilation of the aorta proximal to the AAA repair over time. Although these aneurysms in the paravisceral or thoracic aorta are often small, their incidence along with that of graft-related complications confirms the need to periodically check patients who have undergone AAA repair.

Specifically, we evaluate patients twice in the first year after open AAA repair and annually thereafter. The evaluation includes a physical exam of the femoral and popliteal arteries, a duplex ultrasound of the aortic graft, and a chest x-ray. A contrast CT scan of the aorta is obtained every 5 years following open AAA repair. **Postoperative surveillance following EVAR is changing with an increased reliance on duplex ultrasound compared to contrast CT scan.** In our practice, patients who have undergone an uncomplicated EVAR receive one contrast-enhanced CT scan and an aortic duplex in the month following the procedure. If there is no endoleak we repeat the duplex in 3 and 6 months and the CT scan at the one-year mark following EVAR. If the one-month postoperative CT shows a type II endoleak, the CT is repeated at 3 and again at 6 months, assuming there is no enlargement of the aneurysm. Identification of a type I or III endoleak or aneurysm enlargement (>3 mm) is an indication for a formal aortogram to more thoroughly evaluate the endograft and the dynamics of the aneurysm. Most endoleaks and graft-related complications following EVAR can be treated with endovascular techniques.

THORACOABDOMINAL AORTIC ANEURYSM

Thoracoabdominal aortic aneurysm (TAA) is defined as simultaneous aneurysm involvement of the thoracic and abdominal aortic segments. TAAs represent <10% of degenerative aortic aneurysms and are classified based on a scheme reported by E. Stanley Crawford (Fig. 15.6). Natural history data on TAAs reveals a negligible rupture risk for aneurysms <4 cm. In contrast, 5-year rupture risk is nearly 20% for TAAs between 4 and 6 cm and 33% for those >6 cm. Therefore, the threshold for open repair has traditionally been an aneurysm diameter of 6 cm in healthy patients or for aneurysms that have expanded 1 cm in a year's time. Open repair of thoracoabdominal aortic aneurysms was the only option for treatment until 2005, when the FDA approved a commercially available thoracic aortic stent graft. Although the role of thoracic endovascular aneurysm repair (TEVAR) in the treatment of thoracic aneurysms (TA) and TAA has yet to be fully defined, its introduction as a less invasive option has generated considerable enthusiasm.

I. Preoperative evaluation. In addition to history and physical, a contrast-enhanced dynamic CT scan of the aorta is required. Because of the tortuosity of the thoracic aorta it is important that measurements of diameter be made perpendicular and not tangential to the aortic centerline axis. Accurate measurements can best be obtained using axial centerline software with 3D reconstructions, which allows for sizing of diameter and assessments of length within the aneurysm. Although contrast aortography was historically mandatory prior to TAA repair, advances in CT imaging have allowed this invasive preoperative test to be performed selectively. One indication proposed by some for preoperative aortography is localization of the great radicular artery (**i.e., artery of Adamkiewicz**) which is felt to be useful in decreasing the risk of perioperative spinal cord ischemia. This artery arises from a T_9 to T_{12} intercostal artery in 75% of patients and is the main blood supply to the anterior spinal artery. The utility of preoperative localization of

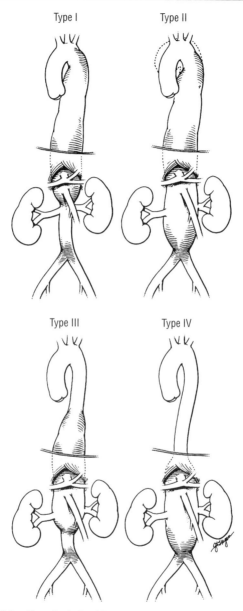

Figure 15.6. Crawford classification of thoracoabdominal aortic aneurysms. (From Crawford ES, Crawford JL, Safi HJ. Thoracoabdominal aortic aneurysms: Preoperative and intraoperative factors determining immediate and long-term results of operations in 805 patients. *J Vasc Surg.* 1986;3:389-404, with permission.)

this artery in reducing the incidence of cord ischemia has not been universally accepted and most groups rely on other perioperative adjuncts to avoid this often devastating complication.

II. Operative principles. The open operative approach to TAA follows one of two distinct methods: (1) **clamp-and-sew** with adjuncts used to minimize end organ ischemia, or (2) **distal aortic perfusion with sequential clamping** of the graft. Both use a left thoracoabdominal approach, and the choice is influenced by the experience of the surgical, anesthesia, and intensive care teams. The following are adjuncts used individually or together during TAA repair to reduce morbidity.

    A. Distal aortic perfusion is achieved with left atrial to femoral artery bypass utilizing a Bio-Medicus pump (Medtronics, Minneapolis, MN, U.S.A.). This technique provides distal perfusion to the lower extremities and visceral arteries during aortic graft placement, and may benefit the heart by unloading the left ventricle during aortic cross-clamp.

    B. Regional spinal cord hypothermia (mean 26°C) using an epidural catheter with infusion of cold saline reduces the metabolic rate and demand of the spinal cord. Temperature and pressure may be monitored simultaneously with a separate intrathecal catheter.

    C. Cerebrospinal fluid drainage improves perfusion pressure of the spinal cord when pressure is greater than 10 to 15 cm H_2O. This technique is commonly used perioperatively and for 1 to 3 days following the operation.

    D. Renal cooling. Direct application of ice and infusion of renal preservation solution (4°C lactated Ringer's with mannitol and methylprednisolone) into the renal artery after opening the aorta reduces local metabolic demands and stimulates diuresis.

    E. In-line mesenteric shunting. After performance of the proximal anastomosis an arterial perfusion catheter is placed from the proximal graft to the celiac or superior mesenteric artery ostia. This allows prograde, pulsatile perfusion to the viscera while the remainder of the graft is being placed.

III. Postoperative course. Operative mortality of TAA repair averages 10% but is much higher in urgent or emergent cases. Other factors that are associated with higher morbidity and mortality are preoperative renal dysfunction (Cr 1.8 mg/dL), intraoperative hypotension, intraoperative transfusion requirements, the development of postoperative spinal cord ischemia, and hypothermia (<35°C).

    Respiratory failure is the most common complication following TAA repair (25-45%). Risk factors are active smoking, baseline pulmonary disease, and division of the phrenic nerve during thoracoabdominal exposure. The incidence of **spinal cord ischemic complications** ranges from 4% to 16% in large series following all types of TAA. This can be as high as 30% in patients with extensive type I and II TAA (Fig. 15.6). **Renal failure** can be expected in 5% to 20% of patients following TAA repair and increases the risk of mortality nearly tenfold. A survival of 55% at 5 years can be expected following elective TAA repair with cardiac events representing the leading cause of death. Rupture of another aneurysm accounts for 10% of late deaths emphasizing the importance of lifelong aneurysm surveillance.

AORTIC DISSECTION

Dissection is a common vascular catastrophe affecting the aorta and is distinct from degenerative aneurysms. Dissection results from an aortic defect that allows a false lumen to form between the intima and adventitia. The **DeBakey classification** of aortic dissection includes types I and II, which involve the ascending aorta, and type III, which involves only the descending aorta (Fig 15.7). The **Stanford classification** includes type A, involving the ascending aorta, and type B, involving only the descending aorta. **Complications of dissection include aortic valve insufficiency, aneurysm formation, aortic rupture and visceral, renal or peripheral ischemia**.

I. Preoperative evaluation. Aortic dissections present as tearing chest or back pain in patients between the ages of 50 and 70 years. A history of hypertension is present in 80% to 90% of patients. The physical exam should be mindful of branch arteries from the aorta, which may be rendered ischemic by the dissection plane. End organ ischemia can present in the cardiac, visceral (i.e., mesenteric or renal), or extremity distribution. Initial diagnostic tests should include an EKG and chest radiograph, but the diagnosis of aortic dissection is made by contrast-enhanced dynamic CT. Gadolinium-enhanced MRA has also been found to be effective in most institutions but generally takes considerably longer to obtain than CT. Contrast aortography is generally reserved for individuals in whom an intervention is planned and not simply as a diagnostic modality.

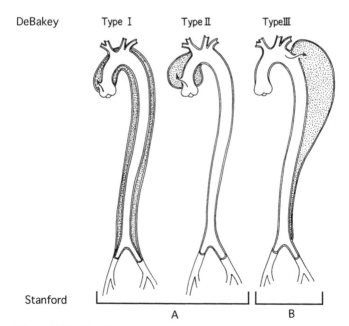

Figure 15.7. Classifications of aortic dissection.

II. Management. A critical initial step in the management of aortic dissection is to decrease the mean arterial pressure and contracting force of the heart. This is achieved foremost with intravenous beta-blockade. Sodium nitroprusside can be useful as a secondary agent but only after the patient has been started on a beta-blocker and stabilized, so as not to cause untoward vasodilation with a compensatory increase in heart rate and contractility. Nearly all patients with dissections involving the ascending aorta (DeBakey, types I and II; Stanford type A) require emergent surgery to prevent death from cardiac tamponade or aortic regurgitation with heart failure. This involves replacement of the ascending aorta and aortic valve via a median sternotomy. **DeBakey type III or Stanford type B dissections can be managed medically in the acute setting 80% of the time.** Surgery via a left thoracoabdominal approach is reserved for the 10% to 20% of patients who develop complications of the dissection over the mid and long term. **Complications from type B dissections that constitute indication for intervention include development of end organ ischemia, aortic expansion with aneurysm formation, aortic rupture, and refractory or recurrent pain.**

III. Postoperative course. Patients with Stanford A dissections have a higher likelihood of death in the first 24 to 48 hours after onset than patients with Stanford B dissections. However, the operative mortality of Stanford B dissections is higher (30% to 50%) if an operation becomes necessary due to failure of medical management. Stanford A dissections carry an operative mortality of approximately 10% to 15%. A 5-year survival of 75% to 85% exists in patients who leave the hospital alive following aortic dissection.

FEMORAL ARTERY ANEURYSM

True femoral artery aneurysms (FAAs) usually are found in male patients who have AAAs and or aneurysms of the popliteal artery. In contrast to AAAs, the natural history of femoral artery is not expansion and rupture but rather distal embolization and thrombosis, which occur in about 30% of FAAs. In these instances patients present with acute limb ischemia requiring urgent intervention. For these reasons elective surgical repair is warranted in most cases when FAAs are discovered.

I. Preoperative evaluation. Because the majority of patients with FAAs will have an associated AAA or popliteal artery aneurysm, the preoperative evaluation must include careful palpation of the abdominal aorta and popliteal arteries. Duplex ultrasound of these areas is also indicated as a more sensitive test to detect concurrent aneurysm disease. In general, contrast arteriography is indicated prior to operative intervention to define distal runoff and delineate involvement of the profunda femoris and superficial femoral arteries. In reality, similar anatomic detail may now be obtained in certain institutions with contrast-enhanced CTA or even MRA in combination with duplex ultrasound.

II. Operative principles. Three factors govern the choice of operation for common FAAs: (1) location of the origin of the profunda femoris artery, (2) patency of the superficial femoral artery, and (3) patency of the aneurysm itself.

A. In **type 1 FAAs** in which the profunda femoris orifice is distal to the aneurysm and all vessels are patent, the simplest and most successful repair is a vein or synthetic graft interposition for the resected aneurysm.

B. In **type 2 FAAs,** the profunda femoris arises from the aneurysmal sac. We cannot overemphasize the importance of **maintaining patency of the profunda femoris when such aneurysms are repaired.** In most instances, such aneurysms are resected and an interposition graft (vein or prosthetic material) is sewn to the superficial femoral artery. A small side-arm graft is then constructed to the profunda femoris artery.

C. When the superficial femoral artery is **chronically occluded,** it is ligated and an end-to-end anastomosis of the graft to the profunda femoris artery is performed.

IV. Postoperative follow-up. After FAA repair, patients should be followed annually. Duplex ultrasound is an ideal method to monitor grafts and to discover other aneurysms. Newly discovered aneurysms of the abdominal aorta or popliteal arteries should be corrected as indicated.

POPLITEAL ARTERY ANEURYSMS

Like other peripheral aneurysms, popliteal artery aneurysms have a natural history of embolization and thrombosis. In a recent study by the Mayo Clinic, 60% popliteal artery aneurysms undergoing repair presented with symptoms (39% chronic ischemia and 21% acute limb ischemia), while 40% were asymptomatic. Large popliteal artery aneurysms may also present as a pulsatile mass behind the knee, which may obstruct the popliteal vein or compress the tibial nerve. Popliteal aneurysms at greatest risk for thromboembolic events have three characteristics that guide indications for elective repair: **(1) size greater than 2 cm, (2) intraluminal thrombus on duplex, and (3) decreased pedal pulses or evidence of distal embolization indicating symptoms and compromised runoff.**

I. Preoperative evaluation. Like patients with femoral artery aneurysms, these patients must be carefully examined for other aneurysms, especially in the aortoiliac location. In the same series from Mayo, approximately 50% of patients had bilateral popliteal aneurysms, 50% had AAAs, and almost 10% had aneurysms in the thoracic or paravisceral aorta. Preoperative imaging of the extremity should define not only the location and extent of the PAA but also delineate the below-the-knee runoff. Special consideration should be given to the condition of the superficial femoral artery and the distal runoff in order to plan an effective operative approach. This information can be obtained with contrast arteriography of the extremity. However, with the increasing sensitivity of CTA and MRA in some institutions, these modalities may be combined with duplex to provide all the necessary preoperative anatomic information in some situations.

II. Operative principles. The preferred surgical treatment for popliteal artery aneurysms is the medial approach, which allows exposure of the above- and below-the-knee popliteal artery. This approach allows proximal and distal ligation of the aneurysm followed by greater saphenous vein bypass. **One should not be fooled into assuming that the distal superficial femoral artery will be a normal artery suitable as an inflow ves-**

sel. In up to two-thirds of cases, the superficial femoral artery above the knee is diseased and not suitable for inflow. Therefore, origination of the vein bypass must come from the common femoral artery in the groin in these cases.

Historically, simple ligation and bypass of the aneurysm from the medial approach has been effective in treating popliteal artery aneurysms. There is some evidence that ligation alone results in continued pressurization and even expansion of the popliteal aneurysm from patent side branches feeding into the ligated aneurysm. Some practitioners now advocate opening the aneurysm after ligation to oversew any back-bleeding vessels to eliminate this possibility. In about 15% of cases, a posterior approach to the popliteal artery aneurysm is used and is particularly useful for large aneurysms causing symptoms of compression. This approach, which is performed through a single incision with the patient prone, allows for more complete decompression of the aneurysm and popliteal space. In these cases larger aneurysms should be opened, the thrombus removed, and a portion of the sac resected to prevent compressive symptoms from the mass effect of the aneurysm.

Popliteal artery aneurysms that present with acute thrombosis and acute limb ischemia are best treated with an attempt at preoperative catheter-directed thrombolysis. If initiated early enough after the onset of symptoms, this preoperative adjunct significantly increases the chance of a successful surgical reconstruction in the ensuing 24-48 hours. Catheter-directed thrombolysis is described in Chapter 11 and involves placement of an infusion catheter (i.e., soaker hose) into the thrombosed aneurysm and administration of a thrombolytic agent such as TPA. This technique improves the infrapopliteal outflow and has decreased the limb-loss rate associated with thrombosed popliteal artery aneurysm from 30% to 10%.

Recent reports have described the endovascular treatment of popliteal artery aneurysms using a self-expanding covered stent. In fact, in select groups of patients, the short-term success of this technique appears acceptable. However, its broad application is limited by yet-to-be-defined anatomic criteria of the femoral and popliteal arteries and established long-term effectiveness. Currently, the standard treatment for popliteal artery aneurysms is open repair and the endovascular approach is reserved for select patients who are not operative candidates.

III. Postoperative follow-up. Patients treated for popliteal artery aneurysms should be reevaluated annually, not only to assess the bypass with duplex but also to check for the development of elsewhere in the arterial system.

SELECTED READING
Abdominal Aortic Aneurysm

Aneurysm Detection and Management (ADAM) Veterans Affairs Cooperative Study Group. Immediate repair compared to surveillance of small abdominal aortic aneurysms. *NEJM.* 2002;346: 1437-1444.

Armstrong PA, Back MR, Bandyk DF, et al. Optimizing compliance, efficiency and safety during surveillance of small abdominal aortic aneurysms. *J Vasc Surg.* 2007;46:190-196.

Blankensteijn JD, de Jong SE, Prinssen M, et al. (Dutch Randomized Endovascular Aneurysm Management (DREAM) Trial Group. Two-year outcomes after conventional or endovascular repair of abdominal aortic aneurysms. *NEJM*.2005;352:2398-2405.

Conrad MF, Crawford RS, Pedraza JD, et al. Long-term durability of open abdominal aortic aneurysm repair. *J Vasc Surg.* 2007;46: 669-675.

DeRubertis BG, Trocciola SM, Ryer EJ, Pieracci FM, et al. Abdominal aortic aneurysms in women: Prevalence, risk factors and implications for screening. *J Vasc Surg.* 2007;46:630-635.

Dillavou ED, Muluk SC, Makaroun MS. Improving aneurysm related outcomes: Nationwide benefits of endovascular repair. *J Vasc Surg.* 2006;43:446-452.

U.K. Small Aneurysm Trial Participants. Mortality results for randomised controlled trial of early elective surgery or ultrasonographic surveillance for small abdominal aortic aneurysms. *Lancet.* 1998;352:1649-1655.

Thoracoabdominal Aortic Aneurysm

Chuter TAM, Rapp JH, Hiramoto JS, Schneider DB, Howell B, Reilly LM. Endovascular treatment of thoracoabdominal aortic aneurysms. *J Vasc Surg.* 2008;47:6-16.

Conrad MF, Cambria RP. Contemporary management of descending thoracic and thoracoabdominal aortic aneurysms: endovascular versus open. *Circulation.* 2008;117:841-852.

Conrad MF, Crawford RS, Davison JK, Cambria RP. Thoracoabdominal aneurysm repair: A 20-year perspective. *Ann Thorac Surg.* 2007;83:S856-861.

Peripheral Artery Aneurysm

Curi MA, Geraghty PJ, Merino OA, et al. Mid-term outcomes of endovascular popliteal artery aneurysm repair. *J Vasc Surg.* 2007; 45:505-510.

Diwan A, Sarkar R, Stanley JC, et al. Incidence of femoral and popliteal artery aneurysms in patients with abdominal aortic aneurysms. *J Vasc Surg.* 2000;31:863-869.

Harbuzariu C, Duncan A, Bower TC, Kalra M, Gloviczki P. Profunda femoris artery aneurysms: association with aneurismal disease and limb ischemia. *J Vasc Surg.* 2008;47:31-35.

Huang Y, Gloviczki P, Noel AA, et al. Early complications and long-term outcome after open surgical treatment of popliteal artery aneurysms: Is exclusion with saphenous vein bypass still the gold standard? *J Vasc Surg.* 2007;45:706-715.

CHAPTER 16

Renal Artery Diseases

Vascular providers are frequently asked to comment on or manage different forms of renal artery disease with a wide range of etiology, pathophysiology, and natural history. **From renal artery aneurysms to fibromuscular dysplasia (FMD) to atherosclerotic occlusive disease, all forms of renal artery disease have two common endpoints of clinical concern; one related to blood pressure elevation and the other to deterioration of renal excretory function.** Renal artery disease either from atherosclerosis or fibromuscular dysplasia is the most common cause of secondary hypertension and is present in about 5% of the elderly population. A recent study of patients referred to a university vascular laboratory identified significant occlusive disease in nearly a quarter of patients, a finding that was more common in those receiving two or more blood pressure medications. In the context of all patients with hypertension, renovascular occlusive disease is responsible for only about 5% of cases. While this percentage seems low, the growing number of Americans with hypertension (31% of the U.S. population or 65 million individuals in 2000) makes the prevalence of this vascular disease process significant, especially in an aging population.

Tremendous gains have been made in the understanding of the natural history of renal artery disease although issues surrounding the indications for and timing of renal artery intervention (open or endovascular) remain somewhat unsettled. The topic of renal artery intervention remains a major clinical challenge in large part because of advancing technologies on all sides of the matter (diagnostic, pharmacologic, and endovascular). There is little question that renal artery occlusive disease accelerates the development of hypertension through activation of pressor systems and, if severe enough, ultimately results in ischemic damage to renal excretory function. Untreated hypertension results in end-organ damage affecting the heart, brain, peripheral vascular, and ophthalmologic systems, as well as the kidneys themselves.

Except for a subset of pediatric patients with renovascular hypertension, most patients referred to the vascular provider for evaluation of renal disease are elderly with chronic hypertension and other comorbidities such as diabetes mellitus. The benefit of an extensive anatomic workup of the renal arteries in these patients is not always clear, as antihypertensive drug therapy has been shown to be quite effective. Medications that block the renin-angiotensin system, either conventional angiotensin-converting enzyme inhibitors (ACE inhibitors) or the newer angiotensin-II receptor blockers (ARBs) have become first-line therapy. And when combined with beta-receptor blockers or calcium channel blockers these medications suffice in treating hypertension even in the presence of renal artery disease in most patients.

The challenge comes when patients require more than 2 or 3 medications to control hypertension or have deterioration of renal function or kidney size. Imaging of the renal arteries and selection of appropriate patients for renal revascularization in this group is really at the center of the clinical challenge. Unfortunately, treatment decisions in these patients are not always guided by high levels of clinical evidence, although this is an area of intense interest and clinical study. **One trial that is underway is the Cardiovascular Outcomes in Renal Atherosclerotic Lesions (CORAL) study, which randomly assigns subjects with proven, high-grade, renal artery lesions to optimal medical management with and without renal stenting.** Understanding the best role for renal artery intervention depends greatly on how such well-designed clinical trials are conducted.

This chapter aims to summarize basic principles related to renovascular hypertension and renal artery disease and reviews indications for and basic principles of the diagnostic evaluation. Indications for renal artery interventions, open and/or endovascular, are also discussed, including techniques and periprocedural care.

I. Renin-angiotensin system. To logically manage renovascular hypertension, one must review the relationship of the kidney to blood pressure control. By adjusting sodium and water retention and through the release of vasoactive factors, the kidney functions as an endocrine organ helping to maintain blood pressure through several mechanisms. A hemodynamically significant obstruction or stenosis of the renal artery or an overall decrease in blood volume decreases blood flow to the kidney. This decrement in blood flow is "viewed" by the kidney as hypovolemia or hypotension and initiates a response from that kidney that involves release of local and circulating factors. **Specifically, baroreceptors in the juxtaglomerular apparatus of the kidney detect decreases in renal blood flow and respond by releasing the enzyme renin. Renin cleaves the serum globulin angiotensin I, forming the vasoactive peptide angiotensin II, which increases renal blood flow by several mechanisms.** Angiotensin II stimulates adrenal release of aldosterone, causes systemic vasoconstriction, and exerts an antidiuretic, antinatriuretic action on the kidney (i.e., fluid or volume retention). Angiotensin II also causes vasoconstriction of the efferent arterioles of the juxtaglomerular apparatus, decreasing flow from this system and producing a subsequent rise in pressure. The result is sodium and water retention, expansion of extracellular fluid volume, and an increase in systemic blood pressure. One very effective class of medications used to treat hypertension includes several that inhibit conversion of angiotensin I to angiotensin II (ACE inhibitors) or directly block the angiotensin II receptor (ARBs).

II. Diagnostic evaluation of the renal arteries should be performed only in appropriate clinical circumstances. As was noted previously, 5-10% of patients with hypertension have some form of renal artery disease resulting in a functional renal artery stenosis. This association occurs more often in hypertensive children and young adults, who more commonly have aortic coarctation, congenital renal artery stenosis, or fibromuscular dysplasia. In this population of young individuals with significant hypertension, diagnostic evaluation of the renal arteries is warranted early in their evaluation to look for congenital abnormalities or FMD.

In contrast, elderly adults are most commonly affected by essential hypertension, and routine diagnostic evaluation of the renal arteries is not necessary early in the course of their workup. In these cases, even though at risk for atherosclerosis and renal artery disease, initiation of one or two medications along with risk factor modification is usually effective in reducing blood pressure. A thorough history and physical exam should be performed and routine lab tests, including serum creatinine and creatinine clearance, should be performed. If there is no indication from the history, physical, or lab testing that the renal arteries are involved, basic medical management (e.g., one or two medications) may be initiated without diagnostic evaluation of the renals. If this strategy, which includes risk modification and exercise, is not effective at achieving a desirable blood pressure within 3 months, diagnostic evaluation of the renal arteries should be performed.

Diagnostic tests of choice to identify and measure renal artery disease vary among institutions. However, initial evaluation should begin with noninvasive tests such as duplex ultrasound, CTA, and MRA. The vascular provider should be mindful that only duplex spares the patient from the nephrotoxic effects of contrast needed with CTA and MRA, and is therefore the preferred diagnostic test. Invasive renal artery arteriography should be performed sparingly and reserved for cases in which an intervention is planned. Alternatively, angiography is indicated for instances in which noninvasive studies are inconclusive or in disagreement, and the information regarding renal artery anatomy is imperative in clinical decision-making process.

A. Screening tests. Duplex ultrasound is the primary noninvasive test of choice in screening for renal artery disease. Renal duplex requires the patient to fast in order to reduce the amount of bowel gas interference with the study. Evaluation of the renal arteries with duplex also requires an experienced vascular technologist and about 45 to 60 minutes of time (Chapter 6). Another noninvasive option for evaluation of the renal arteries is gadolinium-enhanced **magnetic resonance angiography**. MRA has the advantage of imaging the entire aorta and branch vessels and can often provide quite remarkable images. MRA is especially useful in cases of renal artery aneurysms and FMD. However, quality of MRA is often institution-specific and some vascular specialists see MRA as overestimating the degree of renal artery occlusive disease. Furthermore, MRA is relatively expensive, and is not always tolerated by patients who may be claustrophobic. In our practice, we use MRA as a backup for renal duplex imaging that provides inconclusive or equivocal results. Similar to MRA, CTA of the renal arteries can provide exceptional images of the aorta, main renal arteries, and renal hilum. Unfortunately, the contrast necessary to achieve such imaging carries a significant nephrotoxic effect and often precludes use of this noninvasive imaging modality. We rarely use dedicated CTA to image the renal arteries in the setting of suspected renovascular hypertension and save this modality for patients with renal artery aneurysms or congenital renal abnormalities in younger patients who have normal renal function.

Two functional tests for renovascular hypertension that are currently used sparingly, are the captopril test and captopril renal scanning. The captopril test involves oral administration of captopril, an ACE inhibitor, after baseline measurement of plasma renin activity and blood pressure. Renovascular hypertension should be suspected when the post-captopril plasma renin level is excessively high. Some older studies indicate that the sensitivity of this test approaches 100%, with a specificity of 90%. However, the test is less accurate in the presence of renal insufficiency. Criteria for a positive captopril renal scan include a reduction in glomerular filtration rate and a delay in the time to peak clearing of the radionuclide.

B. Arteriography carries the nephrotoxic risk of contrast material and should be performed only when an intervention is planned or when noninvasive studies are inconclusive or in disagreement and information regarding renal artery anatomy is imperative in clinical decision making. The more selective use of renal arteriography is an advance in the management of this vascular condition and is a testament to improvements in noninvasive vascular imaging (e.g. duplex and MRA) and an improved understanding of which patients benefit from renal intervention.

When performed, renal arteriography should include (a) an abdominal aortogram, (b) selective renal artery injections in different planes, and (c) a celiac artery injection with a lateral view if the splenic or hepatic arteries are being considered for open splenorenal or hepatorenal bypass. The amount of contrast should be minimized in all patients with suspected renovascular disease, and imaging adjuncts such as CO_2 aortography and intravascular ultrasound (IVUS) often aid in this objective.

C. Renal vein renin determination is mentioned mostly as a historical note as few vascular specialists continue to use this test in day-to-day practice. Renal vein renin determination has fallen out of favor because of its invasive nature, technical requirements, and often nonspecific findings. The concept behind renal vein renin measurements is as follows: The presence of a renal artery stenosis on an imaging test does not establish its functional importance (e.g., whether it is causing renin release and hypertension). To explore this question, a comparison of renin from venous samples taken from each renal vein and the inferior vena cava above and below the renal veins provides insight into the significance of a renal artery stenosis. Since a kidney that is truly ischemic will produce increased amounts of renin, a renal vein ratio of at least 1.5:1.0 should be present if the renal artery stenosis is significant.

Different aspects of renin determinations complicate the ability to achieve meaningful results. Antihypertensive medications such as beta-blockers, which suppress renin secretion as well as variations in sodium intake, affect renal vein renin assay and often result in nonlateralization of renal vein renins (i.e., an indeterminate finding). One way to stimulate a difference in renal vein renins is captopril administration after baseline renins are collected. Renin levels are again collected 30 minutes after captopril and a post-captopril renal venous ratio of 3 increases the sensitivity of the test. Despite the past value of renal vein renins, their use in everyday clinical practice has diminished in recent years.

III. Indications for invasive intervention. Because of the effectiveness of medical management of renal artery disease and the absence of clear benefit in treating certain renal artery disease, the indications for intervention, open or endovascular, have been highly scrutinized. The bottom line is that not all renal artery abnormalities, blockages or otherwise, need to be treated with a procedure. In fact it is probably the minority, and any planned intervention, open or endovascular, should be well thought out.

A. Renovascular hypertension that is refractory to medical treatment is the most common indication for intervention. In our practices we stress the fact that patients with renovascular hypertension need intensive blood pressure control and cardiovascular risk management (Chapters 7 and 8) before and after any intervention. **Such management requires close attention and follow-up after intervention to assess for clinical and technical adequacy (i.e., whether the blood pressure improved and the revascularization is patent).** In most cases the patient is best served by a multidisciplinary team, which may include vascular and hypertensive specialists and nephrologists.

Success of renal artery revascularization for hypertension depends on the etiology of the disease and the age of the patient. The best results, open or endovascular, have been reported in younger patients (<50 years old) with fibromuscular dysplasia or focal atherosclerotic lesions and preserved renal function. Additionally, renovascular hypertension caused by bilateral disease often responds more dramatically with a better long-term result than patients with unilateral disease. Long-term cure of hypertension occurs in only about 10% of patients while around 70% of patients will have an improvement in their blood pressure as defined by the need for fewer antihypertensive medications. **In contrast, older patients with chronic hypertension and diabetes, both of which damage the renal parenchyma over time (e.g., hypertensive nephropathy and diabetic nephropathy), have less convincing improvements.**

In most cases today the initial treatment modality is endovascular angioplasty with or without stent placement. The most favorable renal disease treated with endovascular means is FMD of the renal artery. In this setting percutaneous transluminal balloon angioplasty is technically successful in more than 95% of cases and provides a very durable treatment. In cases of FMD, angioplasty without stent placement is preferred and may even provide satisfactory treatment in patients where the FMD extends into the first order renal artery branches. The endovascular approach to renovascular hypertension caused by atherosclerotic occlusive disease includes placement of balloon expandable stents in nearly all cases. Because much of this disease is felt to originate in the lumen of the aorta, care is taken to overlap the stent into the aorta slightly to account for and adequately treat this disease.

B. Preservation of renal function through renal artery surgery or angioplasty has also received considerable attention and clinical studies using both methods have been reported. **The trick is to identify the patients who are most likely to benefit from invasive therapy to preserve renal function and then to perform the therapy without causing a decrement in renal performance.** Certainly, consideration should be given to patients with bilateral high-grade renal stenoses or a severe stenosis of a solitary functioning kidney (e.g., prior nephrectomy or nonfunctioning contralateral kidney).

Recent studies have pointed out the utility of measuring and following renal size over time with duplex as an indicator of renal deterioration. The normal size of the adult kidney, measured as the length from the superior to the inferior pole, is 10 to 14 cm. Kidney lengths are usually an average of 3 or 4 measurements to account for slightly oblique and therefore less accurate views. Renal size of less than 10 cm suggests atrophy and should be investigated with additional studies (e.g., serum creatinine, creatinine clearance, MRI/ MRA). Furthermore, a decrement in size of more than 1-2 cm over a 2-year period indicates significant loss of renal parenchyma and should also be further evaluated.

Renal resistive index (RRI) measured by duplex has been advocated by some as an indicator of intrinsic or perenchymal renal function, independent of large vessel renal disease. As such, RRI has been shown in some studies to identify patients who may respond favorably to large vessel revascularization, open or endovascular. The formula for RRI is as follows: RRI =Peak systolic velocity – End diastolic velocity / Peak systolic velocity. The normal RRI is 0.6 to 0.7 and an index of >0.8 is highly resistive which suggests significant intrinsic renal disease often from chronic hypertension or diabetes. In cases of high resistive indices (i.e., RRI >0.8), large-vessel reconstruction is unlikely to improve renal function as the workings of the kidney parenchyma are fundamentally lost. Conversely, those with a lower renal-resistive index have preserved intrinsic renal function that may improve following treatment of main renal artery occlusive disease. Although appealing as a noninvasive indicator of those who may respond to renal angioplasty or open revascularization, RRI has not borne out to be useful in all clinical studies.

In a recent study of patients with renovascular disease who were treated with either medical management or angioplasty and stenting, stenting was found to provide midterm improvement in blood pressure control. The benefit in blood pressure control in this particular study was not sustained in the long term however; renal stenting was found to slow the rate of decline in renal dysfunction. The results of this study are indicative of others, namely that there is a real benefit to revascularization for preservation of renal function in a subgroup of patients with renal artery occlusive disease. Five clinical factors that should be considered prior to renal revascularization and are associated with success (e.g., preservation of renal function) are:

1. Nondiabetic patients
2. Bilateral severe stenoses
3. Renal size >9.5 cm
4. RRI <0.8
5. Serum creatinine <2.5 mg/dl

C. Surgical correction of aneurysm or occlusive disease of the aorta may necessitate preservation of a main or accessory renal artery. Accessory renal arteries <3 mm in size can usually be ligated without significant loss of renal function, while larger accessory arteries should be preserved. Maintaining patency of accessory renal arteries may require reimplantation or bypass during open aortic surgery or modification of endovascular techniques to avoid covering the arteries of interest.

D. Other renal artery problems requiring renal artery reconstruction include renal artery aneurysms or renal artery trauma, which can result in dissection, aneurysm, or arteriovenous fistula. Renal artery aneurysms >2 cm in largest diameter should be repaired when discovered, as they are thought to cause hypertension, distal embolization, and/or thrombosis. CTA is the study of choice to characterize renal artery aneurysms and injuries. Rupture of a renal artery aneurysm is thought to be more likely during pregnancy, so women of childbearing age with aneurysms should be considered with a lower threshold for elective repair. Embolism to the renal artery presents with acute flank pain and often hematuria. Renal arteriovenous fistulas are difficult surgical problems, especially when they are in the renal parenchyma and should be treated with endovascular techniques (e.g., coil embolization or small covered stent) depending upon location. Intrarenal arteriovenous fistulas may also be treated with endovascular coil embolization.

IV. Surgical options. Improvement of blood pressure and preservation of renal function are the primary goals of any operation on the renal arteries. Nephrectomy is done only when no other method of saving a good kidney appears possible and that kidney appears to be responsible for significant hypertension (i.e., a **pressor kidney**). **Open renal artery reconstruction falls into two categories, bypass and endarterectomy**. A variety of autogenous and synthetic graft materials are available for renal artery bypass procedures, while endarterectomy has the advantage of not requiring a bypass conduit. Figures 16.1 and 16.2 illustrate preferred methods of renal artery revascularization. Autogenous grafts, such as those of saphenous vein are preferable to synthetic materials. Factors that generally increase the risk of operative morbidity and mortality are elevated baseline creatinine levels (>3 mg/dL), increased age, and associated cardiac dysfunction. Operative mortality from open renal artery revascularization is between 3-5%.

A large contemporary series of open renal artery reconstruction at Wake Forest University showed that a majority of patients undergo bilateral renal artery repair and nearly half (41%) have renal reconstruction as part of an open aortic repair for either aneurysm or occlusive disease. The indication for treatment in this series was renovascular hypertension and 85% of patients had hypertension cured or improved with an overall improvement in renal function in this select group. In a second

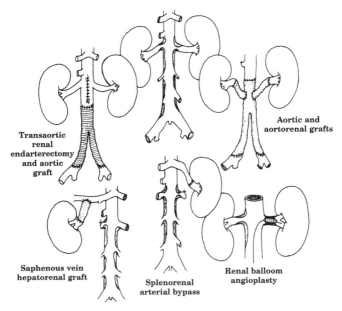

Figure 16.1. Options for renal revascularization for atherosclerotic disease.

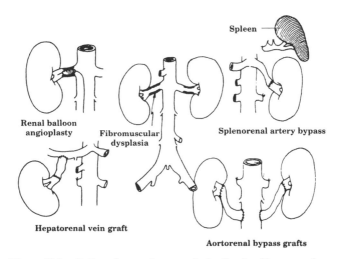

Figure 16.2. Options for renal revascularization for fibromuscular disease.

more recent study from Massachusetts General Hospital, which examined open renal artery reconstruction for preservation of renal function, the operative approach was as follows: aortorenal bypass (38%), extra-anatomic bypass (e.g., hepatorenal or splenorenal bypass) (38%), and endarterectomy (24%). Similar to the Wake Forest report 32% underwent combined aortic and renal reconstruction. Long-term preservation of renal function was noted in 70% of patients with improved results in patients with lower baseline creatinine levels (<3.2 mg/dL) and those undergoing bilateral repair.

V. Preoperative preparation. Before renal artery revascularization, blood pressure and renal function must be stabilized as much as possible.

A. Blood pressure. Most of these patients have significant hypertension, which increases the risk of myocardial and cerebrovascular events. As was stressed earlier, solid treatment and control of hypertension before and after the revascularization is a central tenant of success. One consideration is to reduce or stop diuretic therapy 24 to 48 hours prior to the operation so that chronically contracted intravascular volume can be corrected slowly. Beta-blockers should not be abruptly stopped since discontinuation may result in tachycardia and myocardial ischemia.

B. Renal function. About one-third of patients undergoing renovascular surgery have chronic renal insufficiency (creatinine >2 mg/dL) and several factors can cause deterioration in their creatinine clearance prior to hospitalization and during preoperative evaluation.

> **1.** Vigorous diuretic therapy can cause intravascular volume contraction and prerenal azotemia (i.e., elevation of serum creatinine).
>
> **2. ACE inhibitors or ARB therapy disturbs renal blood flow autoregulation by decreasing efferent arteriolar resistance, which is needed to provide a perfusion gradient to the glomerulus.** In theory, use of these medications in those who also have inflow stenosis to the kidney (e.g., renal artery stenosis) can worsen serum creatinine. It turns out that only a small percentage of patients with renovascular disease do not tolerate ACE inhibitors or ARBs. Starting an ACE inhibitor or an ARB must be done cautiously in all patients and should include checks of blood pressure and serum creatinine, but a minority of patients will not tolerate the therapy. **The solid level of clinical evidence for the benefit of ACE inhibitors in reducing overall cardiovascular morbidity and mortality outweighs the limited risk of renal dysfunction.** In those who manifest renal dysfunction with initiation of therapy, the ACE inhibitor should be stopped and the creatinine will return to baseline in 7 days.
>
> **3.** Another frequent cause for an acute rise in serum creatinine is **contrast nephropathy related to arteriography or CT angiography.** The vascular provider must be mindful when ordering and performing imaging studies. Fortunately, with hydration and observation, most episodes of contrast nephropathy will resolve over several weeks.

Renal revascularization should be delayed until creatinine levels return to baseline following such an event.

VI. Open operative principles.

A. Incisions. Proper operative exposure is one of the most important aspects of renal artery surgery. A midline xiphoid-to-pubic bone incision provides good access to both renal arteries. An upper transverse or subcostal incision may be used but does not provide good exposure of the distal aorta or iliac system. A left splenorenal arterial anastomosis can be constructed through a low, left thoracoabdominal incision (bed of the tenth rib) or a left subcostal incision.

B. Proximal renal lesions. For central lesions, the midline retroperitoneum is opened over the aorta. On the left side, the renal vein can be mobilized by ligation and division of the **adrenal, gonadal, and left renolumbar branches of the left renal vein.** On the right side, the vena cava must be mobilized and retracted to expose the proximal right renal artery.

C. Middle or distal lesions. For middle or distal lesions on the right side, the duodenum must be reflected by a Kocher maneuver to expose the distal right renal artery. On the left side, the splenic flexure of the colon can be mobilized in a similar fashion.

D. Renal protection. Several steps can be taken to reduce the effect of transient ischemia and then reperfusion on the kidney(s).

1. Intravenous hydration with a balanced salt solution (e.g., Ringer's lactated solution, 100 to 125 mL/h) is started several hours before surgery.

2. Heparin (5,000 units) is given intravenously before clamping the renal artery.

3. Mannitol (12.5 to 25.0 g) is administered early in the procedure. If a good diuresis is not achieved with mannitol then intravenous furosemide may be used.

4. The kidney may also be cooled with 200 to 300 mL of a renal perfusate if anticipated renal ischemic time is greater than 45 minutes. We use a combination of 1 L of Ringer's lactated solution, 18 g mannitol, 20 mg heparin, and 500 mg methylprednisolone chilled to 3°C in saline slush.

5. Low-dose (2 to 3 μg/kg/min) dopamine causes renal vasodilatation, which may help minimize vasomotor nephropathy. We start dopamine intravenously in the operating room before renal artery clamping and continue it for at least 12 to 24 hours following the reconstruction.

E. Type of anastomosis. The proximal anastomosis is constructed first. Then, the distal anastomosis is made end-to-end by the spatulation technique. The suture material is usually 6-0 or 7-0 polypropylene. For a particularly difficult anastomosis, the suture line is interrupted. Low-power magnifying loops and a high-intensity headlight are essential in most renal artery reconstructions.

F. Intraoperative assessment of graft patency. The simplest method to ascertain blood flow is the examination of the graft or renal artery with a sterile continuous-wave Doppler. Biphasic signals should be present. Intraoperative duplex ultrasound has proven to be a quick and reliable method for detecting technical problems after renal artery grafting or

endarterectomy. Significant problems are detected in about
10% of reconstructed arteries and most of these are correctable and result in outcomes that are similar to those of
patients with normal intraoperative ultrasound studies.

VII. Postoperative care. In the immediate postoperative
period, intravascular volume must be carefully maintained to
ensure adequate urine output. It may require use of a Swan–
Ganz pulmonary artery catheter for a brief period of time to
monitor filling pressures to ensure adequate volume repletion.
Low-dose dopamine is continued for renal vasodilation, and
dobutamine is administered to patients with marginal cardiac
output (<3 L/m^2). Generally, we strive to maintain a urine output of 1 mL/kg/h. Some patients have a massive or hyper diuresis (>200 mL/h) and require urinary replacement (0.5 mL of
crystalloid per milliliter of urine) for 12 to 24 hours to avoid volume depletion. Diuretics are usually not necessary and should
be avoided in the first 24 hours. When a question arises about
the early patency of the reconstruction, we obtain a renal duplex
ultrasound, which can also be obtained prior to discharging the
patient from the hospital. Any subsequent recurrence of hypertension or deterioration of renal function requires a repeat ultrasound and/or angiographic study. Percutaneous transluminal
angioplasty may be performed on an anastomotic stenosis in an
attempt to salvage a failing graft. Open reoperation of a stenotic
or thrombosed renal graft can achieve a successful result in only
about 50% of patients.

**VIII. Renal balloon angioplasty and stenting is the initial
choice for renal intervention except in cases in which
open aortic surgery is necessary.** Because of its minimally
invasive nature and associated low morbidity and mortality the
endovascular approach to renal artery disease has increased.
Physicians who treat hypertension and renal insufficiency must
be informed about this technique and understand which patients
are optimal candidates for intervention. **As a vascular specialist, one should embrace the premise that just because
renal artery stenting can be performed does not mean
that it *should* be performed.**

Typically, endovascular renal artery intervention is accomplished through a transfemoral approach using only a 6 French
sheath (Chapter 11). Selection of the renal artery is facilitated
by preshaped guide catheters, such as the renal double curve
(RDC) or the Cobra I or II (CI or CII). Once the renal artery has
been identified, selection of the orifice can be accomplished using
a 0.035-inch hydrophilic wire and 4 or 5 Fr catheter or in some
cases simply a 0.014-inch wire with a distal embolic protection
device (Chapter 11). Renal interventions over a wire with distal
embolic protection have been shown in some small series to
reduce the damaging effects of distal embolization from the atherosclerotic lesion into the kidney parenchyma. Although not
clearly shown as beneficial, intervention with distal embolic protection represents a technological development that, as is the
case with smaller profile devices and newer generations of
stents, has advanced this therapy. Most atherosclerotic renal
artery lesions are treated with a premounted, balloon expandable stent on a 0.014-inch over-the-wire delivery system. IVUS is
also used as an adjunct to evaluate renal stenosis and renal

artery diameter in some cases. Use of IVUS may in certain situations minimize use of contrast material by evaluating the post-stent position and expansion, eliminating the need for completion arteriography.

Despite advancements in the technical approach to renal artery occlusive disease, not all renal artery lesions should be treated. There is a complication rate associated with balloon angioplasty and stenting (1-2%) and in certain patient populations a lack of evidence supporting long-term benefit. **Given the increased enthusiasm and financial incentives to treat renal stenoses, the onus is on the vascular specialist to ensure that good patient selection occurs and that only appropriate patients are treated.** Additionally, the vascular specialist will be tasked with performing further clinical study to better characterize patients who benefit from angioplasty and stenting versus those better served with maximal medical treatment and risk-factor reduction.

SELECTED READING

Arthurs Z, Starnes B, Cuadrado D, Sohn V, Cushner H, Andersen C. Renal artery stenting slows the rate of renal function decline. *J Vasc Surg.* 2007;45:726-31.

Balk E, Raman G, Chung M, et al. Effectiveness of management strategies for renal artery stenosis: a systematic review. *Ann Intern Med.* 2006;145:901-912.

Cherr GS, Hansen KJ, Craven TE, et al. Surgical management of atherosclerotic renovascular disease. *J Vasc Surg.* 2002;35:236-245.

Garovic V, Textor SC. Renovascular hypertension: current concepts. *Semin Nephrol.* 2005;25:261-271.

Hansen KJ, Edwards MS, Craven TE, et al. Prevalence of renovascular disease in the elderly: A population-based study. *J Vasc Surg.* 2002;36:443-451.

Labropoulos N, Ayuste B, Leon LR. Renovascular disease among patients referred for renal duplex ultrasonography. *J Vasc Surg.* 2007;46:731-737.

Marone LK, Clouse WD, Dorer DJ, et al. Preservation of renal function with surgical revascularization in patients with atherosclerotic renovascular disease. *J Vasc Surg.* 2004;39:322-329.

Pearce JD, Craven BL, Craven TE, et al. Progression of atherosclerotic renovascular disease: A prospective population-based study. *J Vasc Surg.* 2006;44:955-963.

Stanley JC, Criado E, Upchurch GR, Jr., Brophy PD, Cho KJ, Rectenwald JE. Pediatric renovascular hypertension: 132 primary and 30 secondary operations in 97 children. *J Vasc Surg.* 2006;44:1219-1229.

Tagle R, Acevedo M, Xu M, Pohl M, Vidt D. Use of endovascular stents in atherosclerotic renovascular stenosis: blood pressure and renal function changes in hypertensive patients. *J Clin Hypertens.* 2007;9:608-614.

Textor SC. Renovascular hypertension in 2007: where are we now? *Curr Cardiol Rep.* 2007;9:453-461.

Van Jaarsveld BC, Krijnen P, Pieterman H, et al. The effect of balloon angioplasty on hypertension in atheroclrotic renal-artery stenosis. *NEJM.* 2000;342:1007-1114.

CHAPTER 17

Mesenteric Ischemic Syndromes

Intestinal ischemia comprises a small portion of all peripheral vascular problems. Although aortic atherosclerosis may involve the origins of the mesenteric arteries, intestinal collateral blood flow usually is adequate enough to prevent symptomatic, chronic intestinal ischemia. Likewise, arterial emboli can obstruct mesenteric arteries, but more commonly they flow by the visceral vessels and lodge in the leg arteries. Consequently, these anatomic and hemodynamic features make intestinal ischemia less common than chronic claudication or acute ischemia of the lower extremities.

For several reasons, acute or chronic intestinal ischemia remains one of the most challenging problems of peripheral vascular surgery. Diagnosis is frequently entertained based upon clinical suspicion or a lack of other clear etiology for the patient's problems. It is not unusual for someone who has complained of nonspecific abdominal pain to have had a detailed evaluation of their gastrointestinal tract, and yet be referred for consideration of arterial insufficiency very late in their course. Failure to recognize that a patient has some form of intestinal ischemia is one of the main reasons for poor results obtained with intervention. Patients often are operated on too late to salvage the ischemic intestine or, many times, to save the patient's life. Even when intestinal ischemia is recognized and treated expeditiously, many patients still succumb because of serious underlying medical problems. The best surgical results have been achieved in patients with chronic intestinal angina who undergo intestinal revascularization before severe weight loss or acute thrombosis occurs.

In this chapter, we emphasize early recognition of intestinal ischemia. **Delay in diagnosis represents one of the primary failings in the care of these patients.** Also, we highlight features of treatment and some of the decision making needed in the proper care of these patients.

MESENTERIC ARTERY ANATOMY

Certain anatomic features of the mesenteric circulation determine symptoms and influence management of intestinal ischemia (Fig. 17.1). The celiac axis supplies the foregut, the superior mesenteric artery (SMA) the midgut, and the inferior mesenteric artery (IMA) the hindgut. Although the three major mesenteric arteries supply specific territories, they normally intercommunicate by excellent collateral channels. These collaterals enlarge when a proximal mesenteric artery is stenotic or occluded. The primary collateral pathways between the celiac and superior mesenteric arteries are via the gastroduodenal artery to the pancreaticoduodenal arcade that connects with the superior mesenteric artery. The inferior mesenteric artery has two main sources of collateral flow when it is obstructed

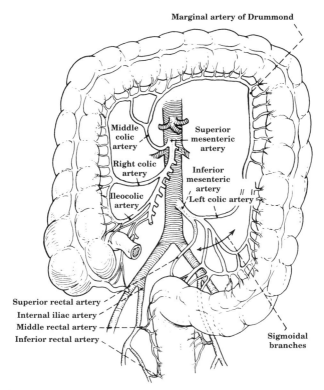

Figure 17.1.   Anatomy of the colonic arterial supply. When the inferior mesenteric artery is diseased or occluded by atherosclerosis, viability of the left colon may depend on collateral flow from the superior mesenteric artery via the marginal artery of Drummond.

(Fig. 17.2). The middle colic branch of the superior mesenteric artery connects around the transverse colon to the marginal artery of Drummond, a continuation of the left colic branch of the inferior mesenteric artery. In some instances a more direct connection in the left mesocolon develops more centrally from the marginal artery. This is known as the Arc of Riolan, or meandering mesenteric artery (Fig. 17.3). The inferior mesenteric artery also receives collateral flow via the middle hemorrhoidal artery, a branch of the internal iliac artery. These abundant collateral channels for mesenteric circulation explain the clinical observation that **intestinal angina usually does not occur until at least two of the three main mesenteric arteries have severe occlusive disease.**

CLINICAL PRESENTATION

Intestinal ischemia is classified as either chronic or acute. However, the presentations may overlap, since chronic intesti-

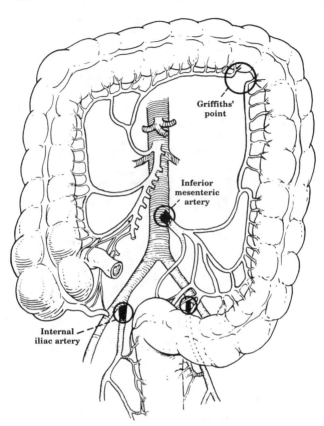

Figure 17.2.   Critical arterial inflow points for the left colon. If occlusive disease or operative reconstruction obliterates flow through both internal iliac arteries and the inferior mesenteric artery, the colon may become severely ischemic. Colonic ischemia is more than likely in this situation if the superior mesenteric-inferior mesenteric-collateral connections are not developed or injured at Griffiths' point.

nal stenosis can progress to acute thrombosis and intestinal infarction.

I. Chronic mesenteric ischemia (CMI) often eludes early diagnosis because the chronic abdominal pain is attributed to some other GI disorder. Frequently, the patient has undergone a negative diagnostic evaluation of the gallbladder, liver, and entire GI tract with CT, contrast swallows and enemas, and upper and lower endoscopies. Because of progressive weight loss, some patients are mistakenly thought to have cancer. Certain clinical features, however, should raise suspicion of chronic intestinal ischemia. Characteristic symptoms are abdominal pain and significant weight loss.

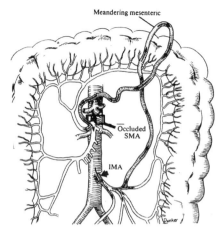

Figure 17.3. Direct connection in the mesocolon between SMA and IMA separate from the marginal artery of Drummond. When developed for purposes of collateral flow this is known as the Arc of Riolan or the meandering mesenteric artery. SMA, superior mesenteric artery; IMA, inferior mesenteric artery.

A. Classically, the **chronic abdominal pain** is intermittent and postprandial. It usually is localized to the epigastrium and has a dull ache, crampy, or colicky quality that begins 30 to 60 minutes after eating and may persist for a few hours. Patients may have associated abdominal bloating or diarrhea.

B. Involuntary weight loss eventually occurs because the patient associates eating with pain. Consequently, a "food fear" develops. While actually avoiding food altogether is rare, oral intake often is modified until liquids become the primary nutrient.

C. Physical findings of chronic intestinal ischemia are limited primarily to **weight loss** and an **abdominal bruit**, which is present in over half of individuals. Since the weight loss usually is insidious over several months and many patients with atherosclerosis have abdominal bruits, the significance of these nonspecific findings often is overlooked when the patient initially presents.

D. Chronic intestinal ischemia should be suspected in any adult who has chronic abdominal pain, progressive weight loss, other signs of generalized cardiovascular disease, and a negative workup for more common GI disorders. Some 70% of patients with CMI have been diagnosed with peripheral vascular disease in other territories. They are usually younger than standard aneurysmal or occlusive disease patients (midsixties), are smokers, and over half are women. These features collectively should lead to the following simple questions of patients suspected of having peripheral vascular disease: (1) Do you have abdominal pain after meals? (2) Have you experienced significant weight loss in the past one or two months?

II. Acute mesenteric ischemia (AMI) has three main etiologies: thrombosis of an arterial stenosis, embolism, and nonocclusive small-vessel insufficiency. Very rarely, venous mesenteric thrombosis may occur. Although the initial symptom for all these etiologies is abdominal pain, the clinical setting often suggests the most likely underlying cause. The frequency of each etiology may vary among medical centers, but generally acute intestinal ischemia is caused by thrombosis in 40% of cases, embolism in another 40%, and intestinal hypoperfusion in 20% of cases.

  A. Severe generalized abdominal pain that is disproportionate to the physical findings remains the classic presentation of acute intestinal ischemia. Nausea, vomiting, or diarrhea may follow shortly after the onset of symptoms and are very common. Although the abdomen may have diffuse tenderness, bowel sounds may be heard and peritoneal signs usually are absent. The only early laboratory abnormality may be a mildly elevated white blood cell count. With these findings the clinician must entertain the possibility of AMI and undertake steps to alleviate it. Aggressive radiologic and surgical intervention at this point can salvage the ischemic intestine in about 50% of such patients.

  Significant leukocytosis and acidosis with elevated serum lactic acid are late findings and herald a more protracted ischemic course. If intestinal ischemia remains unrecognized, physical findings will change as intestinal necrosis develops. Bloody diarrhea may occur, although often it is not present. Hypovolemia becomes evident as fluids are sequestered in the ischemic intestinal wall and surrounding tissues. Fever, peritoneal signs, and shock occur as sepsis becomes established. When intestinal ischemia has advanced to this point, the likelihood of salvaging the ischemic intestine of the critically ill patient is less than 15% to 20%.

  B. The **clinical setting** and the patient's past medical history usually suggest the probable etiology of acute mesenteric ischemia. If chronic intestinal angina preceded acute symptoms, thrombosis of a mesenteric artery stenosis is the most likely etiology. Emboli should be suspected when atrial fibrillation is present or if the patient has had previous cerebral or lower-extremity thromboembolism. Nonocclusive mesenteric ischemia (NOMI) occurs in the setting of low cardiac output. The most common predisposing conditions for nonocclusive, mesenteric ischemia are myocardial infarction, congestive heart failure, renal or hepatic disease, hemodialysis, certain drugs, classically digitalis and diuretics, or any major operation that leads to hypovolemia or hypotension in a patient with atherosclerosis. This type of nonocclusive, acute mesenteric ischemia is being recognized more commonly.

DIAGNOSTIC TESTS

When acute or chronic intestinal ischemia is suspected, the most reliable diagnostic method is arteriography. This remains the gold standard. **Early angiographic diagnosis is the most important principle of successful management of acute intestinal ischemia.** An arteriogram with lateral views of the aorta to show the mesenteric artery origins is the definitive method. The angiographic catheter also has become an important route for delivering vasodilating drugs and thrombolytic agents to the mesenteric circulation by selective mesenteric artery catheterization. Today, arteriography may also facilitate percutaneous treatment by angioplasty and stenting.

The evaluation of possible chronic mesenteric ischemia usually includes other diagnostic tests before angiography is done—commonly endoscopy or barium studies of the upper and lower GI tract. Abdominal ultrasound and CT scanning may also reveal hepatobiliary disease or occult tumors such as cancer of the pancreas or lymphoma of the retroperitoneum. With newer multichannel, multislice, CT, this may also serve as a screening tool for significant visceral segment atherosclerosis and visceral arterial stenosis. The same can be said of contrast-enhanced MRA, however, this technology tends to overcall the degree of narrowing.

Duplex scanning is a very accurate and helpful noninvasive method of interrogating mesenteric blood flow patterns. It allows for noninvasive determination of stenoses and changes in flow before and after a test meal. Similar to other arteries, velocity and waveform parameters are used to discriminate between normal subjects and those with visceral artery stenosis. General findings on fasting examination suggesting ≥70% stenosis include: **Celiac PSV >200cm/s, EDV >55 cm/s, reversed hepatic/splenic arterial flow; SMA PSV >275cm/s, EDV >45 cm/s**. While the absolute criteria may vary between vascular laboratories and the usefulness and sensitivity of postprandial testing is controversial, there is no doubt this examination, performed by experienced technicians, is an invaluable tool. The extent of diagnostic workup for patients presenting with chronic abdominal pain obviously must be individualized, yet recent advances in CTA, MRA, and duplex scanning has provided a relatively quick, easy, and effective way to discriminate those who should have arteriography.

MANAGEMENT

Treatment for mesenteric ischemia also can be organized into the two broad categories of chronic and acute ischemia.

I. Chronic mesenteric ischemia can be relieved only by correction of the occlusive lesions. There is no effective medical therapy. Surgical correction has been the most common technique, although balloon angioplasty and stenting has also been successful.

A. One aspect of perioperative care, **nutritional repletion,** deserves special emphasis. Since chronic mesenteric ischemia leads to progressive weight loss, some patients are chronically malnourished and have no nutritional reserves for a major abdominal operation. In general, one should not delay mesenteric artery surgery for prolonged nutritional repletion but proceed expeditiously to intestinal revascularization before the patient with progressive chronic ischemia suffers an acute catastrophic bowel infarction. We strongly recommend that such catabolic patients receive parenteral nutrition before and after elective surgery. It is not uncommon for these patients to have atrophied bowel mucosa due to the chronic ischemia.

Even after revascularization, adaptation may take several days to weeks. Nausea, vomiting, and colicky pain may be precipitated by full early feeding. Parenteral nutrition with early, slow enteral feedings are essential. Enteral feeding may most easily be accomplished postoperatively with naso-enteric tubes as the patient recuperates. Trophic level feeds should be instituted at 10-20 cc/hour with a very slow advancement to a full nutritional goal.

B. There are two basic surgical options for mesenteric revascularization: bypass grafting or endarterectomy. Over the years, different authors have preferred one technique over the other. Either supraceliac (antegrade) or infrarenal (retrograde) aortomesenteric bypass grafting is the procedure of choice for most patients (Fig. 17.4). The direct retrograde configuration has been hindered with the problem of graft kinking and, therefore, a lazier c-loop graft of reinforced prosthetic should be used. The optimum method of mesenteric revascularization, however, highly depends on the number of vessels occluded and the condition of the abdominal aorta in each patient. Indeed, the optimal number of vessels to be revascularized is controversial. Some centers espouse single vessel (SMA) and others multiple vessel (usually SMA and celiac) reconstruction. Transaortic endarterectomy has also been successful for multiple, focal visceral occlusive lesions at the origins of the mesenteric arteries. Tailoring orificial endarterectomy of the celiac axis, with a smaller prosthetic graft acting as a celiac patch that is distally anastomosed to the SMA, has the benefit of a smaller graft profile and minimal supraceliac aortic manipulation or sewing. Combined infrarenal aortic replacement with retrograde prosthetic bypasses to mesenteric arteries appears to be the technique of choice when either severe aortic occlusive or aneurysmal disease coexists with chronic mesenteric ischemia. However, combining mesenteric revascularization and aortic replacement carries a high mortality rate (10% to 20%) in these cachectic patients. In contrast, limiting the operation to some type of aortomesenteric grafting or endarterectomy alone minimizes mortality (3% to 10%).

Regardless of which method of revascularization is selected, early relief of intestinal angina is achieved in over 90% of patients. Graft patencies reveal primary rates of 60-80% with primary-assisted 5-year patencies of over 90%. Symptom recurrence occurs in roughly 10-20% over the 3 to 5 years following operation. Late survival in this patient subgroup burdened with atherosclerosis is 60-75% at 5 years. In general, we believe the best long-term results have been obtained by revascularization of at least two occluded or stenotic vessels. Yet others believe this to come at a cost of extra morbidity and mortality owing to the more significant dissection, fluid loss, and operative time. Since revascularization of a single mesenteric occlusion often offers relief to most patients, complete revascularization must be weighed against the patient's overall condition, prognosis, and other technical factors.

Chronic or acute intestinal ischemia also may be the result of sacrificing the IMA at the time of infrarenal aortic grafting.

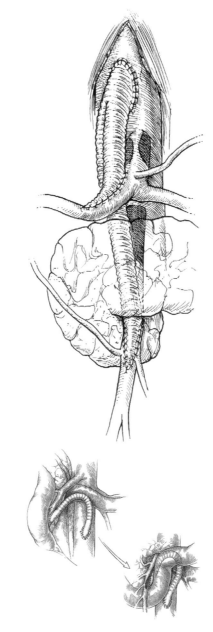

(A)

(B)

Figure 17.4.   **(A)** Antegrade two-vessel aortomesenteric bypass.
(B) Retrograde c-loop reinforced ePTFE single-vessel aortomesenteric bypass.

Revascularization of the IMA should be performed when the SMA is occluded and a large (>3.5 to 4.0 mm) IMA is present. Also, if the IMA shows poor back bleeding at the time of aortic reconstruction, or an IMA pressure is transduced at <40 mm Hg, strong consideration should be given to IMA reimplantation.

Another less common form of CMI is **median arcuate ligament syndrome**, whereby this structure compresses and creates a functional stenosis of the celiac axis. Over time this can injure the artery, leading to an accompanying atherosclerotic lesion. Some extrinsic compression of the celiac axis by the median arcuate ligament is common, particularly in women, but most experts question its functional importance. Certainly, a celiac stenosis may be critical when occlusive disease of the superior mesenteric and inferior mesenteric arteries is present also. Division of the median arcuate ligament with either patch angioplasty of the celiac stenosis or an interposition graft may alleviate symptoms. Another interesting circumstance in which a single stenosis may lead to CMI symptoms is when either a celiac or SMA stenosis occurs after pancreatic resection or complex hepatobiliary surgery in which the pancreaticoduodenal arcade is disrupted.

Recent interest in endovascular therapies has provided less invasive alternatives for the treatment of CMI. Over the last decade, percutaneous angioplasty and stenting have been employed in the mesenteric vessels with varying success. Typically these are found in small, institutional experiences, as this disease process is rare. Several surrounding caveats can currently be addressed. As opposed to other arterial beds, the benefit of reduced morbidity and mortality with endovascular means does not seem to be as pronounced. Although early improvement of CMI symptoms appears equivalent to that of open operation when using percutaneous methods, there are suggestions that midterm symptomatic recurrence and recurrent stenoses are more common with this less invasive option. At this point it is practical to consider endovascular therapy as a potential alternative, particularly in those with comorbidities affecting their open surgical candidacy. Also, some have championed its use in those with mesenteric stenoses and symptoms of unclear etiology almost as a diagnostic procedure.

II. Successful management of **acute mesetneric ischemia (AMI)** usually begins with arteriography to define the mesenteric anatomy. CTA has become so refined, however, that these issues are frequently identified on CTA and the absolute need for arteriography has been lessened (Fig. 17.5) Optimal therapy for acute mesenteric ischemia cannot be determined unless the clinician knows whether the problem is thrombotic, embolic, or hypoperfusion-related. This may sometimes be confusing and the answer may not be apparent until during therapy or afterward.

A. Thrombosis usually is apparent on imaging by obstruction of the superior mesenteric artery at its origin from the aorta. This is usually the most clinically relevant artery in-

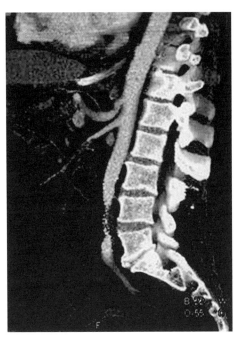

Figure 17.5.   Computed tomography arteriography image revealing superior mesenteric artery (SMA) embolus beyond the first several branches. This is seen as contrast attenuation compared to the aorta and more proximal SMA.

volved by thrombosis. Systemic heparin is indicated to prevent clot propagation. Broad-spectrum antibiotics covering intestinal flora are administered. It is common for these patients to have a history of symptoms consistent with CMI suggesting mesenteric stenoses.

Emergency abdominal exploration should be undertaken to assess bowel viability and to revascularize the obstructed artery. Resection of nonviable intestine without revascularization of the remaining small bowel is associated with a high incidence of further intestinal infarction and death. Generally the bowel should be revascularized before intestinal resection. This allows for interrogation of the bowel with known perfusion in order to assess viability. An exception to this rule is resection before revascularization when a segment of intestine is grossly gangrenous or perforated and the abdomen is considered contaminated. Thrombosis of the SMA should be suspected with significant palpable atherosclerotic burden at its origin and no continuous-wave Doppler signal. A single aortomesenteric bypass is sufficient in these seriously ill patients. The simplest procedure is usually a retrograde infrarenal aortomesenteric or an ileo-mesenteric bypass to the SMA. When bowel contamination is present, a vein graft is preferable to a synthetic material.

Clinical judgment of intestinal viability may be enhanced by fluorescein examination of the GI tract. The test is performed by injection of 2 ampules (1,000 mg) of sodium fluorescein through a peripheral vein and immediate examination of the bowel under an ultraviolet Wood's light in a darkened operating room. A viable bowel has a smooth or uniform fluorescence. Nonviable bowel has decreased, patchy, or no fluorescence. A continuous-wave Doppler can be used to interrogate the mesentery and antimesenteric border of the bowel. Peristalsis usually suggests viability. When it appears that the bowel may survive, it may be left alone and a second-look operation performed within 24 hours to reassess the intestinal viability. Not infrequently, the patient's physiologic status is best served by revascularization, bowel resection, discontinuity with open abdomen, ICU resuscitation, and a second-look operation and restoration of intestinal continuity. **Second-look operations should be routine if *any* bowel had questionable viability at the initial operation.**

B. Emboli usually lodge a few centimeters beyond the origin of the SMA at the level of the first jejunal branches sparing the proximal jejunum (Fig 17.6A). Emboli are usually cardiogenic in nature. The SMA is the mesenteric artery in which emboli are most likely to lodge, due to its acute take-off from the aorta. Operative differentiation suggesting embolism over thrombosis can be suggested by new onset of cardiac arrhythmia, ischemic sparing of the proximal jejunum, and a soft SMA origin and surrounding aorta (Fig. 17.6B). Standard therapy remains similar to the management of thrombosis, except embolectomy is performed by a mesenteric artery arteriotomy and Fogarty® embolectomy catheter (Edwards Lifesciences Corp., Irvine, CA). Some prefer a transverse arteriotomy. The weight of the edematous bowel, however, may lead to tearing of the arteriotomy. We prefer a longitudinal arteriotomy with patch angioplasty closure. Should inflow be poor and inadequately established with embolectomy due to arterial stenosis, bypass is now readily done. Again, vein grafts should be used if there is significant contamination of the abdomen. Milking back the thrombus of the SMA branches, branch embolectomy and on-table direct thrombolytic therapy and heparin are all options to reduce thrombus burden and improve flow after SMA main trunk embolectomy. Emphasis should be made on temporizing damage control surgery with abdominal vacuum packing, resuscitation and second-look operation.

Still, by adhering to the above-mentioned principles, between 10% and 15% of those with AMI will have midgut infarction at exploration and only comfort measures will have to be instituted. Of those in whom operative measures and salvage are pursued, approximately half will require bowel resection at initial operation and the other half subsequent bowel resection at second look. Some may require more review operations until bowel viability is finalized.

The role of endovascular therapy, such as catheter-directed SMA thrombolytic therapy possibly with angioplasty and stenting is described but not well defined. However, follow-up

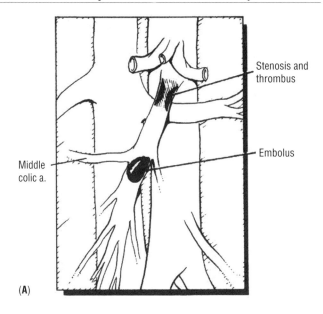

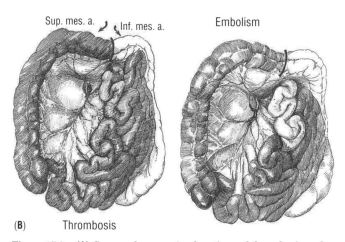

Figure 17.6. **(A) Commonly occurring locations of thrombosis and embolism in the superior mesenteric artery (SMA). (B) Note the spared proximal jejunum in-gut ischemia due to acute embolization, as opposed to that with involved proximal jejunum due to acute thrombosis of SMA stenosis.**

abdominal exploration is still advised if this is done, even if the patient appears physiologically sound. Future clinically evident bowel infarction is morbid, but can be avoided.

C. Nonocclusive mesenteric ischemia (NOMI) generally is seen in critically ill patients who have low cardiac output.

They often are poor risks for any surgery and many times are so labile that transport to the angiographic suite or operating room is a major undertaking in itself. Their arteriograms show peripheral mesenteric vasoconstrictions and a "chain of sausages" appearance, but with no large-vessel occlusions. Noninvasive ischemic colitis appears to be mediated primarily by a remarkable sensitivity of the colonic vasculature to the renin–angiotensin axis.

The best results with this group of patients have been achieved by measures to improve cardiovascular hemodynamics and to vasodilate the mesenteric vasculature. The recommended splanchnic vasodilator therapy is papaverine. Catheter-directed papaverine at 30-60 mg/hour can be accomplished percutaneously, in an attempt to incite this vasodilation. The catheter is placed in the SMA. In general, when peritonitis develops, abdominal exploration is necessary, but very poor outcomes are expected. If a vasopressor is needed to increase blood pressure, dopamine would be the drug of choice, since it reduces renal and mesenteric vascular resistance.

D. Mesenteric venous thrombosis is an extremely rare entity. It may be incited by hypercoaguable states, low mesenteric flow states such as congestive heart failure, cirrhosis, or Budd-Chiari syndrome. Intra-abdominal inflammatory conditions such as diverticulitis may also predispose the patient to this condition. Smoking and prior venous thromboses also appear to place patients at a higher risk. **Seventy percent of these thromboses involve the superior mesenteric vein proper with one-third in the splenic vein and one-third with thrombus burden in the portal vein**. CT venograhy and mesenteric venography are used for diagnostic purposes. Duplex may help. Generally, full anticoagulation is instituted. Abdominal exploration is indicated for peritonitis. There are poorly defined roles for open thromboembolectomy and on-table direct thrombolysis. Similar results have been obtained with surgery and anticoagulation alone.

SELECTED READING

Atkins MD, Kwolek CJ, LaMuraglia GM, et al. Surgical revascularization versus endovascular therapy for chronic mesenteric ischemia: A comparative experience. *J Vasc Surg.* 2007;45: 1162-1171.

Hebert GS, Steele SR. Acute and chronic mesenteric ischemia. *Surg Clin N Am.* 2007;87:1115-1134.

Jimenez JG, Huber TS, Ozaki CK, et al. Durability of antegrade synthetic aortomesenteric bypass for chronic mesenteric ischemia. *J Vasc Surg.* 2002;35:1078-1084.

Landis MS, Rajan DK, Simons ME, et al. Percutaneous management of chronic mesenteric ischemia: Outcomes after intervention. *J Vasc Interv Radiol.* 2005;16:1319-1325.

Mitchell EL, Moneta GL. Mesenteric Duplex Scanning. *Persp Vasc Endovasc Ther.* 2006;18(2):175-183.

Park WP, Cherry KJ, Chua HK, et al. Current results of open revascularization for chronic mesenteric ischemia: A standard for comparison. *J Vasc Surg.* 2002;35:853-859.

ParkWP, Gloviczki P, Cherry KJ, et al. Contemporary management of acute mesenteric ischemia: Factors associated with survival. *J Vasc Surg.* 2002;35:445-452.

Rhee RY, Gloviczki P, Mendonca CT, et al. Mesenteric venous thrombosis: still a lethal disease in the 1990s. *J Vasc Surg.* 1994;20: 688-697.

CHAPTER 18

Upper-Extremity Vascular Disorders

In the spectrum of vascular diseases, upper-extremity arterial problems, including vasospastic disorders, are relatively uncommon. When pain, numbness, coolness, or ulcers involve the fingers or hand, patients generally seek early medical attention. Such symptoms restrict many normal activities and quickly raise the patient's fear of permanent loss of hand function.

The underlying causes of arm ischemia and vasospastic disorders are diverse. For simplicity, they may be organized into the broad groups of emboli, atherosclerotic or aneurysmal occlusions, trauma, and small-vessel arterial occlusive disease. In the initial evaluation the clinician must determine which group the patient fits into and then diagnostic tests can be selected to define the specific underlying etiology. This chapter emphasizes principles of management after a clinical diagnosis has been established.

COMMON CLINICAL PRESENTATIONS

Although there are multiple etiologies for upper-extremity arterial ischemia, including vasospastic disorders, the clinical presentations are relatively few.

I. Raynaud's phenomenon is a description of a clinical presentation or syndrome that suggests vasospasm. The underlying causes are numerous (Table 18.1). Certain clinical features help differentiate Raynaud's phenomenon from other vasospastic disorders, such as acrocyanosis and livedo reticularis (Table 18.2).

Table 18.1. Etiologies of Raynaud's phenomenon

Systemic diseases or conditions
Collagen vascular diseases (e.g., scleroderma)
Cold hemagglutination or cryoglobulinemia
Myxedema
Ergotism
Macroglobulinemia

Nerve compressions
Carpal tunnel syndrome
Thoracic outlet syndrome

Occupational trauma
Pneumatic hammer operation
Chain saw operation
Piano playing
Typing

Arterial occlusive disease

Table 18.2.   Differentiation of vasospastic disorders

Characteristics	Raynaud's phenomenon	Acrocyanosis	Livedo reticularis
Sex	Primarily women (70–80%)	Primarily women (90%)	Men or women
Age	Young adults (15–35 years)	Young adults (15–35 years)	Any age
Color change	Pallor, cyanosis, rubor	Diffuse cyanosis	Mottled cyanosis or rubor
Location	Fingers, toes, sometimes face	Usually hands, sometimes feet	Usually legs, sometimes arms
Duration	Intermittent	Continuous	Continuous
Effect of cold exposure	Increased symptoms	Increased symptoms	Increased symptoms
Skin ulceration	Occurs when collagen vascular disease (e.g., scleroderma) is present	None	Rare

A. Raynaud's phenomenon defines an episodic vasocon-striction of the small arteries and arterioles of the extre-mities. The episodes generally are initiated by cold exposure or emotional stimuli. The symptoms of acrocyanosis and livedo reticularis are constant, although they may increase with expo-sure to cold.

B. The phenomenon usually follows a predictable sequence of color changes in the digits and/ or hand: pallor (i.e., white), followed by cyanosis (i.e., blue), and then rubor (i.e., red). The pallor occurs when skin perfusion is minimal due to intense vasoconstriction of small arterioles in the hand and digits. As cutaneous flow resumes, it is sluggish, beginning with poorly saturated blood leading to the bluish color of cyanosis. Finally, when cutaneous flow resumes, a hyperemic or reperfusion phase occurs causing the skin to be warm and ruborous. Attacks usually are accompanied by numb discomfort of the fingers although pain generally is not severe unless ulcerations are present. In contrast, acro-cyanosis occurs mainly in women and is characterized by con-tinuous bluish discoloration of the hands and occasionally of the lower extremities. Livedo reticularis also is a continuous vasospastic condition consisting of a mottled or reticulated reddish-blue discoloration of the lower extremities and occa-sionally of the hands.

C. Raynaud's phenomenon is localized to the fingers, toes, and occasionally nose and ears. Attacks are limited most commonly to the upper extremities and rarely involve only the toes.

D. The chance of ulceration or gangrene of the tips of the digits depends on the underlying etiology.

1. Raynaud's disease is the term applied to Raynaud's phenomenon that has no clear association with any systemic disease. It rarely results in tissue necrosis and usually occurs in young females (70% of cases). It has been suggested that, before the diagnosis of primary Raynaud's disease is made, the following criteria should be met:

1. Bilateral, symmetric Raynaud's phenomenon is present
2. There is no evidence of large vessel arterial occlusive disease
3. There is an absence of gangrene or significant trophic changes
4. Symptoms should be present for a long period, usually 2 years, without evidence of any other systemic disease associated with Raynaud's phenomenon.

2. Raynaud's phenomenon is the term applied when a local or systemic disease appears to be the precipitating factor for this complex of symptoms. In rare cases Raynaud's phenomenon can also occur in relation to large vessel arterial occlusive lesions in the upper extremity. Gangrene or ulceration of digits is more common in these patients, especially when they have scleroderma, which is the most common collagen vascular disease associated with Raynaud's phenomenon. Raynaud's phenomenon is the initial symptom in 30% of cases and eventually affects 80% of patients with scleroderma. The other common rheumatic diseases associated with Raynaud's phenomenon include mixed collagen vascular disease (80%), systemic lupus erythematosus (30%), dermatomyositis/polymyositis (20%), and rheumatoid arthritis (10%). It must be remembered that Raynaud's phenomenon may exist for years before some underlying systemic collagen vascular, immunologic disease, or large vessel occlusive disease is diagnosed.

3. Acrocyanosis is not associated with skin ulceration. **Livedo reticularis** may occur with ulcerations, generally when some systemic disease (e.g., periarteritis nodosa) is present or atherosclerotic microembolism is evident.

II. Tissue necrosis includes gangrene and poorly healing ulcerations of the digits. It is not uncommon for patients to dismiss small ulcers caused by microemboli as inconsequential bruises or sores of the finger, not recognizing their more serious etiology. If Raynaud's phenomenon precedes the onset of tissue necrosis, other symptoms and signs of underlying systemic disease should be sought. In the absence of Raynaud's phenomenon, evidence of large-vessel occlusive disease, emboli, or small-vessel arterial occlusive disease associated with occupational trauma must be sought.

A. Large-vessel occlusive disease of the arm usually is localized to the subclavian or axillary arteries and is commonly caused by atherosclerosis, often at the origin of the left subclavian. A less common etiology of proximal upper-extremity arterial occlusion is thrombosis of an axillary artery aneurysm caused by years of crutch use. Chronic subclavian artery trauma related to thoracic outlet syndrome also may eventually lead to vessel damage with stenosis, embolization, or occlusion. Extensive acute deep venous thrombosis of the arm (i.e., axillo-subclavian or effort thrombosis) can cause severe venous hypertension or venous gangrene, which may be initially mistaken for arterial ischemia. Finally, postmastectomy irradiation of the axillary area can result in radiation-induced axillary-subclavian arterial stenosis years after radiation treatment.

B. Emboli to the digits may originate from the heart or the subclavian, axillary, or brachial arteries. Additionally, radial or ulnar artery trauma usually from indwelling arterial lines can lead to embolization into the digital arteries. In cases of significant arm ischemia caused by arterial emboli the heart is the origin about 50% of the time, while abnormalities in the arterial network of the arm (i.e., subclavian, axillary, and brachial arteries) are responsible for the other half of cases. The proximal upper-extremity arteries may develop atherosclerotic ulcerative plaques or aneurysms that result in embolization. Poststenotic subclavian aneurysms associated with thoracic outlet compression or axillary aneurysms caused by chronic crutch use also may cause embolism to the hand.

C. Small-vessel arterial disease associated with occupational hand trauma may cause significant hand and/or digit ischemia. Occupations involving repetitive vibration or trauma to the fingers or palmar surface of the hand predispose some individuals to spasm, thrombosis, or aneurysms of the ulnar, radial, or digital arteries. The ulnar artery is especially susceptible to local trauma over the hypothenar eminence, where it is fairly superficial and easily compressed against the underlying pisiform and hamate bones. **The term hypothenar hammer syndrome has been applied to this form of posttraumatic digital ischemia.** Activities that may lead to hand ischemia are operation of the pneumatic hammer, lathe, or chain saw. In industry, the term **vibration-induced white finger** has been applied to posttraumatic digital ischemia.

III. Arm claudication is an unusual presentation of arm ischemia. In general, exertional arm fatigue is more commonly caused by neurologic compression at the cervical spine or thoracic outlet. Because of excellent collateral blood flow around the shoulder, subclavian occlusive disease often is asymptomatic or only mildly symptomatic (Fig. 18.1). However, active adults, especially manual laborers, may experience arm claudication from subclavian or brachial artery stenosis.

DIAGNOSTIC TESTS

Patient history and physical examination provide most of the information necessary to diagnose the general type of upper-extremity arterial disease. The following tests may be performed to confirm the clinical impression, to identify underlying etiologies, and to monitor therapy.

I. Doppler velocity flow detection. The continuous-wave Doppler is a simple means for assessing arm perfusion when pulses are not palpable. The axillary, brachial, radial, ulnar, palmar, and digital arteries can easily be checked for the presence and quality of Doppler signal. Biphasic or triphasic arterial signals are normal, while monophasic or dampened signals suggest

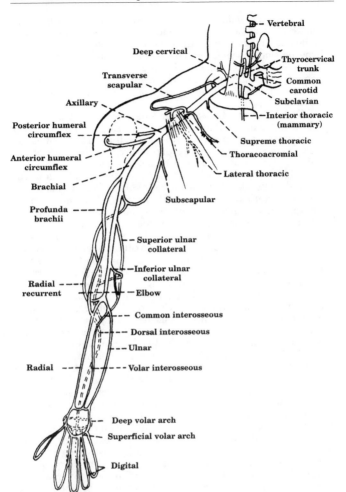

Figure 18.1.   Arterial anatomy of the upper extremity. The collateral circulation of the arm is well developed, and, consequently, proximal large-vessel occlusion seldom results in distal extremity necrosis and amputation.

significant arterial obstruction. Upper-arm and forearm blood pressures can be measured with a routine blood pressure cuff and the Doppler unit, and in cases of suspected claudication arm pressures should be obtained at rest and after 2 to 5 minutes of exercise.

II. Digital plethysmography or laser Doppler flow patterns may provide more detail in the evaluation of digital ischemia and vasospastic disorders. Flat or diminished (<5 mm) pulse volume recordings (PVRs) confirm severe digital flow reduction and are predictive of poor healing in the presence of ulceration. PVRs using digital cuffs and/or laser Doppler flow measurements can be repeated to assess for changes in digital blood flow after initiation of treatment, either operative or nonoperative.

III. Duplex ultrasonography provides excellent visualization of most upper-extremity arterial segments. The main limitations are the proximal subclavian arteries, especially on the left, which is covered by the bulky clavicle. As with other arterial segments, duplex provides both a B-mode image of the vessel in question as well as an assessment of blood flow (i.e., velocity) through the segment.

IV. Arteriography. Arteriography is helpful in defining the severity and extent of large vessel occlusive disease of the upper extremity although it is not indicated in all such cases. Specifically, arteriography defines the location of the occlusive disease and provides information regarding the runoff to the forearm and hand. Arteriography is not necessary to diagnose vasospastic disorders but may be useful to rule out large-vessel occlusive disease when Raynaud's phenomenon is complicated by finger ulcers. When performed, arteriography must show the entire upper-extremity vasculature from its origin (i.e., innominate on the right and subclavian on the left) to the digital arteries. Failure to obtain complete upper-extremity arteriography is a common reason for a missed diagnosis such as digital occlusions due to an ulcerated atheroma in the proximal subclavian artery.

V. Digital temperature recovery time following emersion of the hands in a cold ice-water bath (i.e., cold immersion test) can help establish the diagnosis of Raynaud's phenomenon. The physiologic principle behind the test is simple, as is the technique. Digital cutaneous blood flow is linearly related to digital skin temperature over a wide range. Normally, digital skin temperature recovers to normal within 10 to 15 minutes after cold exposure. In contrast, digital skin temperature in patients with Raynaud's phenomenon does not recover for at least 20 to 25 minutes after cold stimulus. The accuracy of the test is improved when the following guidelines are followed for measuring the digital temperature recovery time:

1. The patient should sit in a warm (24°C ± 2°C), quiet room for at least 30 minutes before the test.
2. Baseline digital pulp temperatures are taken with a thermistor probe
3. The hand is immersed in an ice-water mixture for 20 seconds, removed, and dried
4. Digital temperatures are checked every 5 minutes for 30 to 45 minutes
5. A temperature-time graph can be constructed to show the digital temperature versus recovery time
6. Controls for a particular laboratory should be established for comparison.

VI. Systemic disease workup. Since systemic diseases so often underlie vasospastic disorders and upper-extremity ischemia, a number of screening laboratory tests should be considered. A platelet count should be done, since thrombocytosis can mimic Raynaud's phenomenon. An elevated sedimentation rate should raise suspicion of a systemic illness. Since serum protein abnormalities may be associated with vasospasm, a

serum protein electrophoresis should be performed and cryo-
globulins, macroglobulins, and cold agglutinins should be
checked. Basic immunologic tests should include antinuclear
antibody, rheumatoid factor, and lupus erythematosus tests. If
scleroderma is suspected, a skin biopsy in an affected area may
confirm the diagnosis or a barium esophagogram may reveal
characteristic esophageal dysfunctions.

MANAGEMENT

In our experience, these guidelines have provided the best assurance of relieving upper-extremity ischemia, including vasospastic disorders. Where there are areas of controversy, we offer
several different points of view.

I. Vasospastic disorders.

   A. Raynaud's disease or primary Raynaud's usually can
   be satisfactorily managed by nonoperative methods. Tissue
   necrosis rarely is a problem; consequently, the patient needs
   assurance that loss of fingers or their function is not likely to
   occur if the following guidelines are observed.

   **1. Avoidance of any tobacco use and protection from
   cold exposure** are the fundamentals of initial treatment.
   Tobacco leads to vasoconstriction, a fact that can be documented by comparing baseline digital PVRs to tracings
   taken immediately after the patient smokes several cigarettes. The basics of protection from cold exposure include
   warm gloves and footwear during cold weather and gloves
   when working with refrigeration. Maintaining core body
   temperature by wearing warm clothing over the trunk also
   helps. For many patients, these simple measures are
   enough to prevent symptoms from occurring.

   2. When vasospasm is not satisfactorily relieved by these
   simple measures, **medical options** are available and usually provide some benefit. The best results are obtained with
   calcium channel blockers such as nifedipine or the alpha-
   receptor blocker prazosin. For some patients, the longer-act-
   ing form of nifedipine causes fewer side effects, which can
   include headache, dizziness, palpitations, flushing, and
   edema. **Recent evidence suggests that the medication
   sildenafil (Viagra, Pfizer, Inc.) improves microcircu-
   lation and symptoms of Raynaud's that are otherwise
   refractory to vasodilator therapy.**

   3. Thermal biofeedback has demonstrated good results
   in many patients in whom anxiety and stress play a role in
   the initiation of vasospastic attacks. After biofeedback
   training, 80% to 90% of patients can avert an attack of Raynaud's phenomenon, and some can actually increase skin
   temperature as much as 4°C.

   4. The role of **surgical or thoracoscopic sympathectomy** for Raynaud's disease is limited. Few patients should
   need sympathectomy, since conservative management controls symptoms in at least 80% of patients. Reasonable candidates for sympathectomy are those patients whose
   vasospastic attacks have become progressively debilitating,
   especially when trophic or ulcerative changes have
   occurred. Approximately 50% to 60% of such patients with
   primary Raynaud's phenomenon and no underlying sys-

temic collagen vascular or immunologic disease will have improvement after sympathectomy, although the early favorable results may not last more than 3 to 6 months.

B. Raynaud's phenomenon or secondary Raynaud's due to some underlying systemic disease or large-vessel occlusive lesions often is a more difficult problem to manage than primary Raynaud's disease. Tissue necrosis with exceptionally painful digital ulcers can be a chronic problem in such patients. The fundamentals of therapy remain avoidance of tobacco, protection from cold, and treatment of calcium channel blockers. Sympathectomy is far less effective than it is for primary Raynaud's disease. In fact, only 20% to 30% of patients with scleroderma and Raynaud's phenomenon improve after sympathectomy, so we rarely recommend sympathectomy in these patients. **In instances where secondary Raynaud's is clinically significant and associated with large-vessel occlusive disease (e.g., subclavian, axillary, or brachial arteries) such lesions should be treated to maximize perfusion to the arm and hand. This is especially true in cases where noninvasive testing confirms significant ischemia in the forearm and hand or there has been tissue loss in the digits.**

C. Acrocyanosis does not lead to tissue loss, so treatment is directed at relieving cold-induced symptoms. The conservative management described for primary Raynaud's disease usually is sufficient.

D. Livedo reticularis is also manageable in most cases by conservative treatment. Digital ulceration may occur when livedo reticularis is associated with periarteritis nodosa, lupus erythematosus, or cholesterol embolization. In such cases, sympathectomy may be considered, although results have been variable.

E. Cold hypersensitivity may be seen after recovery from frostbite. The affected area may become bluish and have an associated burning pain with even mild cold exposure. The problem seems to be a variant of **reflex sympathetic dystrophy or causalgia (i.e., sympathetically maintained pain).** Initially, the medical treatment described for Raynaud's disease should be undertaken. For severe cases, regional sympathectomy may provide lasting relief, especially if it is done before pain becomes chronic.

II. Threatened limb loss. Although vasospastic disorders may cause ulcerations of the tips of the digits, the hand and arm seldom become ischemic. Severe hand ischemia usually is associated with large-artery occlusions, emboli, or trauma.

A. Acute ischemia generally requires emergency surgical intervention. The history and physical exam usually will identify the cause. If there is a delay for medical stabilization or arteriography we administer heparin systematically to the patient to prevent thrombus propagation. Patients who develop brachial artery occlusion after cardiac catheterization should undergo immediate brachial thrombectomy and repair of the access site often under local anesthesia. Although the patient's hand may initially be relatively asymptomatic, a chronic brachial artery occlusion in these situations can cause bothersome arm claudication in active individuals. Thus, urgent brachial artery repair is preferable to delayed surgery as it can be accomplished with minimal risk and achieve return of distal pulses in nearly all patients.

B. An arterial embolus to the upper-extremity arterial circulation is the most common cause of acute arm ischemia. The most common source of such emboli is the heart and most often the embolus lodges in the brachial artery at the takeoff of the profunda brachius artery. These emboli can nearly always be successfully extracted with local exploration and limited Fogarty® catheter (Edwards Lifesciences Corp., Irvine, CA) embolectomy. Thromboemboli lodged in more proximal arterial segments such as the subclavian axillary can also be approached through the proximal brachial or distal axillary artery with passage of the Fogarty® embolectomy catheter (Edwards Lifesciences Corp., Irvine, CA) proximally. In cases of proximal subclavian or axillary artery emboli, transfemoral arteriography with placement of a catheter in the subclavian artery may provide useful diagnostic information and even therapeutic options. Distal forearm emboli are more completely removed by a more distal brachial artery cutdown, allowing for selective passage of a small Fogarty® embolectomy catheter (Edwards Lifesciences Corp., Irvine, CA) down each of the ulnar and radial arteries. In cases where the emboli or subsequent thrombus (i.e., clot) has extended into the distal digital arteries adjuvant thrombolytic agents may be helpful in restoring distal outflow or runoff. If, in such cases, the distal emboli or thrombosis is relatively chronic, local thrombolytic therapy is less likely to help. Importantly, if the source of the embolus is not the heart but instead an atherosclerotic lesion in the proximal subclavian or axillary artery, these will require open operative or endovascular treatment to remove the source of the emboli.

C. Large-artery occlusions in the upper-extremity circulation require treatment, either open or endovascular, as they cause significant symptoms. Proximal subclavian stenoses are preferably treated with angioplasty and stenting using a balloon-expandable stent. If the proximal subclavian artery is occluded and/or not amenable to endovascular treatment, a carotid-to-subclavian bypass or reimplantation of the subclavian artery into the common carotid artery are very effective options with low associated morbidity and mortality. Subclavian artery thrombosis secondary to thoracic outlet syndrome will require resection of the first rib and any cervical rib in conjunction with arterial repair. In contrast, **axillo-subclavian vein thrombosis** secondary to thoracic outlet compression (i.e., effort thrombosis) is treated by catheter-directed thrombolytic infusion and anticoagulation followed by first-rib resection. The timing of the first-rib resection is somewhat controversial. Some recommend early resection after thrombolysis while others prefer to anticoagulate the patient with warfarin for 6 to 8 weeks prior to resection, to allow the surface of the vein to heal. Thrombosed axillary artery aneurysms are best treated with open operative reconstruction using an interposition graft of saphenous vein or prosthetic material. Saphenous vein is the best conduit for brachial, radial, and ulnar revascularizations.

III. Arm claudication. As discussed earlier, incapacitating arm claudication is fairly uncommon because of the rich collateral blood flow to the arm. For the few patients who need revascularization, the options, open and endovascular, described above for threatened limb loss are also applicable to relieve claudication.

LONG-TERM PROGNOSIS

The long-term prognosis for most arterial problems of the upper extremity is good. Nonoperative treatment is successful in many patients. Therefore, unless the viability of the extremity is acutely threatened, a period of conservative treatment and observation should generally be followed. **The patients with the worst prognosis generally are those with Raynaud's phenomenon secondary to progressive collagen vascular disease or those with extensive distal small-vessel occlusion secondary to recurrent emboli or thrombosis.**

SELECTED READING

Aleksic M, Hackenkamp J, Gawenda M, Brunkwall J. Occupation-related vascular disorders of the upper extremity–two case reports. *Angiology*. 2006;57:107-114.

Bhatt SP, Handa R, Gulati GS, et al. Peripheral vascular disease in systemic lupus erythematosus. *Lupus*. 2007;16:720-723.

Cooke JP, Marshall JM. Mechanisms of Raynaud's disease. *Vasc Med*. 2005;10:293-307.

Fries R, Shariat K, von Wilmowsky H, Bohm M. Sildenafil in the treatment of Raynaud's phenomenon resistant to vasodilatory therapy. *Circ*. 2005;112:2980-2985.

Sanders RJ, Hammond SL, Rao NM. Diagnosis of thoracic outlet syndrome. *J Vasc Surg*. 2007;46:601-604.

Suter LG, Murabito JM, Felson DT, Fraenkel L. Smoking, alcohol consumption and Raynaud's phenomenon in middle age. *Am J Med*. 2007;120:264-271.

Taylor LM. Hypothenar hammer syndrome. *J Vasc Surg*. 2003; 37:697.

Thune TH, Ladegaard L, Licht PB. Thoracoscopic sympathectomy for Raynaud's phenomenon–a long term follow-up study. *Eur J Vasc Endovasc Surg*. 2006;32:198-202.

Wigley FM, Flavahan NA. Raynaud's phenomenon. *Rheum Dis Clin North Am*. 1996;22:765-781.

CHAPTER 19

Venous Disorders and Venous Thromboembolism

A spectrum of chronic venous disorders, from simple varicose veins to venous stasis ulcers, afflicts at least 20% to 25% of the population. Varicose veins are one of the most common vascular problems seen in office practice. Most varicose veins are the result of a congenital or familial predisposition that leads to loss of elasticity in the vein wall and the absence or incompetence of venous valves. These primary varicosities generally progress downward in the saphenous system. Prolonged standing, obesity, and pregnancy make all leg varicosities more symptomatic.

Most patients who have had femoropopliteal deep vein thrombosis will develop some degree of **post-thrombotic syndrome.** Thrombosis damages deep venous valves and often leaves them incompetent. The musculovenous pump can no longer reduce ambulatory venous pressures. Consequently, the patient has chronic venous hypertension in the leg when he or she stands with high venous pressures transmitted through perforating veins from the deep to superficial venous system. In 20% to 50% of patients with symptoms and signs of chronic venous insufficiency, no history of deep venous thrombosis (DVT) is obtainable. The classic physical findings are a chronically indurated ankle, dark stasis pigmentation around the ankle, and skin ulceration in some patients. The exact means by which this chronic venous hypertension causes stasis skin changes and ulceration is still unclear. Evidence suggests that local capillaries leak fibrinous protein that is not adequately removed by fibrinolysis. A liposclerosis occurs and local tissue oxygen diffusion may be impeded. The result is tissue necrosis and skin ulceration. **Skin ulceration seldom occurs unless the popliteal vein valves are incompetent.**

Post-thrombotic syndrome or primary deep valvular incompetence can be especially disabling for active ambulatory workers, since leg dependency increases pain and swelling and impedes ulcer healing. Fortunately, proper elastic leg support, skin care, and, in some situations, surgery can alleviate chronic venous insufficiency enough that patients can remain comfortable and active. In patients with chronic iliofemoral venous obstruction, venous capacitance is increased at rest and cannot compensate during exercise. The result is severe thigh pain and a sensation of tightness with vigorous exercise, dubbed **venous claudication.** Leg symptoms are more common in patients with chronic venous obstruction than in those who have recanalized veins with incompetent valves. A surprising observation is that 5 to 10 years after lower-extremity DVT, over 80% of patients will develop some symptoms of chronic venous insufficiency (edema, pain, ulceration).

The current clinical approach to acute venous thromboembolism focuses on prevention, rapid diagnosis, and treatment. A better understanding of the pathophysiology of DVT and pulmonary embolism (PE) has resulted in more aggressive preventive measures. The limitations of the physical examination in accurate diagnosis of venous thromboembolism have culminated in the development of efficient, noninvasive methods for detection. Newer anticoagulant medications and regimens offer alternatives for prevention and treatment. Finally, clinical trials will define the role of catheter-directed thrombolysis in the treatment of DVT.

The basic pathophysiology and natural history of venous disorders are summarized in Chapter 2. A description of the initial lower extremity venous examination is found in Chapter 5. This chapter focuses on the principles of medical, catheter-based, and surgical therapy.

I. **Chronic venous disorders.**

A. **The CEAP classification** scheme (see Table 2.1) has been adopted worldwide in order to standardize and facilitate communication about chronic venous disorders. Venous disease is defined by clinical class (C), etiology (E), its anatomic (A) distribution in the veins, and the pathologic mechanism (P) of development (reflux or obstruction or both).

1. Clinical presentation of venous disorders relies upon physical examination. C1 disease is evidenced by telangiectasias and/or reticular veins, commonly referred to as **spider veins**. Varicose veins are distinguished by diameter <3 mm and their characteristic protuberance and are seen in C2 disease. Progression to edema and skin changes from venous hypertension is seen with C3 and C4 disease, respectively. Skin changes may be mild such as eczema or erythematous dermatitis. **Lipodermatosclerosis** is a localized chronic inflammation and fibrosis of the skin and subcutaneous tissues of the lower leg, occasionally associated with scarring of the Achilles tendon. Lymphangitis and cellulitis should be differentiated by local signs and systemic features. **Atrophie blanche, or white atrophy, refers to the smooth, stellate scarring that can occur with venous stasis**. The most severe clinical manifestation is venous ulceration. A healed ulcer is seen in C5 disease. An active ulcer with a full thickness skin defect, most frequently in the ankle region, defines C6 disease.

2. The **etiology** of the venous disease is also used for classification. Venous disease may be congenital, as in **Klippel-Trenaunay syndrome,** which appears to be a fetal developmental abnormality. The classic clinical triad includes (a) port-wine stains, (b) hypertrophy of soft tissue and bone with overgrowth of the extremity, and (c) varicose veins. Because of the benign course of this disease, the majority of these patients do not have surgery and do well with conservative therapy. Occasionally, a more aggressive operative approach may be necessary in patients with large, symptomatic varicosities, especially if hemorrhage or ulceration has occurred. It is important to rule out deep venous hypoplasia, which can be present in these patients, prior to any treatment of superficial varicosities. **Venous disease may also be primary from the degeneration of valves or secondary as a result of damage from prior thrombosis (post-thrombotic).**

3. **Anatomically,** venous disease can roughly be classified as superficial, deep, and/or perforating veins. The affected veins cannot be accurately defined by physical exam alone. Duplex ultrasound is necessary if precise identification of the involved veins is desired (Chapter 6).

4. The **pathophysiology** of venous disease is from reflux, obstruction, or a combination of the two. Reflux can develop primarily or as a result of post-thrombotic degeneration of valves. Obstruction is most commonly a post-thrombotic event, and may occur when the affected vein is only partially recanalized. The residual webs and synechiae prevent normal venous flow. **May-Thurner syndrome** is a congenital obstruction of the left iliac vein by the anatomic crossover of the right iliac artery. In some patients, this impingement may result in pain (venous claudication), edema, and a predisposition toward developing left iliofemoral venous thrombosis. It is interesting that over 20% of the population demonstrates this compression in cadaver studies, but only a minority becomes symptomatic.

B. **Diagnosis**

1. **Clinical presentation.** Varicose veins present with unsightly bulges on the lower extremity and often with associated achiness or heaviness in the legs with prolonged standing. Symptoms may not correlate well with the degree of anatomic defect. Occasionally, a patient will abrade a varicosity, which may cause a rather impressive hemorrhage. A more common complication of varicose veins is superficial thrombophlebitis, which may cause considerable pain and disability but rarely leads to PE. Longstanding varicose veins may also result in chronic ankle induration, stasis dermatitis, and, occasionally, leg ulcerations. As was previously noted, post-thrombotic syndrome is found in patients with a history of DVT leading to deep venous insufficiency and/or obstruction. This syndrome is manifested by skin changes, edema, and ulceration of the lower extremity.

2. **Noninvasive venous testing** is very helpful in the diagnosis of both acute and chronic venous disease as described in Chapter 6. Duplex ultrasound is the mainstay of diagnosis. Reflux in the superficial and deep veins can be determined by prolonged valve closure times (>0.5 seconds). Perforator incompetence is determined by reversed or outward flow (deep to superficial) in the perforating veins of the leg. **Duplex has greater than 95% accuracy in the detection of acute venous thrombosis, and can also recognize the signs of chronic thrombosis, such as recanalization, collaterals, and more echogenic clot.** Plethysmography can provide a global assessment of the limb's venous function and is generally applied as an adjunct to Duplex in more severe cases of chronic venous insufficiency. CT and MR venography are particularly useful in evaluation of the central veins, which are less accessible by ultrasound. However, both CT and MR can only determine anatomic abnormalities and provide no physiologic evaluation. MR is the test of choice for characterization of venous malformations. Invasive venography is

generally reserved for those patients with chronic venous insufficiency or congenital disorders in order to evaluate for venous reconstruction. Ascending venography provides a roadmap of the limb and central drainage, such that obstructive lesions can be identified. Descending venography can localize incompetent valves and assess the severity of the reflux.

C. Treatment.

1. Nonoperative treatment is appropriate for the majority of chronic venous disorders. The symptoms may range from mild (varicose veins) to severe (ulcers). Patients should be reassured that the presence of chronic venous disease is neither life- nor limb-threatening. In our experience these are frequently the unspoken concerns of our patients. Even severe venous ulceration is usually superficial and does not threaten the limb in the absence of superimposed infection or arterial insufficiency. Chronic venous insufficiency is incurable, thus it is important that the patient understands that the goal of treatment is to minimize symptoms and prevent ulcer recurrences.

The following measures will promote venous health for patients with chronic venous diseases:

1. Compression therapy with graduated stockings
2. Elevate the feet and legs for 10 to 15 minutes whenever possible
3. Walk to improve the musculovenous pump of the calf
4. Avoid trauma to varicose veins
5. Weight reduction for obese patients
6. Avoid prolonged standing or sitting
7. Consultation with vascular and wound care specialist at the first signs of ulceration or cellulitis
8. Maintain skin integrity, avoiding cracking and eczema, with proper emmolients

a. Compression therapy is the mainstay of medical treatment for all chronic venous disorders. Graded elastic stockings are available in a variety of strengths, lengths, and styles. Strengths of 20–30 mm Hg are most commonly prescribed for varicose veins and milder venous disorders. The stockings alleviate many of the symptoms of leg achiness, heaviness, and swelling. Although below-the-knee stockings are suitable for most patients, some women with varicose veins prefer a high-quality sheer panty hose with graduated pressure from the ankle to waist. Several companies offer specialized venous stockings and hosiery [e.g., Sigvaris (Ganzoni and Cie, AG, St. Gallen, Switzerland), Jobst (Beiersdorf–Jobst Inc., Charlotte, NC, U.S.A.), and Medi (Medi USA Inc., Whitsett, NC, U.S.A)].

Patients with post-phlebitic syndrome and deep venous insufficiency are often affected by **ambulatory venous hypertension**. In such patients venous pressures decrease only 20–30% during exercise compared with a 70% decrease in the setting of normal venous function. Venous pressures are highest in the most dependent portion of the leg at the ankle, where most post-thrombotic changes occur. Although chronic venous hypertension cannot be corrected by elastic leg support, elastic leg support can prevent some of the leg edema. For these patients, strengths ≥30–40 mm Hg are desirable. Below-the-knee stockings are generally sufficient in most patients for several reasons. First, post-thrombotic problems nearly always occur below the knee, where venous pressures are highest. Thigh swelling seldom is a problem after acute DVT has resolved. Second, support hose that comes above the knee often binds or constricts the popliteal space, especially if the hose slip down the leg. Third, patients generally do not like a heavy support hose that covers the entire leg. Many patients who are given full-length or pantyhose-type heavy support hose will wear them only when visiting their physician for a check-up. However, some patients with vena cava occlusion and severe leg swelling to the waist will need full-leg heavy support hose and will wear them without complaint.

Compliance with compression therapy is particularly important for patients with active or healed venous ulceration. **Active venous ulcers heal at an average of 5 months in 97% of compliant patients compared to 55% of patients who are non-compliant**. Continued compression therapy also significantly reduces the incidence of ulcer recurrence. Several suggestions should be offered to the patient to ensure the proper and comfortable use of heavy support hose. First, the hose should be put on in the morning, prior to ambulation. Otherwise, early leg swelling may begin before the elastic support can control it. This routine usually requires that the patient bathe or shower before going to bed at night. Second, heavy hose may be difficult to slide on the leg, especially for patients who have difficulty applying the stockings due to hand arthritis or poor conditioning. Special stocking-donning devices are commercially available. The stocking can be loaded onto the donning device, which stretches it sufficiently for easier application. A silky liner or light nylon hose worn beneath the heavy stocking can also make application easier. Third, elastic support hose must be properly fitted, or the patient will not wear them. Patients with large or unequal leg size may need custom-fitted stockings. We encourage patients to contact the fitting shop for adjustments if their new hose do not fit satisfactorily. We also periodically recheck patients in the outpatient clinic to ensure that their hose fit properly. In general, most heavy elastic support hose will need to be replaced every 6 to 12 months.

b. Leg elevation remains a simple and effective method of alleviating ankle edema. Patients with post-thrombotic syndrome should elevate their legs above the level of the heart for 10 to 15 minutes every 2 to 4 hours during the day. This recommendation may seem impractical for the working individual, but most workers are allowed breaks during their normal work hours

at which time elevation can be done. Periodic leg elevation allows most patients to remain comfortable during
work. An explanatory note from the physician to the
patient's employer often avoids any problem that the
patient may encounter by periodically sitting down on
the job.

c. Skin care is important if dermatitis, local infection,
and ulceration are to be prevented. Scaly pruritic skin of
the foot or ankle may indicate fungal infection, which is
managed by a topical fungicide such as Baza® antifungal
cream (2% miconazole nitrate, Coloplast Corp., Mari-
etta, GA) or Lotrimin® (1% clotrimazole, Schering-
Plough Corporation, Kenilworth, N.J.). Eczematous
stasis dermatitis may be alleviated by a topical steroid
cream, such as hydrocortisone cream 1%. Routine leg
washing should be done with warm water and a mild
soap. We discourage soaking the leg, since this may mac-
erate friable skin and increase swelling due to dependency of the extremity. Non-perfumed emmolients such
as Aquaphor® or Eucerin® (Beiersdorf, Wilton, CT) should
be used to treat dry, cracked skin to prevent further
breakdown, ulceration, and cellulitis.

**d. Venous ulcers classically occur in the lower
third of the leg above the ankle, referred to as the
"gaiter distribution."** Most frequently, ulcers occur at
the medial malleolus adjacent a medial ankle perforator. Less commonly, they occur on the lateral or posterior
calf at the site of the lateral ankle perforator or the mid-
posterior calf perforator (Fig. 19.1). The treatment of
venous ulcers utilizes all of the principles listed previously, however, supplementary measures may be needed
to treat refractory ulcers. A compressive bandage should
be applied over the ulcer dressing (Fig. 19.2). A rigid
bandage can provide a greater amount of continuous
compression than a stocking, and is a good adjuvant
technique for nonhealing ulcers. **The Unna boot is the
most well known of these rigid bandages**. The
three-layered boot is applied by a medical professional.
The innermost layer is a medicated paste gauze that
contain calamine, zinc oxide, glycerin, sorbitol, and magnesium aluminum silicate. The second layer is gauze,
followed by an outer elastic compression wrap. The boot
hardens and can be left on for a week, although more
frequent checks (e.g., every 2–3 days) of the leg should
be performed in diabetic patients or those with resolving cellulitis. The advantage of a boot is that continuous
compression is applied and patient compliance is
enforced. An absorbent dressing can be applied to the
ulcer before applying the boot. The Profore system
(Smith and Nephew, London, U.K.) is a four-layer, commercially available bandage that works by the same
principles and is also effective for venous stasis ulcers.

Meticulous wound care is a critical part of the treatment
of venous ulcers. A nurse or midlevel provider dedicated
to the performance of wound care and able to devote time
to counseling is an invaluable asset. The vascular special-

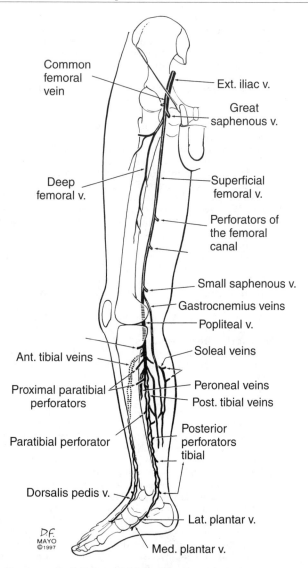

Common femoral vein

Ext. iliac v.

Great saphenous v.

Deep femoral v.

Superficial femoral v.

Perforators of the femoral canal

Small saphenous v.

Gastrocnemius veins

Popliteal v.

Ant. tibial veins

Soleal veins

Proximal paratibial perforators

Peroneal veins

Post. tibial veins

Paratibial perforator

Posterior perforators tibial

Dorsalis pedis v.

Lat. plantar v.

D.F.
MAYO
©1997

Med. plantar v.

Figure 19.1. Location of the major lower-leg perforators. The perforating vein sites on the medial leg, especially the upper, middle, and lower posterior tibial perforators (formerly called Cockett perforators), are common locations for post-thrombotic venous ulcers. Ulcers seldom occur at the posterior and lateral venous perforators.

ist must be committed to supervising the wound care for these patients who require lifelong maintenance. Various ointments, salves, and dressings are available for compre-

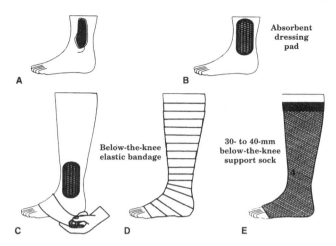

Figure 19.2. Application of a compressive bandage for a venous ulcer. **(A)** The ulcer should be washed with warm water and mild soap. In general, topical antibiotics should be avoided since they may cause topical allergic reactions. For grossly infected ulcers, the infection should be controlled before the bandage is applied. **(B)** A soft absorbent pad should be placed over the ulcer. **(C, D, E)** The leg from the foot to the knee is wrapped with a compressive dressing: an Unna's paste boot bandage, and Ace wrap, or a 30 to 40 mm below-the-knee support stocking.

hensive wound care. Clean, granulating wounds should be treated with a hydrogel or hydrocolloid dressing to maintain a moist healing environment, and wounds with large amount of necrotic tissue should undergo manual sharp debridement. Treatment with an enzymatic debriding ointment such as collagenase or papain and urea may also be beneficial, but some patients experience discomfort or burning with application. Wounds with large amounts of serous drainage should be treated with application of absorbent dressing or powder, such as calcium alginate. All of these dressings can be applied underneath a compression stocking or boot although we would caution not to use the Unna Boot or Profore systems in the setting of active infection or cellulitis. In such cases, more frequent changes of the wound will be necessary (e.g., once or twice daily). **If the ulcer appears infected, evidenced by foul odor, surrounding cellulitis, or increased drainage, a biopsy for quantitative culture can be taken, although superficial wound swabs are discouraged as a multitude of flora will grow from every open wound**. Local cellulitis usually responds to a 5- to 7-day course of an empiric oral antibiotic, such as a cephalosporin.

2. Invasive therapies can be used to treat chronic venous disorders that are refractory to compression therapy or in patients who are unable or unwilling to comply with compression. Indications for treatment include (a) cosmetic concerns, (b) symptoms of achiness, heaviness, pain or edema, (c) bleeding from friable varicose veins, (d) recurrent superficial thrombophlebitis, and (e) venous ulceration. The type of treatment is guided by the severity and location of venous reflux and/or occlusion, as defined by the preintervention duplex. Additional tests (plethysmography, venograms) are obtained in more complex cases, such as those that have had prior venous operations or may require venous reconstruction. Duplex is unnecessary in patients with only spider veins. All patients should obtain well-fitted compression hose, which are worn for at least several weeks after treatment of varicose veins and indefinitely for patients with history of venous ulceration. Preoperative prophylaxis against DVT with 5,000 units of subcutaneous heparin should be considered in patients at higher risk for periprocedural DVT. Risk factors include older age, obesity, hormone replacement or oral contraceptives, smoking, and history of previous DVT.

a. Sclerotherapy is the injection of a sclerosing agent into the varicose vein to damage its endothelium to cause an aseptic thrombosis, which organizes and closes the vein. We use sclerotherapy as primary treatment for **spider veins, reticular veins, and smaller varicosities** (<6 mm). Sclerotherapy can also be used to obliterate small residual varicosities that persist after treatment of great saphenous reflux. In contrast, sclerotherapy is not as durable a treatment for large (8 to 12 mm) varicosities that cascade down the entire lower extremity from a completely incompetent great saphenous vein. **Sclerotherapy will have limited long-term success in patients with untreated saphenous or deep system reflux**, therefore patients with more significant C2 and greater disease should first be evaluated by duplex ultrasound. Complications of sclerotherapy include hyperpigmentation, skin necrosis, thrombophlebitis, and allergic reactions.

The essentials of safe and effective sclerotherapy are as follows:

(1) Relative contraindications to sclerotherapy include use of anticoagulants, ABI <0.7, veins on the foot; veins in fat legs where perivenous reactions may cause painful fat necrosis, and history of strong allergic conditions.

(2) No more than 0.5 mL of the sclerosant (sodium tetradecyl sulfate 0.25% to 3%, hypertonic saline (23.4%), or sodium morrhuate) should be used in any one injection site. A small-gauge (size 25, 26, or 30) needle is used to inject four to six locations at one injection session. Detergent-based agents can also be mixed with room air to make a foam. Foam sclerotherpay has been used to treat larger varicosities as well as C1 disease.

(3) The injection is done while the patient is reclining, not standing. The sclerosant is retained in the vein segment by compressing it above and below the injection site for about one minute. The injection is stopped if the patient complains of severe local pain, since this suggests extravasation of the sclerosant outside the vein. **It is particularly important to have the leg elevated when using foam sclerotherapy to avoid migration of air into the deep venous system or centrally**.

(4) A compressive elastic bandage is applied and the patient is actively ambulated immediately. This ambulation helps the musculovenous pump of the calf to wash out any sclerosant that may have leaked into the deep venous system. Patients are asked to wear the compressive bandage or compression stockings for at least one week following an average injection in small veins.

b. Surgical and endovascular treatment of varicose veins. The treatment of saphenous vein reflux is indicated for symptomatic varicose veins (aching, hemorrhage, superficial thrombophlebitis). The best surgical candidates are active, healthy patients who are not overweight. Some patients simply desire removal of the varicose veins for cosmetic reasons. Occasionally, primary varicose veins lead to leg ulcers. In addition, there is evidence that correction of the superficial reflux in patients with combined superficial and deep reflux improves venous hemodynamics. **In a large randomized controlled trial (ESCHAR), eliminating superficial reflux in combination with compression therapy reduced venous ulcer recurrence, although healing rates were not improved compared to compression alone**.

(1) Saphenous vein stripping is the traditional method for treating saphenous reflux. Before the operation, the correct limb is marked with an indelible felt-tipped pen or other nontoxic dye while the patient stands. If stab phlebectomy is planned, the sites of varicose clusters are marked with an *X*. The surgeon or surgeon's assistant should do this marking and be sure that the patient agrees with the veins to be removed. A small incision is made at the groin and the saphenofemoral junction is exposed and ligated along with each of its five or six tributaries. Starting from the groin, a disposable stripper is passed through the vein. The distal vein is tied to the stripper and then removed by pulling the vein through its subcutaneous tunnel. Whether to strip to the knee or to the ankle level is somewhat controversial given the proximity of the saphenous nerve to the vein at and below the knee. Stripping the vein to the ankle has a higher rate of saphenous nerve injury and the decision depends on the degree of disease in the below-knee great saphenous vein. At the ankle, the great saphenous vein should be exposed medially and slightly anterior to the medial malleolus. Careful exposure at the ankle includes identifying and separating the saphenous nerve from the vein to lessen the incidence of nerve injury resulting in numbness in the foot.

(2) **Endovenous ablation** is a relatively new technique for treating superficial saphenous vein reflux. **Laser and radiofrequency ablation (RFA) are the two available methods and are less invasive than traditional vein stripping**. The entire procedure is performed under ultrasound guidance. The great saphenous vein is accessed percutaneously, a sheath placed over the wire into the vein and the laser or radiofrequency fiber positioned in the vein just distal to the saphenofemoral junction. We begin the ablation 1.5 to 2 cm distal to the junction, as beginning closer can lead to transmission of energy into the deep venous system and increase the risk of DVT. A good rule is to position the fiber just distal to the superficial epigastric vein, as this allows the stump of the saphenous vein to drain rather than acting as a potential "blind stump" for thrombosis. Dilute tumescent anesthesia is injected around the saphenous sheath for analgesia and to insulate the skin and adjacent nerves against injury. Endovenous ablation can be performed in an office setting with minimal sedation. **The initial success of endovenous RFA and laser ablation for treating saphenous reflux has been comparable to surgical stripping. Continued freedom from reflux is seen in 84% of patients at 5 years with RFA and greater than 93% at 2 years with laser.**

(3) **Stab phlebectomy** may be used in combination with stripping or endovascular ablation in order to treat tributary varicosities (Fig 19.3). In many cases, these are the only varicosities that the patient sees, as the saphenous vein itself may not bulge. Since these procedures are, in part, cosmetic; the skin incisions should be very small "stabs" over the premarked varicosities. A crochet hook or specially designed vein hook is then used to elevate the varicosity, which is then grasped with a hemostat and plucked out. Some surgeons remove only these obvious varicosities and preserve the great saphenous trunk. This approach is reasonable if the great saphenous vein is competent by duplex. However, most patients with large, symptomatic lower-limb varicose veins have a diffusely incompetent great saphenous vein and will be at high risk for recurrent varicosities if this underlying problem is untreated. Finally, skin incisions are closed with adsorbable subcuticular sutures or Demabond with or without Steri-Strips.

(4) **Post-procedural care.** After any procedure to treat varicosities, the leg is wrapped in a compressive gauze bandage with an elastic wrap from the toes to the groin. As most vein surgery is performed in the outpatient setting, the patient is instructed to keep the operated leg elevated for a night. The next

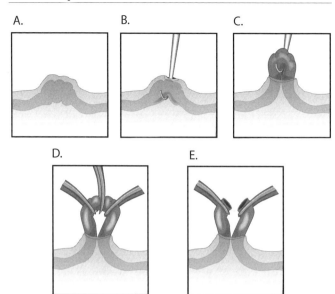

Figure 19.3.   **The technique of stab phlebectomy to excise varicose tributaries. (A, B)** The varicosity is visualized and a small stab incision is made directly over it. The dermis is undermined. **(C)** A crochet hook or specially designed ven hook is used to elevate the vein. **(D)** Once above the skin, the vein is grasped with hemostats and divided with scissors. **(E)** Each end is romoved by taut traction on the hemostat.

morning, the dressings are removed and a new below-the-knee elastic bandage or stocking is applied. The patient should ambulate every 2 hours for 5 to 10 minutes, beginning on the first postoperative day.

After endovascular ablation, patients are encouraged to ambulate immediately. The patient should return in 2 to 3 days for a duplex, to ensure no interval development of DVT and to reconfirm successful ablation of the vein. The patient is rechecked in the office after 2 to 4 weeks. Below-the-knee elastic support stockings are continued for a minimum of 2 weeks. For some patients, this support is continued for several more weeks to alleviate mild leg swelling and dependent heaviness that may follow lower-extremity venous procedures.

(5) Complications. Wound cellulitis, hematomas, and bruising can occur after vein stripping or endovenous ablation. Bruising and pain are more common after laser than radiofrequency ablation. Below-the-knee stripping or inadequate tumescence with ablation procedures can increase the risk of saphenous nerve injury resulting in temporary paresthesias or numbness in the foot. Recurrent reflux can present through the saphenous vein or through accessory veins years after ablation and neovascularization after saphenous stripping can result in new pathways of reflux and varicosities. DVT is the most dreaded postoperative complication after endovenous ablation and for this reason most patients undergo surveillance duplex several days and again one month after the procedure. Overall, the incidence of DVT is less than 1% and occurs in the calf veins more commonly than in the common femoral vein. Careful positioning of the tip of the fiber caudal to the saphenofemoral junction, adequate tumescent insulation around the saphenous vein, and early ambulation may reduce the risk of DVT.

c. **Subfascial endoscopic perforating vein surgery (SEPS)** can be performed in patients with incompetent perforating veins and venous ulceration. Perforators often occur at the sites of ulceration, and interruption of venous hypertension at this level may be necessary to achieve healing. **Data from the North American SEPS registry demonstrates favorable results, with 88% of ulcers healed at one year after an average of 54 days. However, at 2 years ulcers recur in 46% of post-thrombotic limbs compared to 20% in patients with primary valvular incompetence**. Over two-thirds of these patients underwent concomitant treatment for superficial varicosities (e.g., stripping, stab phlebectomy). No randomized, prospective trial has proven greater benefit of perforator interruption for healing ulcers or preventing recurrence versus best medical therapy (e.g., compression, wound care). In current practice, SEPS may be combined with treatment of saphenous reflux, particularly when large incompetent perforators are present beneath ulcers. Otherwise, SEPS may be applied on a selective basis if the initial treatment of superficial reflux fails to heal the ulcer. Open subfascial ligation using the classic Linton operation has largely been abandoned due to unacceptably high wound complication rates. New methods of treating perforating veins include ablation with a specially designed RFA probe and duplex-guided foam sclerotherapy.

Success with SEPS requires **meticulous attention to the details of surgical technique and postoperative care.** Several principles must be emphasized:

(1) SEPS is indicated in patients with active (C6) and healed (C5) ulcers in the setting of chronic venous insufficiency. Invasive infection and wound necrosis should be under control before the procedure.

(2) Before the operation, duplex is used to ascertain patency and incompetency of both the superficial and deep venous systems. Incompetent perforators are also localized and marked preoperatively with duplex imaging.

(3) Surgery is performed with two ports in the lower leg, one for a camera and one for dissection. Carbon

dioxide is used to insufflate the subfascial space, similar to standard laparoscopic techniques. Perforators are divided under direct vision with clips or a harmonic scalpel.

(4) After surgery, the operated leg should be elevated for 3 hours, after which ambulation is allowed. Essentially, patients undergo postoperative care similar to that following saphenous vein stripping.

(5) Perioperative heparin can be used for patients considered at moderate to high risk for DVT or if bedrest is initiated for any period of time.

(6) If wound healing appears satisfactory at the first dressing change, a compressive elastic Ace wrap is reapplied from the toes to below the knee. This bandage is essential until any sutures are removed. Then, a 30 to 40 mm Hg below-knee compression stocking is prescribed.

(7) Patients who undergo SEPS must understand that they must continue to wear below-the-knee elastic support hose following operation, as the procedure does not correct the deep venous hypertension due to valvular incompetence.

d. Open surgery for chronic deep venous insufficiency is performed at specialized centers and only for severe cases failing best medical therapy. Direct repair of venous valves (valvuloplasty) is most effective for primary venous reflux. Valve transfer (e.g,. axillary to femoropopliteal) may be superior to valvuloplasty for incompetent, severely damaged valves as a result of postthrombotic syndrome. The presence of venous obstruction is associated with more debilitating symptoms (swelling, venous claudication) than reflux alone, and most often occurs as a result of incomplete recanalization after DVT. **Unilateral iliofemoral obstruction can be treated with a crossover femoral-femoral bypass using the saphenous vein (Palma method).** Open venous reconstructions are technically demanding operations with modest long-term success, thus limiting their applicability to well-selected and motivated patients.

Endovascular treatment has been lauded in recent years as a minimally invasive and highly successful modality in patients with chronic iliofemoral obstruction. Perhaps the most common cause of primary venous obstruction is May-Thurner syndrome. This condition results from excessive compression of the left iliac vein by the crossover of the right iliac artery and usually occurs in young women. **In a recent report of 982 iliofemoral stents placed for primary venous obstruction, 6-year patency rates are 79% with assisted primary patency achieving 100%.** Patients with secondary (post-thrombotic) iliofemoral obstruction also have commendable long-term results, although not quite as good as those for primary obstruction.

II. Acute venous thromboembolism.

   A. Prevention. Several prophylactic measures may decrease the incidence of venous thromboembolism, especially in sick patients at bedrest. These preventive measures may be organized conveniently around **Virchow's etiologic triad** for venous thrombosis: stasis, hypercoagulability, and endothelial injury.

1. Stasis. Prolonged immobilization of the lower extremities is perhaps the single most important event that precedes DVT. At bedrest, blood tends to pool in large, valveless venous sinuses of the calf muscles. The soleus venous plexus normally drains anteriorly into the tibial veins. Consequently, if the body is supine, blood pools in the calf muscles unless these muscles contract to empty the calf veins. Historically, ^{125}I-labeled fibrinogen studies show that calf vein thrombosis often begins while the patient is supine on the operating table.

Venous stasis in the calf may be prevented by elevation and intermittent or continuous mechanical compression of the leg. Simply elevating the leg 15 to 20 degrees improves emptying of major leg veins but may not completely empty the soleus venous sinuses. Likewise, graduated compression stockings may hasten flow in the tibial veins but not completely empty the soleus plexus where clots often begin. **Several studies have confirmed that intermittent pneumatic leg compression reduces postoperative DVT, especially in urologic and neurosurgical patients**. However, patients may not be consistently compliant with wearing these devices, finding them uncomfortable, unwieldy, or unimportant. Early mobilization and ambulation should be encouraged in all patients able to bear weight. Finally, one of the simplest, yet most effective, methods of preventing calf vein stasis is to have the patient exercise the legs (plantar flexion) against a footboard for 5 minutes every hour. This exercise not only promotes venous flow but actually may enhance fibrinolytic activity, which clears small clots. We have found that patients will exercise regularly when the importance of these exercises is explained to them and encouragement is given after the operation. Patients at higher risk for thromboembolism generally receive pneumatic compression devices on the lower extremities and/or some type of anticoagulant therapy, such as low-dose heparin or low-molecular weight heparin (Table 19.1).

2. Hypercoagulability. Acute DVT is more likely to occur in patients with some abnormality of coagulation (Chapter 3). Coagulation defects may be acquired or inherited. Low levels of antithrombin III have been found in women taking oral contraceptives. Antithrombin III activity also diminishes while thrombin activity increases with soft-tissue trauma and operative wounding. Increased platelet adhesiveness may be another problem that predisposes certain patients to recurrent DVT. Lupus anticoagulant and anticardiolipin antibodies are acquired as a result of autoimmune activity and may also be identified in patients in the absence of an autoimmune disorder. Recurrent venous thromboembolism has been correlated with congen-

Table 19.1.   Anticoagulants used for thrombotic prophylaxis and disorders

Trade Name	Generic	DVT Prophylaxis	Treatment for Acute DVT
Unfractionated heparin			
	Heparin sulfate	5,000 U s.c. 1–2 h preoperatively; then 5,000 U s.c. q8–12 h	40–80 U/kg IV bolus and 2–18 U/kg/h IV infusion (adjust for aPTT ratio 1.5–2.5x)
LMWH			
Fragmin (Pfizer, New York, NY)	Dalteparin	2,500 U s.c. 1–2 h preoperatively; then 5,000 U s.c. daily	120 U/kg s.c. q12h
Lovenox (Sanofi-Aventis, Bridgewater, NJ)	Enoxaparin	20–40 mg s.c. 1–2 h preoperatively; then 40 mg s.c. q24h or 30 mg s.c. q12h	1.5 mg/kg s.c. q24h or 1 mg/kg s.c. q12h
Direct thrombin inhibitors			
Refludan (Bayer Health Care, Wayne, NJ)[a]	Lepirudin (recombinant hirudin)		0.4 mg/kg IV bolus; then 0.15 mg/kg/hr IV continuous infusion (adjust for aPTT ratio 1.5–2.5x)
Argatroban (GlaxoSmithKline, London, UK)[a]			2 mcg/kg/min IV (adjust to aPTT ratio 1.5–3x)
Anti-Xa inhibitor			
Arixtra (GlaxoSmithKline, London, UK)	Fondaparinux	2.5 mg s.c. q24h	7.5 mg s.c. q24h

LMWH, low molecular weight heparin.
[a]Indicated for anticoagulation in setting of heparin-induced thrombocytopenia

ital deficiencies of protein C and protein S, antithrombin
III, a single point mutation in factor V Leiden causing activated protein C resistance, prothrombin gene 20210A
mutation, and abnormal levels of fibrinogen and plasminogen. **Of these, the most common inherited hypercoagulable state is the factor V Leiden mutation.
Screening for these hypercoagulable states is appropriate in certain patients with recurrent, idiopathic
DVT (Chapter 3).**

Certain patients are at increased risk of DVT and PE.
They usually are referred to as **high-risk patients** and
include those who have experienced (a) previous venous
thromboembolism; (b) lower-extremity trauma (e.g., hip
fracture) and other orthopedic surgery of the hip, knee, or
lower limb; (c) major pelvic operations (e.g., open prostate-
ctomy or gynecologic operations); (d) prolonged bed rest or
extremity immobility (e.g., stroke or back surgery); (e)
acute myocardial infarction; (f) chronic congestive heart
failure; and (g) malignancies (e.g., pancreatic cancer), as
well as those on (h) oral contraceptives. Prophylactic, low-
dose anticoagulation does offer high-risk patients significant protection against venous thromboembolism.

Several anticoagulant agents are available: low molecular weight heparin (LMWH), low-dose unfractionated
heparin, warfarin, and direct Xa inhibitors (fondaparinux).
Of course, the risk of anticoagulant therapy in surgical
patients is bleeding, but major bleeding complications are
rare if therapy is properly delivered and monitored and certain contraindications are observed. **These contraindications include an active peptic ulcer, intracranial or
visceral injury, hemorrhagic diathesis, gastrointestinal bleeding, severe hypertension, and gross hematuria or hemoptysis.**

a. Adjusted-dose warfarin can be an effective prophylaxis for venous thrombosis, however, there is not
widespread acceptance of this strategy. The dosage may
be difficult to regulate and an excessively prolonged prothrombin time is associated with increased bleeding
complications. Recommendations from the American
College of Chest Physicians only include warfarin prophylaxis as an option for elective hip or knee surgery
patients.

b. Unfractionated heparin has received widespread
attention for its use in the prevention of fatal postoperative PE. Compared to those who receive no prophylaxis,
heparin-treated patients experience a 40% reduction in
nonfatal and a 64% reduction in fatal PE. The usual
dosage has been a loading dose of 5,000 units given subcutaneously, 2 hours prior to operation and then 5,000
units every 8 to 12 hours until the patient is ambulatory.
Low-dose heparin enhances antithrombin III activity
with minimal to no change in coagulation tests although
bleeding and wound complications may be slightly
higher in patients on prophylactic heparin. Therefore,
the use of prophylactic heparin should be reserved for
those at increased risk of thromboembolism, including

patients with prior venous thromboembolism, those immobilized for long periods, and those subjected to major surgical procedures.

c. Low molecular weight heparin (LMWH) has three potential advantages over unfractionated heparin: (1) effective prophylaxis with once-daily administration, (2) improved efficacy, and (3) a lower frequency of bleeding. LMWHs have higher bioavailability and extended half-life compared to unfractionated heparin. Compared to unfractionated heparin, LMWH has greater anti-Xa activity compared to anti-IIa activity, which may reduce the risk of bleeding complications without compromising efficacy. Several randomized clinical trials have demonstrated that LMWH is as effective and as safe as unfractionated heparin in the prophylaxis against venous thromboembolism (VTE).

d. Data showing efficacy of **antiplatelet agents or dextrans** for VTE prophylaxis is equivocal and their use for this purpose is not supported by current guidelines.

e. Fondaparinux is a synthetic pentasaccharide that acts exclusively as a factor Xa inhibitor. With a long half-life, dosing is once a day subcutaneously, although renal excretion limits its use in patients with renal insufficiency. Fondaparinux is currently approved for VTE prophylaxis in orthopedic and general surgery patients. This agent has shown improved efficacy compared to LMWH in patients after hip or knee surgery, although bleeding risk may be slightly higher.

3. Vein injury. During elective operations, meticulous attention must be given to the gentle dissection and handling of veins. Large-vein injuries should be repaired by fine lateral suture technique and ligation should be avoided. The surgeon also must avoid prolonged compression of the vena cava or other large veins with retractors or packs. Experimental studies have also documented endothelial tears that occur in extremity veins remote from an elective operative site. These endothelial lesions may become the focus of DVT.

B. Diagnosis. Patient history and physical examination frequently are unreliable in establishing an accurate diagnosis of either acute DVT or PE. **In fact, about 75% of patients who are evaluated for suspected venous thrombosis or PE do not have these conditions.** Since either condition requires systemic anticoagulation, with its potential complications, we recommend the following approach to ensure that an accurate diagnosis is established.

1. Superficial thrombophlebitis generally is recognized by the physical findings of a tender superficial venous cord in the upper or lower extremity. Usually, there is no deep vein involvement. If the process extends to the groin, extension into the deep femoral system may be present. Duplex is the best method to ascertain thrombotic involvement of the common femoral vein, which may occur in 5% to 40% of patients and sometimes in the contralateral leg. It is noteworthy that a given percentage of these patients may be hypercoagulable due to an inherited or acquired condition, and careful personal and family history should be obtained

with this in mind. Superficial thrombophlebitis not infrequently affects a preexisting varicose vein, and vein
removal may be indicated in recurrent cases.

2. DVT is suggested by leg pain, swelling, and tenderness.
Since these findings are not specific for venous thrombosis,
treatment generally should not be started without confirmation by duplex examination. Phlegmasia alba dolens
and phlegmasia cerulea dolens are dramatic clinical presentations of DVT manifested by massive leg swelling with
white or blue discoloration, respectively. Rarely, these may
progress to venous gangrene.

> **a.** Compression **duplex ultrasonography** is highly
> sensitive (sensitivity, 90% to 100%) for detecting proxi-
> mal femoropopliteal vein thrombosis, but is less sensi-
> tive (60% to 90%) for detecting calf-vein thrombosis.
> Noninvasive studies, however, have limitations espe-
> cially in the pelvic veins, below the knee, and in the pro-
> funda femoris vein. Also, duplex may be difficult to
> interpret if the patient had a previous DVT that has not
> recanalized. If the results of noninvasive tests are nor-
> mal, other etiologies for the leg symptoms are investi-
> gated. CTV, MR venography, or invasive venography is
> reserved for those rare patients with equivocal duplex
> results and an elevated clinical suspicion of DVT, such as
> with isolated iliac vein thrombosis.
>
> **b.** Plasma **D-Dimer** is a fibrin-specific product, and
> therefore a marker of fibrinolysis, which may be ele-
> vated with venous thrombosis. The D-Dimer test has
> emerged as a useful screening test to rule out DVT. **In
> outpatients with a low clinical likelihood of DVT
> and a normal D-Dimer level, the negative predic-
> tive value exceeds 99% and duplex is probably
> unnecessary**.

**3. PE is a condition in which thrombus (i.e., clot) has
migrated or embolized through the right heart and
into one of the pulmonary arteries obstructing flow
of unoxygenated blood to that segment of lung.**
Depending upon the size of the pulmonary embolus, it may
cause significant strain on the right heart and often presents with chest pain, dyspnea, and, occasionally, hemoptysis. The source of the emboli is nearly always the leg or
pelvic veins. Similar symptoms may occur with myocardial
ischemia, bronchitis, pneumonia, or pleurisy, so PE must
be confirmed by other tests. Given that the mortality of
untreated PE is great, it is important to maintain a high
index of suspicion and to have a low threshold for pursu-
ing diagnostic testing and early treatment with anticoagulation.

> **a.** Although hypoxia demonstrated on **arterial blood
> gas testing** is common with PE, a low arterial PO_2 is
> not diagnostic. Other laboratory tests may be abnormal
> but often are inconclusive. **Electrocardiographic
> abnormalities** may include a rhythm disturbance and
> ST segment depression or T-wave inversion, particularly
> in leads III, aVF, V1, V4, and V5. These findings are
> indicative of myocardial ischemia associated with acute

PE. **The classic finding of S1, Q3, T3 (S wave in lead I, Q-wave and T-wave inversion in III) is uncommon unless the PE causes acute right heart strain.** In many patients, the only ECG finding is sinus tachycardia. The ECG is most important to rule out an acute myocardial infarction as the cause of chest pain. The chest radiograph may look normal, although in seriously ill patients it may show infiltrates from pneumonitis or atelectasis. An x-ray is therefore important to examine for other potential pulmonary pathology.

b. Ventilation/perfusion lung scanning (V/Q scan) uses a radioisotope to identify areas of disproportionate lung perfusion that may occur as a result of PE. False-positive V/Q tests may occur in patients due to preexisting lung pathology such as asthma, emphysema, chronic bronchitis, pneumonitis, or neoplasm. Consequently, the chest radiograph should be checked before a lung scan to identify any disease process that may affect the scan. In properly performed and interpreted scans, normal results essentially exclude a significant pulmonary embolus. High-probability scans predict the presence of PE in about 90% of patients. However, the majority of V/Q scans fall into the "intermediate probability" category, often necessitating further diagnostic testing. Although V/Q scanning has historically been the screening test of choice for PE, in recent years spiral CT has been popularized due to its speed and specificity. However, some patients are unable to undergo CT due to severe dye allergy, renal insufficiency, or limited hospital resources.

c. Helical CT is a rapid and acute method for the detection of pulmonary emboli. In many institutions, helical CT has become the test of choice for emergency room and hospitalized patients and can be performed and resulted within minutes. CT is able to directly visualize the location of emboli, whether they are in the central, segmental, or subsegmental branches. The appearance of the lung parenchyma and chest structures is noted in addition to the pulmonary vasculature. Whereas V/Q scan results may be clouded by intrinsic lung disease, CT may demonstrate a differential diagnosis (e.g., effusion, pneumonia) to more fully explain the clinical situation. Compared with pulmonary angiography, the traditional gold standard, helical CT has sensitivity and specificity of 90% to 100%. The limitations of CT are mostly in the detection of small subsegmental emboli, although the newest scanners can detect these with great accuracy. By timing contrast injection and performing delayed imaging, CT venography of the legs can also be added to the initial PE scan. This adjuvant imaging provides even greater sensitivity to the examination by identifying deep venous thromboses. The presence of DVT in association with high clinical suspicion for PE, despite negative helical CT for emboli, likely warrants further imaging or empiric anticoagulation.

d. Pulmonary arteriography remains the definitive diagnostic test for PE if V/Q scanning or helical CT scan cannot define a diagnosis. One must remember that most pulmonary emboli resolve over a period of days to several weeks, and, consequently, a pulmonary arteriogram may look normal after a while. Although pulmonary angiography has been the gold standard for diagnosis, it is rarely performed due to a 3% to 4% risk of complications from this invasive procedure.

C. Treatment. In Chapter 2, we emphasize that the natural history of DVT and PE may be altered by anticoagulation. In certain situations, catheter-based and/or surgical intervention also may help the patient. **Specifically, catheter-directed thrombolytic therapy has added another important alternative to managing serious DVT and PE.**

1. Treatment of **superficial thrombophlebitis** depends on the extent of the phlebitis and the general health of the patient. Elastic support, local heat, and an anti-inflammatory medication (e.g., aspirin or a nonsteroidal anti-inflammatory agent) may relieve localized superficial phlebitis. The inflammation results in erythema that resembles cellulitis; however, infection is rarely present and antibiotics are generally not indicated. Resolution may take 7 to 14 days. Anticoagulation is reserved for patients in whom DVT is documented or in whom the phlebitis extends to the saphenofemoral junction and deep venous extension seems likely. If the thrombophlebitis is confined to superficial veins and the patient is a good operative risk, excision of the thrombosed vein and ligation and stripping of the greater saphenous vein may be curative and may shorten the time of disability. Likewise, the patient with recurrent superficial thrombophlebitis can benefit from removal of the affected vein. Rarely, suppurative thrombophlebitis can result from an intravenous line infection, and should be treated with antibiotics, warm compresses, and occasionally resection or open drainage of the vein to prevent septicemia.

2. For **established DVT,** standard therapy is initiated with a form of heparin followed by a longer course of warfarin (Table 19.1). The goal of anticoagulation is to prevent the propagation of thrombus or embolism to the pulmonary circulation. Anticoagulation does not dissolve the present clot, but allows the patient's inherent fibrinolytic system to eliminate the thrombus over months.

a. Continuous heparin infusion has been associated with fewer bleeding complications than intermittent intravenous therapy. The patient is systemically heparinized with an intravenous bolus of 5,000 to 10,000 units (100 units/kilogram), followed by a continuous infusion based on a weight-based protocol (usually 1,000–1,500 units/h). Although the ideal method of monitoring heparin therapy is debatable, an activated partial thromboplastin time test (aPTT) is the standard in most hospitals. Anticoagulation is considered adequate when these test values are at least 1.5 to 2.0 times the pretreatment values. It is extremely important to achieve therapeutic levels within 24 hours, as subtherapeutic levels have been associated with recurrent thromboembolism in randomized trials. There is a common misconception that an aPTT greater than twice normal (usually >100 seconds) is associated with more bleeding complications. On the contrary, clinical trials demonstrate a lack of association between a supratherapeutic aPTT (ratio of 2.5 or greater) and the risk of clinically important hemorrhage. **Recent clinical trials indicate that the length of heparin therapy can be shortened to 5 days without loss of effectiveness or safety if oral anticoagulants are started on the first or second day of treatment for DVT or PE.**

Platelet counts should also be checked at least every other day, since heparin may induce thrombocytopenia. **Heparin-induced thrombocytopenia (HIT)** generally is recognized at least 3 days after onset of therapy, and appears more commonly in patients with prior heparin exposure. HIT occurs with an incidence of 1% to 5% with UFH and can result from an immune reaction to the heparin-platelet complex. **A smaller percentage of patients with antiplatelet antibodies experience profound platelet aggregation and clumping that can lead to the devastating syndrome of HIT with thrombosis.** This condition can result in paradoxical arterial and venous thrombosis despite heparin therapy. In any patient with a decreased platelet level on heparin, antiplatelet antibodies should be checked. The treatment of HIT is to stop all heparin, including heparin flushes and heparin-coated lines, as this condition is not a dose-dependent phenomenon. **If continued anticoagulation is necessary, alternative agents such as recombinant hirudins or argatroban can be used (Table 19.1 and Chapter 3).**

b. LMWH has been proven in clinical trials to be equally effective as UFH in the treatment of DVT. LMWHs have several advantages over UFH. Their bioavailability is better due to lesser plasma protein binding. The dosage is a convenient once or twice per day, subcutaneously, with no need for monitoring of levels. LMWHs act more specifically on factor Xa, rather than thrombin, which may lessen the risk of bleeding. LMWHs are weight-based and do not need monitoring, which avoids the frequent blood draws that are needed for monitoring UFH. **The incidence of heparin-induced thrombocytopenia with LMWH is ten times less than with unfractionated heparins.** Outpatient treatment is also practical for selected cases of first-time, uncomplicated DVT in conjunction with the initiation of warfarin therapy. Unfractionated heparin should be used for complicated venous thrombosis, suggested by significant symptoms, large thrombus burden, or recurrent thrombosis. In these more complicated cases of DVT, admission to the hospital allows for leg elevation, observation for phlegmasia, and consideration of catheter-directed thrombolysis in appropriate candidates. A meta-analysis of the literature has concluded that **the relative risk of recurrent thromboembolic events with initial LMW heparin compared with standard heparin is similar (odds ratio of 0.85), but bleeding risk and mortality rates favor LMWH group (odds ratio 0.71 and 0.57, respectively).**

c. Oral anticoagulation with warfarin is started during heparin therapy and is continued for 3 to 6 months. During this period, the deep veins usually recanalize slowly. Since warfarin inhibits coagulation by inhibiting liver synthesis of vitamin K–dependent clotting factors (II, VII, IX, X), which have long half-lives, anticoagulation with oral agents requires several days of therapy before the patient is anticoagulated. Additionally, warfarin inhibits the synthesis of the anticoagulant protein C, which has a fairly short half-life causing a relative prothrombotic state during the first several days after starting warfarin. Heparin therapy during these first few days keeps the patient anticoagulated until eventually all of the vitamin K–dependent factors have been effectively inhibited.

To standardize the PT for oral anticoagulation, the World Health Organization has developed an international reference (INR) thromboplastin from human brain tissue and has recommended that the PT be expressed as this INR. With the past conventional use of rabbit brain thromboplastin reagents, a PT ratio of 1.3 to 1.5 (16 to 20 seconds) corresponds to an INR of 2.0 to 3.0. Clinical trials support less intense oral warfarin therapy (INR of 2.0 to 3.0) for most conditions requiring anticoagulation.

As previously mentioned, when warfarin is started, protein C levels fall more quickly than the other vitamin K–dependent factors resulting in a transient prothrombotic state. Patients with underlying protein C deficiency may be particularly at risk for warfarin-induced skin necrosis, which appears typically on the breasts, buttocks, and thighs. The safest method of instituting warfarin therapy is the nonloading technique, administering an average dose (we suggest 5 to 7.5 mg) orally each day until INR is in the therapeutic range. Dose alterations can be made, keeping in mind that a particular dose of warfarin is not reflected until the peak effect 36 to 72 hours later. A heparin "bridge" should be initiated prior to warfarin in order to counteract warfarin's transient thrombogenicity and in order to begin to treat the clinical thrombosis. **The target INR for warfarin should be 2.0 to 3.0 for at least two days before stopping the heparin.** A more prolonged INR places the patient at increased risk of bleeding complications. It may be continued longer or indefinitely in patients with ongoing risk factors for venous thromboembolism. For patients who cannot take warfarin (e.g., pregnant women) full dose subcutaneous LMWH may be administered (usually 1mg/kg daily) for extended periods of time.

d. Leg pain and swelling can range from mild or absent with calf thrombi to severe with larger and more proximal iliofemoral thrombosis. Leg elevation above the level of the heart is important to minimize swelling. Bedrest is no longer considered standard for smaller DVTs, and patients are permitted to ambulate ad lib. Before discharge, patients should be fitted for 30 to 40 mm Hg compression stockings, which are part of a long-term strategy to minimize the morbidity associated with postphlebitic syndrome. **The consistent use of compression hose for several years after proximal DVT is the only therapy proven in randomized trials to reduce the risk of developing symptoms of post-thrombotic syndrome such as skin changes and ulcers.**

e. The role of **catheter-directed thrombolytic therapy for acute DVT** is still debated despite clinical evidence demonstrating its effectiveness in proximal DVT of less than 72 hours in duration. The initial goal of treating DVT is to prevent clot propagation and PE. Although standard treatment with anticoagulation treats this problem, it does not prevent the long-term sequelae of post-thrombotic syndrome. Years afterward, only a minority of patients are completely recanalized, whereas most have residual obstruction and valvular damage. Patients with iliofemoral DVT are particularly at risk for developing severe post-thrombotic syndrome. Intuitively, early lysis of the thrombus would seem beneficial and support for this lies with studies demonstrating that early spontaneous recanalization more often results in preserved valvular function.

The National Venous Registry has reported a large experience from a number of centers using catheter-based techniques of pharmacologic thrombolysis. Complete lysis was achieved in 65% of patients. Among those who had a first-time DVT and experienced complete lysis, 96% maintained a 1 year vein patency. Favorable results are also seen in quality of life questionnaires at follow-up 1 to 2 years later. Thrombolysis is contraindicated in patients with recent internal bleeding (within 2 months), cerebrovascular accidents, or other active intracranial disease. It also may cause serious hemorrhage after recent (within about 10 days) major surgery or obstetric delivery, organ biopsy, and previous puncture of a noncompressible vessel. Although life-threatening complications such as intracranial hemorrhage are rare ($<1\%$), careful patient selection is important to minimize this risk. In addition, thrombolytic therapy must be used only by physicians who are completely familiar with its dosage and contraindications and in a setting in which therapy can be continuously monitored. Catheter-directed thrombolytic therapy for DVT has yet to be compared to standard anticoagulation in a large randomized trial. Long-term follow-up in such a trial would be needed to determine the potential impact on post-thrombotic syndrome.

The technique of venous thrombolysis is most often used in patients with extensive iliofemoral thrombosis and/or phlegmasia cerulea dolens. With the patient in a prone position, the popliteal vein can be accessed via ultrasound guidance, and a sheath is placed in the femoral-popliteal vein. Many clinicians have combined the use of mechanical thrombolysis using one of several commercially available devices with pharmacologic lysis (Chapter 11). The mechanical component allows for debulking of the thrombus, and can hasten the process of thrombolysis and may reduce the amount of thrombolytic needed to achieve an acceptable result. The Angiojet (Possis Medical, Minneapolis, MN) is one mechanical thrombectomy device that functions by creating a Venturi effect to break up and then evacuate the thrombus. A thrombolytic catheter (e.g., "soaker hose catheter") with multiple side holes is then positioned within the clot, and lytic agent can be infused at a continuous rate. Low dose heparin infusion is usually administered through the sheath concomitantly. Venograms are performed over 12-hour intervals to monitor the success of lysis. During this period, patients are monitored in the ICU, with periodic checks of the aPTT and fibrinogen levels. Bleeding at the sheath site may be treated by holding the lytic agent temporarily. Once lysis is complete, venography and intravascular ultrasound should be used to evaluate for residual stenosis. These stenoses are best treated by venoplasty and occasionally stenting.

Subclavian-axillary venous thrombosis may be associated with central venous catheters or thoracic outlet syndrome. If a catheter is present in the affected vein, it should be removed and systemic heparin administered just as for lower-extremity DVTs in order to minimize the risk of PE. Catheter-directed thrombolytic therapy is encouraged in younger patients with thoracic outlet syndrome and effort thrombosis (i.e., Paget-Schroetter syndrome). This may be performed via a lytic catheter inserted through the antecubital or basilic vein into the subclavian vein. Of course, definitive treatment requires surgical correction of the thoracic outlet compression once the vein has been recanalized with the thrombolytic therapy. This operation involves removal of a portion of the first rib, removal of a cervical rib (if present), division of any fibrous or constricting bands, and release of scalene muscle compression (Fig. 5.1 and Chapter 18). The timing of thoracic outlet surgery is controversial. While some advocate delay between thrombolysis and surgical treatment of 2 to 3 months, others prefer to treat the thoracic outlet during the initial hospitalization. Regardless, warfarin should be continued for a period of at least 3 months after the acute thrombosis.

f. Surgical thrombectomy for acute DVT has had less than spectacular results over the years. Nonetheless, patients with phlegmasia cerulea dolens who are not candidates for thrombolysis should be considered for this rarely performed procedure. An arteriovenous fistula is performed at the end of the procedure in order to help maintain long-term venous patency. Surgical thrombectomy is not a substitute for anticoagulation, as full heparinization followed by conversion to warfarin must be continued after the procedure to prevent early rethrombosis.

g. The **management of DVT during pregnancy** begins with the establishment of a solid diagnosis, usually made with duplex, although MRV can be useful for cases of proximal DVT. V/Q scan is the test of choice to rule out PE during pregnancy, as it avoids the radiation exposure associated with CT. **Warfarin crosses the placenta and is contraindicated during pregnancy. Subcutaneous LMW heparin provides an adequate means of full anticoagulation, and has a lower risk of osteoporosis and heparin-induced thrombocytopenia when compared to long-term UFH.** Full anticoagulation is accomplished using LMWH during the pregnancy and then near the time of delivery, the patient is admitted for a "heparin window." The LMWH is stopped and intravenous heparin, which has a short half-life, is started. The intravenous heparin is stopped prior to the delivery and then restarted following the delivery. Temporary vena cava filters have been used in pregnant women at high risk for PE, and must be placed in a suprarenal position in order to prevent compression by the gravid uterus.

3. PE is a potentially life-threatening event from acute DVT. Many patients with clinically silent DVTs experience PE as their initial clinical presentation. Untreated, the mortality of PE is extremely high. In some situations, such as unexplained and rapid cardiopulmonary demise, there may be a role for empiric initiation of treatment (heparin) until diagnostic testing can be completed.

PE also requires systemic heparinization followed by long-term oral anticoagulation. The dosages methods of administration and duration of therapy are the same as those used for acute DVT. Heparin and warfarin are intended to prevent further thromboembolism or clot propagation within the lung. They do little to resolve an existing thrombus. In select patients with massive acute PE, intravenous thrombolytic can be administered. One regimen is 100 mg of tPA intravenously over 2 hours. Emergency pulmonary embolectomy either by percutaneous suction catheter or surgery is indicated for salvageable patients who have documented massive PE and persistent refractory hypotension despite maximum medical therapy. In select patients with chronic organized pulmonary thromboemboli and pulmonary hypertension, elective pulmonary embolectomy also may improve chronic hypoxia and respiratory disability.

Vena cava filter placement is indicated for recurrent PE in patients who are fully anticoagulated or in situations where anticoagulation is contraindicated or not possible. Contraindications to anticoagulation usually include gastrointestinal hemorrhage, recent stroke or neurosurgery, or hemorrhage requiring transfusion after anticoagulation was started. Elderly patients at high risk for falls may also be poor candidates for anticoagulation. **Filters are usually deployed in the inferior vena cava below the renal veins and function by capturing thromboemboli and preventing them from traveling to the pulmonary arteries**. Vena cava filters can be placed percutaneously under fluoroscopic or ultrasound guidance via a femoral or jugular approach.

In general, filter placement is a safe and quick procedure that can be performed in an angiogram suite or at the bedside in the intensive care unit in critically ill patients. Complications of vena cava filters include misplacement, recurrent PE (<5%), caval occlusion or thrombosis, migration, and caval penetration. Relative indications for filter placement have increased with the use of retrievable "temporary" filters. For example, filters have been placed in patients at high risk for venous thromboembolism, such as after major trauma or spinal cord injury and around the time of bariatric surgery. The retrievable filters can be removed with a second percutaneous procedure after a period of presumed thrombogenicity is over. However, long-term complications after permanent filter placement are rare, and the advantages of retrievable filters have yet to be shown in prospective trials.

SELECTED READING

Barwell JR, Davies CE, Deacon J, et al. Comparison of surgery and compression with compression alone in chronic venous ulceration (ESCHAR study): randomized controlled trial. *Lancet.* 2004;363:1854-1859.

Caparrelli DJ, Freischlag J. A unified approach to axillosubclavian venous thrombosis in a single hospital admission. *Semin Vasc Surg.* 2005;18:153-157.

Gloviczki P, Bergan JJ, Rhodes JM, et al. Mid-term results of endoscopic perforator vein interruption for chronic venous insufficiency: lessons learned from the North American Subfascial Endoscopic Perforator Surgery Registry. *J Vasc Surg.* 1999;29:489-502.

Gould MK, Dembitzer AD, Doyle RL, et al. Low-molecular-weight heparins compared with unfractionated heparin for treatment of acute deep venous thrombosis: a meta-analysis of randomized, controlled trials. *Ann Intern Med.* 1999;130:800-809.

Kelton JG. The pathophysiology of heparin-induced thrombocytopenia: biological basis for treatment. *Chest.* 2005;127:9S-20S.

Marston WA, Owens LV, Davies S, et al. Endovenous saphenous ablation corrects the hemodynamic abnormality in patients with CEAP clinical class 3-6 CVI due to superficial reflux. *Vasc Endovasc Surg.* 2006;40:125-130.

Meissner MH, Wakefield TW, Ascher E, et al. Acute venous disease: Venous thrombosis and venous trauma. *J Vasc Surg.* 2007;46 (suppl):25S-53S.

Meissner MH, Gloviczki P, Bergan J, et al. Primary chronic venous disorders. *J Vasc Surg.* 2007;46(suppl):54S-67S.

Meissner MH, Eklof B, Smith PC, et al. Secondary chronic venous disorders. *J Vasc Surg.* 2007;46(suppl):68S-83S.

Mewissen MW, Seabrook GR, Meissner MH, et al. Catheter-directed thrombolysis of lower extremity deep venous thrombosis: report of a national multicenter registry. *Radiology*. 1999;211:39-49.

Min RJ, Khilnani N, Zimmet SE. Endovascular laser treatment of saphenous vein reflux: long-term results. *J Vasc Interv Radiol*. 2003;14:991-996.

Neglén P, Hollis KC, Olivier J, Raju S. Stenting of the venous outflow in chronic venous disease: long-term stent-related outcome, clinical, and hemodynamic result. *J Vasc Surg*. 2007;46:979-990.

Puggioni A, Karla M, Carmo M, et al. Endovenous laser therapy and radiofrequency ablation of the great saphenous vein: analysis of early efficacy and complications. *J Vasc Surg*. 2005;42:488-493.

Stone WM, Tonnessen BH, Money SR. The new anticoagulants. *Perspect Vasc Surg Endovasc Ther*. 2007;19:332-335.

Winer-Muram HT, Rydberg J, Johnson MS, et al. Suspected acute pulmonary embolism: evaluation with multi-detector row CT versus digital subtraction pulmonary arteriography. *Radiology*. 2004;233:806-815.

CHAPTER 20

Hemodialysis Access

In 1972, an amendment to the Social Security Act provided Medicare coverage for patients suffering from end-stage renal disease (ESRD). The magnitude of the current expenditure is impressive, with over $19 billion spent on almost half a million patients with ESRD in 2005. Nearly 350,000 patients are dialysis dependent, with diabetes and hypertension the leading causes of ESRD, respectively. Patients with ESRD also suffer from a higher incidence of comorbid conditions such as chronic anemia, congestive heart failure, peripheral arterial disease, and metabolic bone disease. The five-year life expectancy of a patient on dialysis is merely 25%, with the largest percentage of deaths occurring from cardiac causes. With an aging population of ESRD patients, the magnitude of medical care and economic burden is expected to rise dramatically.

Procedures involving dialysis access are the most common vascular surgical procedures performed in the United States. A well-functioning and durable vascular access is truly a "lifeline" for patients on hemodialysis. Patients with a poorly functioning access or central venous dialysis catheters have increased morbidity and suffer frequent hospitalization for access-related complications such as thrombosis or infection. Management of vascular access requires the coordinated efforts of health care providers and a well-informed patient. The ideal care paradigm uses a multidisciplinary team of nephrologists, surgeons and interventionalists, dialysis nurses and technicians, diabetes educators, dieticians, and social workers. Patients with ESRD should be referred early to a vascular surgeon, prior to initiating dialysis, in hopes of establishing autogenous access (e.g., native arteriovenous fistula). Unfortunately, one of the most predictable aspects of chronic hemodialysis is the need for additional procedures in order to achieve, maintain, or restore access patency. Consequently, this chapter focuses on essentials in the initial evaluation, placement, and revision of hemodialysis accesses.

I. Indications for dialysis.

Chronic kidney failure from a loss of nephrons is measurable by a decrease in the glomerular filtration rate (GFR). A patient's GFR can be estimated from a formula using variables for serum creatinine, age, race, and gender. Chronic kidney failure with a GFR <15 mL/min is considered ESRD and correlates with the need for dialysis. Acute renal failure, which can result from a variety of etiologies, may also require dialysis. Dialysis is indicated when one or more of the following of the following clinical problems are present:

   A. Hyperkalemia (>6 mEq/L), especially when accompanied by ECG or neuromuscular abnormalities, requires immediate dialysis. Dietary restriction and potassium-bonding resins may suffice for lower levels of hyperkalemia.

   B. Fluid overload is another indication for both acute and chronic dialysis. This includes patients who have not responded satisfactorily to fluid restriction and diuretics.

C. Worsening acidosis results from the kidneys' inability to excrete hydrogen and resorb bicarbonate, and represents an indication for hemodialysis.

D. Drug overdose is a less common indication for hemodialysis but one that occasionally arises in an emergency room or critical care practice.

E. Uremic signs and symptoms are the most common indication for chronic dialysis as blood-urea-nitrogen (BUN) and serum creatinine levels rise. Neurologic symptoms related to uremia include lethargy, seizures, myoclonus, and peripheral neuropathy, and it has been shown that mortality and morbidity can be reduced if the BUN level is maintained below 100 mg/dL.

II. Access Planning.

First, whether dialysis is intended to be **temporary** or **permanent** must be ascertained. Patients who develop acute renal failure in the setting of previously normal renal function will often recover over a period of days to weeks. In contrast, patients who develop acute renal insufficiency in the setting of chronic renal failure are likely to require chronic dialysis. Patients with chronic renal failure (GFR <25 mL/min) should be referred to a vascular surgeon, preferably months to a year in advance of dialysis. The goal of initial consultation should be to obtain a thorough history and to perform an examination, with a focus on the potential options for vascular access. This visit should allow enough time for the creation and maturation of an autogenous arteriovenous (AV) fistula, whenever possible. Even when an autogenous fistula is not an option, establishing a rapport between surgeon and patient helps to facilitate realistic expectations regarding the location and durability of future access procedures.

A. A history of all prior access procedures should be recorded. The original date, type (fistula or graft), and location (forearm, upper arm, or thigh) for each access should be noted, in addition to the dates and methods of failure (e.g., thrombosis, infection, failure to mature). It is also important to ask about the number, location, and duration of prior central venous catheters. Patients with a history of indwelling catheter access have a significant probability of central venous stenoses or occlusions in the subclavian, jugular, and/or innominate veins. Right or left handedness is also noted, with preference for access placement given to the nondominant arm. However, even when the dominant arm harbors a more suitable vein the authors prefer an autogenous fistula in this arm rather than a prosthetic graft in the nondominant arm.

  1. Medical comorbidities such as poor cardiac function should be determined, as these can limit the long-term success of hemodialysis access. The choice of anesthesia (general, regional, or local) may also be influenced by the presence of serious comorbidities. Lastly, the presence of diabetes should be noted, as diabetics have overall the worst results with dialysis and pose a higher risk for hand ischemia due to steal from access procedures.

  2. The use of **antiplatelet and anticoagulant medications** should be noted and in some cases these should be held, depending upon the type of medication and/or planned access operation. These medications are particularly important to note, as patients with ESRD typically have platelet dysfunction as a consequence of associated uremia or thrombocytopenia. Generally, aspirin can be continued throughout most if not all access operations, although for those such as a basilic vein transposition that require larger incisions, one may consider stopping aspirin 5 days prior to the case. Because clopidogrel (Plavix) is a more potent antiplatelet agent, it should be held 7 to 10 days prior to elective access operations to reduce the risk of bleeding complications such as hematoma (Chapter 7). Similarly, because warfarin provides full anticoagulation, it should be held prior to access operations, although the anticoagulant effects typically wear off within 4 to 5 days. This can be confirmed by drawing a coagulation panel from the patient prior to the access operation.

3. Smoking negatively influences long-term access patency and all patients should be encouraged to quit preoperatively and provided access to formal smoking cessation programs if available (Chapter 7).

B. Physical examination is the primary determinant for the hemodialysis access site.

1. Surgical scars and location of previous access procedures are noted, including percutaneous or tunneled central venous catheters. **Skin conditions** must be noted for signs of infection or other dermatologic disorders that would impair healing.

2. The axillary, brachial, radial, and ulnar pulses should be palpated and blood pressure recorded in both arms. Decreased pulses or a difference in blood pressure of more than 10 mm Hg may indicate proximal arterial occlusive disease on the side with the lower pressure. The proximal subclavian arteries in the area of the supraclavicular fossa should also be auscultated, as the presence of a bruit would suggest an underlying arterial stenosis. Underlying arterial occlusive disease (i.e., inflow disease) is critical to recognize prior to the access procedure, as once the fistula is created, flow across any proximal arterial disease will increase, resulting in a decrease in pressures. This phenomenon is well recognized and can result in failure of the dialysis access, distal ischemia (i.e., steal), or both.

3. Perfusion of the hand should be thoroughly examined prior to creation of an upper-extremity dialysis access site. Specifically, performance of the **Allen test** provides a good assessment of radial and ulnar artery patency as well as patency of the palmar arch in the hand. This evaluation is especially important when planning for an access configuration that will use the radial artery as the inflow vessel (e.g., radiocephalic fistula). The dominant artery to the hand in more than 85% of patients is the ulnar artery, and confirmation of this indicates that diversion of flow from the radial artery will not significantly reduce perfusion to the hand. If during the Allen test the radial artery is found to be the dominant artery supplying the hand, one should consider using a different inflow vessel.

To perform the Allen test, first the hand should be elevated for a brief period of time. Then, with the patient making a tight fist, the examiner should compress the radial and ulnar arteries simultaneously. Separately, the radial and then the ulnar artery should be released as the examiner observes the opened hand for return of perfusion. If the ulnar artery is the dominant vessel, perfusion (i.e., color) will not return to the hand until it is released.

4. The extremities should be examined for swelling or edema, which would suggest the presence of **central venous outflow obstruction** (e.g., subclavian or innominate veins). Just as arterial inflow disease can be exacerbated by creation of a high-flow AV fistula, a central venous outflow obstruction can become quite symptomatic following creation dialysis access in the effected arm.

5. The **cephalic and basilic veins** should be inspected for patency and size. They should be palpated carefully for compressibility (normal vein) or firm cords (chronic thrombosis). Application of an upper arm tourniquet to increase distal venous filling is sometimes helpful in delineating veins that may be suitable for use in dialysis access configurations.

6. When peritoneal dialysis is being considered, the abdomen should be examined for prior surgical scars. Prior abdominal operations may compromise the placement of a chronic peritoneal dialysis catheter.

C. Noninvasive vascular laboratory testing is a critical part of the preoperative evaluation for hemodialysis access and has been shown to increase effectiveness and durability of access procedures.

1. Duplex ultrasound of the upper-extremity veins should be performed before access configuration is considered. Suitable veins for fistula formation can be identified by ultrasound that may be otherwise under-appreciated on basic physical examination. Additionally, direct and indirect evaluation of the central venous system can be achieved by duplex, which is especially important in individuals who have had prior central venous dialysis catheters. **Studies have shown an increase in the ability of the surgeon to provide autogenous AV fistulas to his or her patients if use of preoperative duplex is maximized**. These same studies report higher patency rates of such fistulas with the use of preoperative duplex, and this modality has also been found to be useful in sorting out patients who have had previous access sites that have failed.

2. Measurement of segmental pressures of the upper extremities can be helpful in select instances if the pulse examination is abnormal or arterial occlusive disease is suspected. Furthermore, formal duplex assessment of arterial flow can provide anatomic and hemodynamic information in complicated cases. In our experience, when bilateral upper extremity blood pressures are equivalent and the Allen test is normal, significant arterial inflow disease is rarely present.

3. Duplex ultrasound of the **central veins** can be performed if a proximal stenosis is suspected based on a history of multiple catheters, arm edema, or prominent venous collaterals. This examination is relatively sensitive for the detection of subclavian venous stenosis or occlusion, although complete visualization is limited by the structure of the thoracic outlet. Central venous stenosis may occur in 10% to 50% of patients with a history of indwelling dialysis catheters.

III. Vascular access options. Hemodialysis works by filtering the patient's blood to remove fluid, electrolytes, and toxins—functions that are normally performed by the kidneys. To achieve this end, the patient must have a dialysis access established that can withstand high flows and repeated trauma from cannulation. Establishing a connection between the arterial and venous system is the most effective way to create such a high-flow circuit. A direct connection between an artery and vein (**i.e., AV fistula**) results in enlargement and thickening of the outflow vein. As the vein matures, it undergoes "arterialization," making it strong enough to support hemodialysis. A prosthetic bridge graft can also be used to connect an artery and vein (**i.e., arteriovenous graft**), so that the graft and not a vein is punctured for dialysis. An extremity is the most accessible and common location for either type of dialysis access.

In 1997, The National Kidney Foundation published evidence-based guidelines on all aspects of vascular access, referred to as Kidney Disease Outcome Initiative (K/DOQI). This consensus statement was revised in 2001 and should be frequently referred to by vascular providers who care for dialysis patients and perform access procedures. Foremost among these recommendations is an emphasis on maximizing the use of AV fistulas. Specifically, the initiative recommends that autogenous AV fistulas make up more than 50% of new, permanent hemodialysis operations (Table 20.1). Historically, the United States has lagged behind Europe in the use of native fistulas for hemodialysis, despite statistical analyses controlling for patient characteristics (e.g., obesity, diabetes, age). These findings suggest that practice patterns in the United States may be the major limitation to use of autogenous fistulas as the preferred access configuration. Nonetheless, there is a consensus among clinicians that autogenous fistulas are preferred over prosthetic AV grafts and catheters for hemodialysis, due to greater durability and fewer complications (Table 20.1).

Table 20.1.   Selected guidelines for vascular access from the K/DOQI work group

1. 50% AVF placement in incident hemodialysis patients (i.e., first-time patients)
2. 40% AVF usage in prevalent hemodialysis patients (i.e., patients who have had dialysis access)
3. Less than 10% prevalent patients with chronic (>3 months) catheter access
4. Order of preference for AV access
   a. Wrist (radiocephalic) fistula
   b. Elbow (brachiocephalic) fistula
   c. AV graft with PTFE or basilic vein transposition

K/DOQI, National Kidney Foundation Kidney Disease Outcome Initiative; AV, arteriovenous; PTFE, polytetrafluoroethylene; AVF, arteriovenous fistula.

A. An autogenous AV fistula is the "gold standard" for hemodialysis access and should be established at least one to two months in advance of initiating dialysis. Following creation of the fistula, a 6- to 8-week interval must elapse to allow maturation before it is ready for cannulation. Despite this interval, about 10% to 30% of fistulas fail to mature, a difficult clinical scenario addressed in 9 of the 38 clinical practice guidelines in K/DOQI. Recommendations are made for optimal vein diameter and time for cannulation as well as direct methods to enhance maturation such as hand exercises, ligation of fistula side branches, and resting the fistula following needle infiltration. Use of preoperative ultrasound mapping is also important to minimize the use of a vein that is too small or inadequate to support flow through the fistula.

A mature AV fistula provides excellent access for hemodialysis and has the highest patency rates; 60% to 90% one year and 40% to 70% over 2 to 3 years. These results are superior to the 40% to 75% one-year patency and 25% to 50% 2- to 3-year patency for prosthetic AV grafts. Patency also varies according to the location of fistula, vein size, and comorbidities such as diabetes. Secondary interventions such as thrombectomy, angioplasty, and revision may improve long-term patency by 20% to 30%. **Prosthetic AV grafts require a higher number of interventions than native fistulas to maintain and restore patency, and infectious complications are higher with grafts and catheters than with native fistulas.** In fact, patients with AV grafts or catheters have a higher mortality than those with an autogenous fistula, with infectious etiologies accounting for the majority of this difference.

Numerous configurations of AV fistulas are possible in the upper extremity. The hierarchy of fistula placement is typically the non-dominant before the dominant arm, and forearm before the upper arm (Table 20.1). However, a more suitable (larger) vein may be selected out of standard sequence. Likewise, concern for arterial insufficiency in the arm should prompt further evaluation or selection of an alternative location (e.g., the opposite arm). Common sites for a native AV fistula in the upper extremity are as follows:

1. The original AV fistula was the **Brescia-Cimino fistula**, which remains popular in clinical practice today (Fig. 20.1A). The anastomosis is constructed between the cephalic vein and the radial artery at the wrist, most often in an end-to-side fashion and is therefore also dubbed a **radiocephalic fistula.** The location of this fistula at the wrist makes it attractive for the initial access procedure, because it does not "burn any bridges" further up the arm. Veins that are 2.5 mm or larger by examination or ultrasound can be selected, although smaller veins can be used if lower maturation rates are accepted. The Allen's test should indicate good ulnar collateral flow to the hand.

2. **Brachiocephalic** fistulas are created in the antecubital region by an end-to-side anastomosis and are often termed a **cephalic vein turndown** (Fig. 20.1B). A few studies have shown superior maturation of brachiocephalic fistulas over those at the wrist. The cephalic vein develops in its superficial location on the lateral aspect of the upper

arm, where it can be readily cannulated once the fistula is mature.

3. A basilic vein transposition is another option for an upper arm fistula (Fig. 20.2). Because the basilic vein lies deep in the medial upper arm, the vein is dissected out and then "transposed" into a superficial, subcutaneous tunnel on the lateral surface of the upper arm. The distal vein is then sewn to the brachial artery. The vein selected for a basilic transposition should be 4 mm or larger in order to provide the best chance of maturation. Because a long incision is required for this operation, regional block or general anesthesia is often used, whereas simple fistulas can be performed with local anesthetic and intravenous sedation. Patients with large arm girth are not good candidates for basilic vein transpositions because the length of transposed vein may not be sufficient to reach the artery. Additionally, wound complications in patients with obese arms are a significant concern, which may lead to selection of another access option.

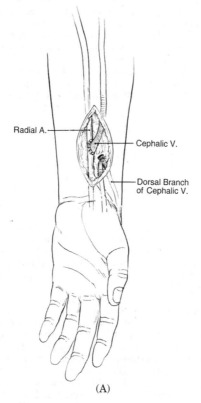

Radial A.

Cephalic V.

Dorsal Branch of Cephalic V.

(A)

Figure 20.1.   (A) The radiocephalic (Cimino) fistula and brachio-cephalic fistula are common forearm and upper arm AVFs, respectively.

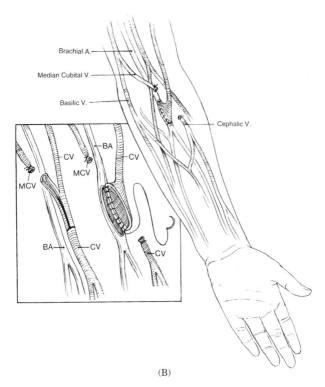

(B)

Figure 20.1. *(continued)* **(B) The anastomosis is constructed from the end of the vein to the side of the artery. After 6 to 8 weeks of maturation, the outflow vein should be dilated and thickened enough to cannulate on dialysis.**

B. An AV graft is constructed by sewing a synthetic polytetrafluoroethylene (PTFE) bridge between an artery and vein in one of many configurations. The authors' first choice is a loop graft placed in the non-dominant forearm, which in the authors' experience has been preferable to a straight forearm graft from the radial artery to an antecubital vein. Straight forearm grafts have a limited area for puncture and provide unique challenges associated with sewing a larger prosthetic graft to an often calcified smaller radial artery. Additionally, these straight grafts appear to have decreased patency compared with forearm loop grafts. The second choice for an upper extremity graft is an upper-arm loop graft between the brachial artery just proximal to the antecubital fossa and the very proximal basilic or axillary vein. The lower extremity is used only when the upper extremities can no longer accept some type of hemodialysis access. Although grafts can be placed in the groin area (e.g., saphenous vein to proximal femoral artery), infection is a greater problem than in the upper extremity, and patency rates are limited.

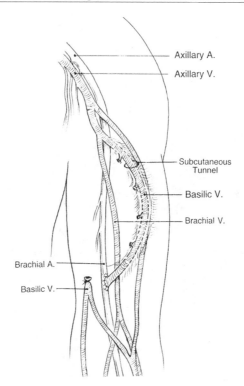

Axillary A.

Axillary V.

Subcutaneous
Tunnel

Basilic V.

Brachial V.

Brachial A.

Basilic V.

Figure 20.2. The basilica vein transposition is another option for an upper arm AVF in patients with suitable vein. The vein is transposed to a more superficial location in a lateral subcutaneous tunnel.

One advantage of prosthetic grafts is that they can be anastamosed to veins that are considered too small for autogenous fistula formation with reasonable patency. Although an autogenous fistula should be created in advance of dialysis in order to allow time for maturation, the same is not true for prosthetic grafts, which can generally be used within 14 days of placement. This advantage notwithstanding, the graft should be examined by the surgeon prior to dialysis, as use prior to graft incorporation can result in subcutaneous hematomas and wound complications. If the patient is not a candidate for an autogenous fistula the AV graft should be deferred until dialysis is imminent because of the risk of failure in the intervening time period.

C. A variety of dialysis catheters are available for acute hemodialysis that provide quick percutaneous access. These catheters may be used for days to weeks depending upon whether or not they are of the long, tunneled configuration or are short and not designed to be tunneled. Infection and central venous thrombosis are common complications associated with this form of hemodialysis and limit its long term and repeated usage. **The internal jugular vein is preferable to the subclavian vein** for the site of access, as chronic subclavian vein catheterization is associated with thrombosis and/or stenosis with risk of dysfunctional hemodialysis access in the upper extremity. Prolonged catheterization through the jugular vein can also lead to innominate vein or superior vena cava stenosis, although it is less common than that following subclavian vein cannulation.

   1. **The most common dialysis catheters** (Shiley, Vas-Cath, or Quinton catheters) are short, noncuffed, dual-lumen catheters placed percutaneously using the Seldinger method.

   2. **Cuffed dialysis catheters** (PermCath or VasCath) are longer, designed to be tunneled under the skin, and placed when prolonged catheterization (>2 to 3 weeks) is anticipated. Initial vein access is similar to the noncuffed catheters, except that these are brought through a subcutaneous tunnel on the chest wall, which offers stability and provides resistance to infection. These catheters are relatively soft and well tolerated by patients and will often function for weeks or even months. Again, central venous thrombosis and catheter infection are the complications that generally necessitate catheter removal.

D. Chronic peritoneal dialysis is another alternative preferred by some patients. This form of dialysis can be performed at home and generally at a lower cost than hemodialysis. The major long-term disadvantage is the possibility of recurrent infection (i.e., bacterial peritonitis). For patients with difficult upper-extremity access for hemodialysis, chronic peritoneal dialysis becomes an important option.

IV. Perioperative care.

A. The indications for dialysis, the type of dialysis, and potential complications should be discussed with the patient and family members prior to the operation. In particular, infection, thrombosis, and ischemic steal syndrome of the hand should be explained. Additionally, the authors find it useful to establish realistic expectations with the patient and his or her family with regards to patency rates and need for repeat procedures, including access attempts at alternative sites.

B. Prophylactic antibiotics (e.g., cefazolin 1 g) given within one hour of the procedure may reduce the risk of infection, especially in cases where a prosthetic graft is being used.

C. Most extremity hemodialysis procedures can be performed under local anesthesia with intravenous sedation. A supplemental axillary block may be necessary, depending upon the location of the access, and general anesthesia may also be preferable in some instances of high upper arm cases (e.g., basilic vein transposition). **It is important for the surgeon to discuss the location of the access and anticipated anesthesia requirements before any such plan is initiated**.

D. Although **anticoagulation** is not mandatory, a small dose of heparin (e.g., 2,000 to 5,000 units) is often used prior to occluding arterial flow and creating the anastomosis. Heparin may reduce the risk of early thrombosis in locations where

344 Section V. Disease-Specific Care

vasoconstriction may initially cause lower flow rates. Protamine may be used to reverse the heparin effect at the completion of the operation in order to minimize bleeding.

E. Skin incisions over a prosthetic AV graft should be constructed so that there is good tissue coverage at the end of the procedure. Whenever possible, skin incisions should not be placed directly over the course of a synthetic graft.

F. When the access has been completed, it is essential to check the **presence of pulses** at the wrist and good perfusion in the hand. Additionally, it is helpful to auscultate flow in the palmar arch with a continuous-wave Doppler unit. The loss or diminution of wrist pulses and the absence of Doppler flow in the palmar arch are harbingers of postoperative hand ischemia.

G. Postoperatively, the extremity should be placed at a **position of comfort.** Generally, it does not need to be elevated. In fact, elevation may exacerbate hand ischemia in patients who have marginal perfusion following placement of the AV circuit. Finally, constrictive bandages or wraps should be avoided, as they may limit flow through the fistula or graft placed in a superficial position.

H. The access should be checked for patency within 6 hours of placement. The two most reliable signs of patency are the presence of a **palpable thrill and audible bruit** heard with a stethoscope over the venous anastomosis and distal vein. A handheld Doppler will not pick up flow over a fresh prosthetic graft because porosity in the graft material and air in the tissues impede the Doppler transmission. Once the graft becomes incorporated into the tissues, a Doppler may be effective.

I. Development or maturation of an autogenous fistula may be aided in some patients by performance of daily exercise of the hand (e.g., squeezing a soft, rubber ball).

J. The hand must be checked for symptoms or signs of **ischemic steal syndrome.** The earliest symptom is numbness of the fingers, although in the setting of severe steal, progressive paresis of the intrinsic muscles of the hands will evolve over 24 hours. An absent radial pulse that was previously present is the key physical finding in such patients. Additionally, patients with hand ischemia will have monophasic or no Doppler signals over the radial, ulnar, and palmar arteries. **If ischemic steal syndrome is present and progressive, early intervention is warranted.** However, many cases of steal are more subtle and develop weeks to months after access placement. In such instances patients may complain of pain or numbness in the hand only during hemodialysis, when episodes of hypotension exacerbate the symptoms of steal.

Although ischemic steal can usually be diagnosed on clinical grounds alone, additional testing can be helpful. Digital photoplethysmography demonstrates dampened arterial waveforms in the fingers in the presence of steal syndrome that improve or return to normal with manual compression of the access site. Arteriography should be reserved for severe or progressive forms of steal and is used to rule out arterial inflow stenoses. **Increasingly, endovascular techniques such as balloon angioplasty are being applied to treat the underlying inflow stenosis responsible for the symptoms of steal.**

During diagnostic arteriography, steal is confirmed when compression of the access results in filling of the forearm and/or digital arteries distal to the access site.

Ligation of the hemodialysis access is a straightforward treatment for ischemic steal, eliminating flow through the fistula or graft and restoring perfusion to the hand. This option, however, leaves the patient without dialysis access and should be reserved for very ill patients or when other options are not feasible. An alternative is to decrease flow through the shunt by "banding," which narrows the flow channel by one of several techniques. Small Weck clips can be applied along the side of the proximal access for approximately 1 cm or a PTFE ring of fixed diameter can be placed around access to narrow its lumen. Wrist pulses will usually increase and Doppler signals of the palmar arch will improve if the banding is effective. Ultimately, banding is imprecise and the ability to achieve a balance between treating steal and occluding the shunt is difficult.

A more effective treatment for ischemic steal is referred to as **distal revascularization and interval ligation (DRIL)** (Fig. 20.3). In the upper extremity DRIL involves bypassing an identified inflow stenosis using a saphenous vein conduit from the proximal to the distal brachial or ulnar artery. The intervening brachial artery segment is ligated to prevent retrograde flow back into the access. This method of bypass restores flow into the forearm and hand beyond the access site while leaving the dialysis configuration intact.

V. Late complications. The most important complications that occur with hemodialysis are chronic hand ischemia, infection, dysfunction, failure (i.e., thrombosis) or formation of pseudoaneurysm along the dialysis channel.

A. Infection is uncommon with an autogenous AV fistula; however, synthetic dialysis grafts are more susceptible. Physical exam findings of erythema, induration, tenderness, and drainage from or around incisional sites are pathognomonic for infection. Occasionally, a patient will present with a fever of unknown origin and minimal signs of local graft infection. In these instances a positive blood culture may indicate a more subtle graft infection and duplex ultrasound may identify fluid around the graft. An indium-labeled white blood cell scan may also localize infection to the graft in more subtle cases. An infected synthetic graft must be removed entirely, although a localized infected segment can occasionally be resected with a new segmental bypass around the infected area.

B. Pseudoaneurysm is another relatively common problem of chronic synthetic AV grafts. These aneurysms occur from repeated puncture over a particular site where the wall of the graft weakens, and duplex is the best way to diagnose and characterize these areas. Pseudoaneurysms can gradually erode through the skin and lead to hemorrhage and should be repaired by resection of the pseudoaneurysm site and grafting around the area.

C. A **dysfunctional AV access** is a common problem referred to the surgeon or vascular interventionalist. Essentially, there are two categories of dysfunctional AV access: (1) improper function since placement (e.g., nonmaturation of an

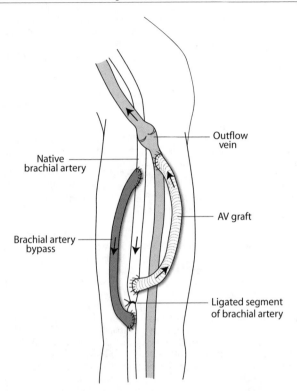

Figure 20.3. The distal revascularization and interval ligation (DRIL) procedure can be used to treat ischemic steal, which occur with an incidence of about 5% with vascular access procedures. In the upper extremity, a brachial–brachial bypass is constructed to restore blood flow to the hand, and the segment of brachial artery between the distal bypass anastomosis and the distal access anastomosis is ligated to prevent steal. Long-term patency of the DRIL is 80% to 90%.

autogenous AV fistula), or (2) a failing access site that had previously functioned well.

    1. Diagnosis. Findings on physical examination or during dialysis can be useful for identifying the dysfunctional access site. Reasons for reevaluation of the access include

        a. Weak or diminished thrill,
        b. Significant arm edema
        c. Prolonged bleeding after needle withdrawal
        d. Increased venous pressures
        e. Poor flows during the dialysis run
        f. Inadequate hemodialysis
        g. Difficulty with cannulation

Although often performed, routine surveillance with duplex ultrasound is not generally recommended after access placement, as this has not been shown to improve long-term patency.

2. Etiology. Failure of an autogenous AV fistula to mature may result from a technical problem; abnormal arterial inflow; or inadequate (small) vein, damaged vein, or central venous stenosis. These causes also account for the majority of early dysfunctional prosthetic AV grafts. In contrast, the late finding of a failing graft is most often caused by myointimal hyperplasia at the venous anastomosis in over 80% of cases. Venous outflow problems, whether in the arm or central vein, tend to cause edema and "pulsatility" in the access that can be appreciated on examination. A very high-pitched bruit may also indicate a venous outflow stenosis.

3. Salvage of a dysfunctional AV dialysis access may be possible under many circumstances. However, revised accesses have a lower long-term patency compared with non-revised accesses, even when proper function is restored. In general, repeated intervention for treatment of a dysfunctional access is the rule, rather than the exception.

The standard test for a dysfunctional AV access is duplex ultrasound followed by a **fistulogram (i.e., an angiogram of the AV fistula)** in certain cases. To perform the angiogram, percutaneous access is obtained to the flow channel and a small sheath is placed, generally using ultrasound or fluoroscopic guidance. Contrast dye is injected in order to examine the entire access, including the inflow and outflow anastomoses as well as a central venogram to look for more proximal obstructive lesions limiting outflow. Duplex ultrasound should be performed prior to the fistulogram to identify and localize hemodynamically significant stenoses.

    a. Endovascular techniques are most commonly used to treat dysfunctional AV dialysis fistula. Myointimal hyperplasia at an anastomosis can be treated effectively in the short- to mid-term with percutaneous angioplasty (PTA) using standard, high-pressure, or even cutting balloons. Short segment stenoses in the outflow vein and central venous stenoses are also amenable to PTA and/or stenting. Frequently, additional interventions are needed in order to maintain patency. The long-term durability of percutaneous treatment for central venous stenosis is poor, reported to be in the wide range of 11% to 70% at one year.

    b. Open surgical treatment is also effective for the treatment of dysfunctional AV access and should be tailored to the underlying problem. Patch angioplasty can be used to treat a stenosis at either the arterial or venous anastomosis. An interposition graft or an extension bypass (jump graft) to more proximal vein can also be used to address venous outflow stenoses. Surgical treatment of central venous stenosis is more durable than endovascular methods, but surgery on the chest harbors much higher morbidity.

D. Thrombosis is usually the endstage of a chronically dysfunctional access, although it may also occur in the absence of previous dysfunction and be due to hypotension, a hypercoagulable condition, or an otherwise ill-defined reason. Once an access site has thrombosed it cannot be used for dialysis unless a high rate of AV flow can be restored within the access. Although prosthetic AV grafts can often be salvaged by thrombectomy (i.e., removal of thrombus or clot), complete thrombus removal from autogenous AV fistulas is less likely and often leads to re-thrombosis. Thrombectomy can be performed by a variety of techniques. Open surgical thrombectomy using a cut-down and retrieval of clot with a Fogarty® thrombectomy catheter (Edwards Lifesciences Corp., Irvine, CA) is often combined with completion angiogram (i.e., fistulogram) to evaluate for any underlying causative lesion. When identified, the stenosis can be treated concomitantly with endovascular techniques or open revision. Purely endovascular techniques are also effective and may include mechanical thrombectomy with specifically designed devices (e.g., Angiojet, Possis, Minneapolis, MN, U.S.A.) or with thrombolytic drugs such as tissue plasminogen activator (TPA). In this setting it is essential to correct any flow-limiting problems (e.g., stenoses) identified in the access configuration following the thrombectomy, in order to prevent early re-thrombosis.

SELECTED READING

Bakken AM, Protack CD, Saad WE, et al. Long-term outcomes of primary angioplasty and primary stenting of central venous stenosis in hemodialysis patients. *J Vasc Surg*. 2007;45:776-783.

Casey K, Tonnessen BH, Mannava K, et al. A comparison of basilic versus brachial vein transpositions. *J Vasc Surg*. 2008;47:402-406.

Eknoyan G, Levin NW, Eschbach JW, et al. Continuous quality improvement: DOQI becomes K/DOQI and is updated. National Kidney Foundation's Dialysis Outcomes Quality Initiative. *Am J Kidney Dis*. 2001;37:179-194.

Gibson KD, Gillen DL, Caps MT, et al. Vascular access survival and incidence of revisions: A comparison of prosthetic grafts, simple autogenous fistulas, and venous transposition fistulas from the United States Renal Data System Dialysis Morbidity and Mortality Study. *J Vasc Surg*. 2001;34:694-700.

Knox RC, Berman SS, Hughes JD, et al. Distal revascularization-interval ligation: A durable and effective treatment for ischemic steal syndrome after hemodialysis access. *J Vasc Surg*. 2002;36:250-256.

McClafferty RB, Pryor RW III, Johnson CM, Ramsey DE, Hodgson KJ. Outcome of a comprehensive follow-up program to enhance maturation of autogenous arteriovenous hemodialysis access. *J Vasc Surg*. 2007;47:981-985.

National Kidney Foundation. K/DOQI. Clinical Practice Guidelines for Vascular Access. *Am J Kidney Dis*. 2000;37(suppl 1):S137-S181, 2001.

Tonnessen BH, Money SR. Embracing the fistula first national vascular access improvement initiative. *J Vasc Surg*. 2005;42:585-586.

INDEX

Note: Numbers followed by the letter *f* indicate figures; numbers followed by the letter *t* indicate tables